learning HUMAN ANATOMY

A Laboratory Text & Workbook

D0780797

learning HUMAN ANATOMY

A Laboratory Text & Workbook

Third Edition

Julia F. Guy, MS, PhD
Assistant Professor
The Ohio State University
College of Medicine and Public Health
Division of Anatomy
Columbus, Ohio

With Illustrations by
Pamela Blackshere Lewis
Susan J. Myers
Gina Lapurga

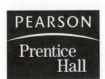

PEARSON

Prentice
Hall

Upper Saddle River, New Jersey 07458

NOTICE

The author[s] and the publisher of this volume have taken care that the information and technical recommendations contained herein are based on research and expert consultation, and are accurate and compatible with the standards generally accepted at the time of publication. Nevertheless, as new information becomes available, changes in clinical and technical practices become necessary. The reader is advised to carefully consult manufacturers' instructions and information material for all supplies and equipment before use, and to consult with a healthcare professional as necessary. This advice is especially important when using new supplies or equipment for clinical purposes. The author[s] and publisher disclaim all responsibility for any liability, loss, injury, or damage incurred as a consequence, directly or indirectly, of the use and application of any of the contents of this volume.

Publisher: *Julie Levin Alexander*
Publisher's Assistant: *Regina Bruno*
Senior Acquisitions Editor: *Mark Cohen*
Associate Editor: *Melissa Kerian*
Editorial Assistant: *Jaquay Felix*
Director of Manufacturing and Production: *Bruce Johnson*
Managing Editor for Production: *Patrick Walsh*
Production Liaison: *Cathy O'Connell*
Production Editor: *Bruce Hobart/Pine Tree Composition, Inc.*
Manufacturing Manager: *Ilene Sanford*
Manufacturing Buyer: *Pat Brown*
Creative Director: *Cheryl Asherman*
Senior Design Coordinator: *Christopher Weigand*
Cover Designer: *Kevin Kall*
Director of Marketing/Marketing Manager: *Karen Allman*
Channel Marketing Manager: *Rachele Strober*
Marketing Coordinator: *Janet Ryerson*
Media Editor: *John Jordan*
Media Production Manager: *Amy Peltier*
Media Project Manager: *Stephen Hartner*
Composition: *Pine Tree Composition*
Printer/Binder: *The Banta Company, VA*
Cover Printer: *Phoenix Color Corp.*

Copyright © 2005 by Pearson Education, Inc., Upper Saddle River, New Jersey 07458

Pearson Prentice Hall. All rights reserved. Printed in the United States of America. This publication is protected by Copyright and permission should be obtained from the publisher prior to any prohibited reproduction, storage in a retrieval system, or transmission in any form or by any means, electronic, mechanical, photocopying, recording, or likewise. For information regarding permission(s), write to: Rights and Permissions Department.

Pearson Prentice Hall™ is a trademark of Pearson Education, Inc.
Pearson® is a registered trademark of Pearson plc
Prentice Hall® is a registered trademark of Pearson Educaiton, Inc.

Pearson Education LTD.
Pearson Education Singapore, Pte. Ltd
Pearson Education, Canada, Ltd
Pearson Education–Japan
Pearson Education Australia PTY, Limited

Pearson Education North Asia Ltd
Pearson Education de Mexico, S.A. de C.V.
Pearson Education Malaysia, Pte. Ltd
Pearson Education, Upper Saddle River, New Jersey

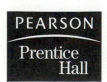

10 9 8 7 6 5 4 3 2 1
ISBN 0-13-143320-2

Contents

UNIT IV   THE ABDOMEN, PELVIS, AND THORAX

Preface

The third edition of *Learning Human Anatomy: A Laboratory Text and Workbook* continues to be a unique resource for introductory human anatomy courses/labs that use human cadavers and human organs (or models) as demonstration tools. The book has been written in an outline format and is designed to help students organize the anatomical material and find information quickly. Much of the text is included within the illustration keys, so the visual image of the *structure,* its *name,* and its *purpose* in an anatomical position can be related. The illustrations continue to emphasize the anatomy that is vital for a one-term, introductory course, or for general review. A reference text will still be required by students who need great amounts of detailed information.

The idea for this book was conceived from a need for a gross anatomy guide for undergraduates; therefore, its treatment of embryology and histology is minimal. Some basic understanding of biology (cell organization and function) is assumed, but not necessary.

Because anatomy is a visual science, the lab experience is vital in understanding three-dimensional relationships. For this reason, the more time spent looking at the structures, relating them to the living body, and forming mental images, the more easily the student will learn the material. Further, it aids the student in understanding the *relationships* and *organization* of the *major structures* within a given *body region*.

To further the understanding of relationships within body regions, this book presents a combined regional and systemic approach to human anatomy. Regionally, the body is divided into four units, as is the book:

- Lower Limb
- Upper Limb
- Head & Neck
- Abdominopelvis & Thorax

Activities and exercises are designed to reinforce each lesson and help students form the mental images and the understanding of positions on their own bodies, which will help in remembering the information. The illustrations are designed to be actively integrated into the student's study and instructions are noted to direct students to make their own colored illustrations. *Clinical comments* make selected information more clinically relevant. In this *third edition* there are several new illustrations as well as additional clinical comments, more functional anatomy, and a few more exercises. When the course is completed and this book is used as designed, the student will own a customized review book, created in part, by the student.

SUPPLEMENTAL LABORATORY CD-ROM SAMPLE INCLUDED

In the back of this book you will find a sample CD that includes one lesson from each of the four units of the book. The lessons were chosen to give an overview of the manner in which different material is presented. The ANATLAB (Anatomy Lab) program parallels the information in the book and provides real cadaver views of the major structures of the body. It is an interactive multimedia tutorial that helps the student visualize the body three-dimensionally. It is unique in its use of narrated cadaver demonstrations that make the information in the lab text come alive. Many of the illustrations that have been so well received by students who used the first and second editions of the book are included within the computer program. These illustrations are often compared to real cadaver images, bones, or x-rays. The computer program supplements the book by providing a cadaver orientation to all the anatomical structures, and by helping with the pronunciation of words. It is a tutorial, so answering the questions within the lesson helps the student really understand the anatomy. Quizzes at the end of each of the 28 lessons and unit quizzes following each of the four units check for mastery of the subject. *The Anatomy Lab* runs on both Windows and Macintosh formats. To purchase, see the order form at the back of this book.

Acknowledgments

I would like to thank my friend and colleague, Susan Turner, PhD, for her ongoing review, counsel, and encouragement. I also wish to express my appreciation for the positive comments and suggestions of the many students who have used this book.

Reviewers

Fredric Bassett, MS
Professor
Health Sciences Division
Rose State College
Midwest City, Oklahoma

Edward W. Carroll, Ph.D.
Clinical Assistant Professor
Department of Biomedical Sciences
Marquette University
Milwaukee, Wisconsin

Suzanne M. Cooke Schreiber
Instructor
University of New Hampshire
Durham, New Hampshire

Marie L. Hornyik, Ph.D., ATC
Assistant Professor
Department of Health and Kinesiology
Purdue University
West Lafayette, Indiana

Jonathan K. Kalmey, Ph.D.
Assistant Professor of Anatomy
College of Medical Sciences
Nova Southeastern University
Fort Lauderdale, Florida

Roberto Lopez-Rosado, MA
Instructor
Department of Physical Therapy
Florida Gulf Coast University
Fort Myers, Florida

Judith L. Schotland, Ph.D.
Assistant Professor
Department of Health Sciences
Boston University
Boston, Massachusetts

Howard Spector, Ph.D.
Lecturer
Oakland University
Rochester, Michigan

John Storsved, HSD, ATC/L
Clinical Assistant Professor
Purdue University
West Lafayette, Indiana

Mark D. Womble, Ph.D.
Associate Professor
Department of Biological Sciences
Youngstown State University
Youngstown, Ohio

Overview of Body Systems and the Lower Limb

With Detailed Introductions to:

· Skeletal System
· Muscular System
· Nervous System
· Cardiovascular System

Introductory Terminology and Orientation to the Body

The language of anatomy must be learned in order to understand the discipline. You will be exposed to new terminology throughout the course so we can communicate accurately as we discuss anatomical structures.

■ OBJECTIVES

1. State the meaning of the important anatomical terms listed.
2. Use the terms of position in describing anatomical structures.
3. Describe the planes that are used in cutting anatomical material.
4. Define the regions of the body.

■ METHODS

1. Study the list of words below. Use your own body to locate body parts and terms of position.
2. Listen for the new words when they are used by the instructor; practice using them yourself.
3. Complete the activities and Exercise 1.

A. GENERAL TERMINOLOGY

1. **Gross Anatomy:** the study of large (gross) structures that can be seen with the naked eye.
2. **Histology:** microscopic study of cells and tissues.
3. **Tissue:** groups of cells that are similar in structure and that function together. The four primary tissues are:
   a. **epithelial**—forms the linings and coverings of free surfaces of the body.
   b. **connective**—supportive and binding tissue found throughout the body. Examples: bone, tendons, cartilage.
   c. **muscle**—contractile tissue for movement.
   d. **nerve**—communication cells capable of sending impulses.
4. **Organ:** groups of tissues that work together to perform a common function. Examples: heart, lungs, kidneys, liver.
5. **System:** a group of organs working together to perform a common function. Examples: circulatory, respiratory, urinary.
6. **Neuroanatomy:** study of the structure of the nervous system.
7. **Embryology:** study of the developing organism from the time of fertilization to birth.

8. **Germ cell layers:** the three layers of embryonic tissue from which all body tissues are derived.
   a. **endoderm**—innermost of three germ cell layers. It will form most of the linings of tubular structures of the body.
   b. **ectoderm**—outer germ cell layer. Derivatives: skin and the nervous system.
   c. **mesoderm**—layer between the endoderm and the ectoderm. Derivatives: muscles and connective tissues.

9. **Fascia:** compact layers of connective tissue that form a fibrous membrane. It invests the whole body, supporting and separating muscles and organs.

10. **Collagen:** the protein that makes up the fibers in connective tissue structures.

11. **Ligaments:** thickened connective tissue (collagen fibers), which serves to hold bones together.

12. **Tendons:** thickened, dense connective tissue that holds muscle to bone.

13. **Aponeurosis:** a broad, flat tendon.

14. **Regional study:** all the structures in an area are studied together. Example: lower extremity includes bones, muscles, nerves, and vessels.

15. **Systematic (systemic) study:** studying a complete system independent of region. Example: learning all the bones of the body.

16. **Anatomic position:** the body is standing erect, face toward observer, with feet together and parallel, the arms at the sides and palms directed forward.

B. DIRECTIONAL TERMINOLOGY

See Figure 1–1A and B (Anterior and Lateral Views).

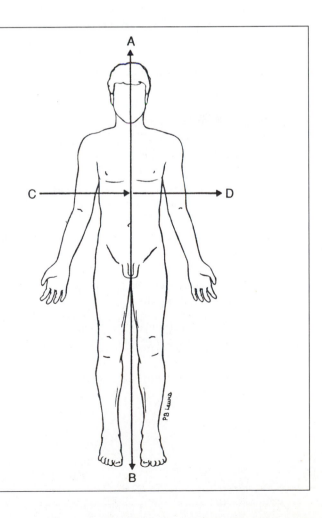

FIGURE 1–1A
ANTERIOR VIEW

1. **Anterior (ventral):** refers to the front surface of the body.

2. **Posterior (dorsal):** refers to the back surface of the body.

3. **Superior (cranial):** nearer the head end, line A.

4. **Inferior (caudal):** farther from head end, line B.

5. **Superficial (external):** nearer the surface.

6. **Deep (internal):** farther from the surface.

7. **Medial:** nearer the mid-plane of the body (C).

8. **Lateral:** farther from the mid-plane of the body (D).

9. **Proximal:** nearest the point of origin. If used with extremities, closer to the attachment. If used with an organ, closer to the organ.

10. **Distal:** farthest from point of origin.

■ **Student Activities**

Using the terms "proximal" and "distal," fill in the blanks to compare the relative positions of the shoulder, elbow, and wrist in Figure 1–1B.

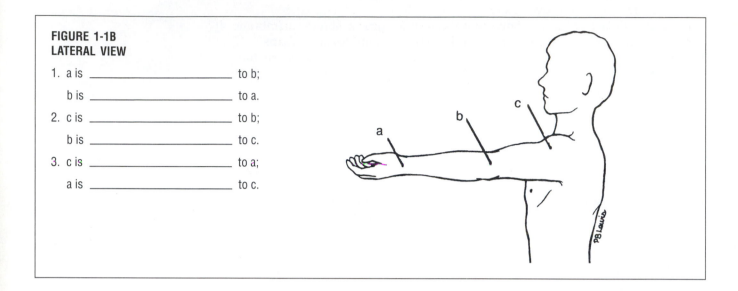

FIGURE 1-1B
LATERAL VIEW

1. a is _____ to b;

   b is _____ to a.

2. c is _____ to b;

   b is _____ to c.

3. c is _____ to a;

   a is _____ to c.

C. PLANES, REGIONS, AND CAVITIES OF THE BODY

To study anatomical material it is often advantageous to look at internal structures by making cuts in specific planes. For instance, a coronal plane would be used in some areas, but a transverse section (cross section) provides a better view of muscles around a bone in the limbs.

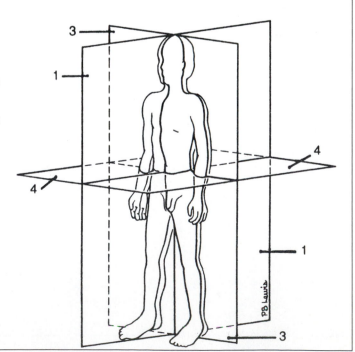

FIGURE 1–2
PLANES OF THE BODY

1. **Median (midsagittal) plane:** a vertical plane that divides the body into right and left halves. *(Color it yellow.)*

2. **Sagittal plane:** (not illustrated) a vertical plane parallel to the median plane.

3. **Coronal (frontal) plane:** a vertical plane at right angles to the median plane. It divides the body into anterior and posterior portions. *(Color it light blue.)*

4. **Transverse plane:** a horizontal plane at right angles to both the median and frontal planes. It cuts the body into superior and inferior portions.

FIGURE 1–3
REGIONS OF THE BODY

1. Head and neck

2. Upper limb

3. Thorax

4. Abdomen

5. Pelvis

6. Lower limb

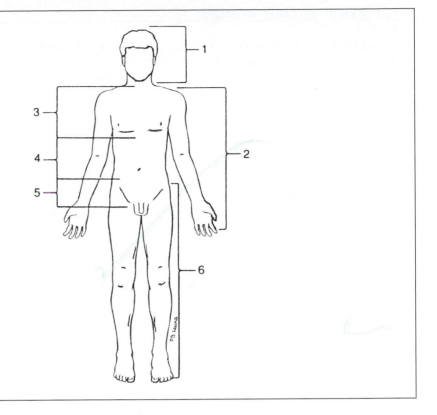

FIGURE 1–4
BODY CAVITIES

Many organs of the body are located in body cavities. Ventrally, a large cavity is subdivided by the diaphragm. Above the diaphragm, the thoracic cavity houses the lungs and the heart; below the diaphragm, the abdominopelvic cavity contains the major organs of digestion, reproduction, and the urinary system.

The cranial cavity houses the brain; the spinal cavity houses the spinal cord and spinal nerves. Together these are referred to as the dorsal body cavity.

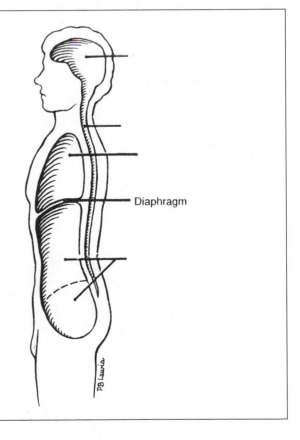

Diaphragm

■ **Label the cavities in Figure 1-4.**

D. OVERVIEW OF BODY SYSTEMS

In order for the body to work as a unified whole, many systems must work together. The anatomy of the systems will be illustrated as we encounter them in the various regions of the body. Figures 1–5 to 1–13 complete the general terminology and introductory overview of the body.

FIGURE 1–5
SKELETAL SYSTEM

Structural Components:
- Bones
- Cartilage
- Tendons
- Ligaments
- Joints

Functions:
- Support
- Protection (organs)
- Leverage in movement
- Produce blood cells
- Storage of minerals

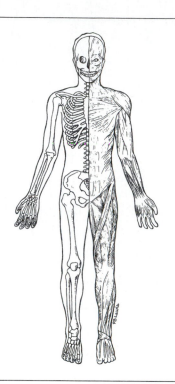

MUSCULAR SYSTEM

Structural Components:
- Skeletal muscle
- Cardiac muscle (heart)
- Smooth muscle (walls of hollow organs)

Functions:
- Movement
- Heat production

FIGURE 1–6
CIRCULATORY SYSTEM

Components:
- Heart
- Blood vessels
- Blood

Functions:
- Transports oxygen and nutrients to the cells, and transports carbon dioxide and wastes away.
- Carries hormones and other substances to areas of the body where they are needed.

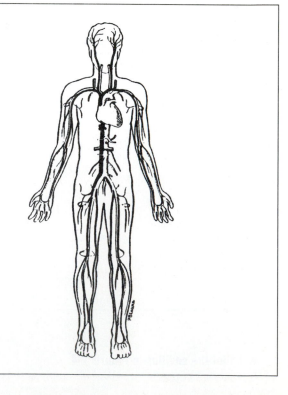

FIGURE 1–7
LYMPHATIC SYSTEM

Components:
- Lymph vessels and nodes
- Spleen
- Thymus gland
- Tonsils

(With red bone marrow, these are structures of the *immune system,* a functional system.)

Functions:
- Returns lymph (formerly interstitial fluid) to the cardiovascular system.
- Filters blood and lymph.
- Produces white blood cells to protect the body from disease.

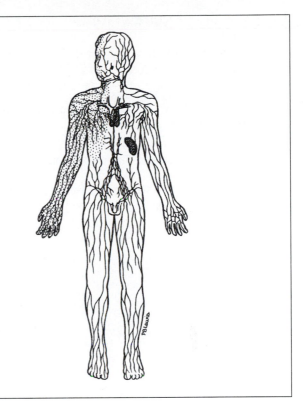

FIGURE 1–8
NERVOUS SYSTEM

Components:
- Brain
- Spinal cord
- Nerves
- Sense organs: eyes, ears, tongue, and sensory receptors in the skin

Function:
- Communication system that detects changes in internal and external body environment and, by way of a nerve impulse, responds by producing some effect in muscle or gland.

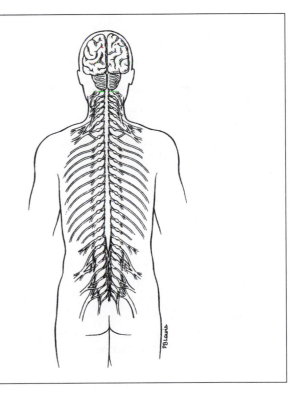

FIGURE 1–9
ENDOCRINE SYSTEM

Components:
- Hormone-producing structures:
- Pituitary, pineal, thyroid, parathyroid, and adrenal glands
- Ovaries, testes, and pancreas

Functions:
- Communications system that uses hormones as chemical messengers.
- Helps maintain homeostasis by regulating body activities.

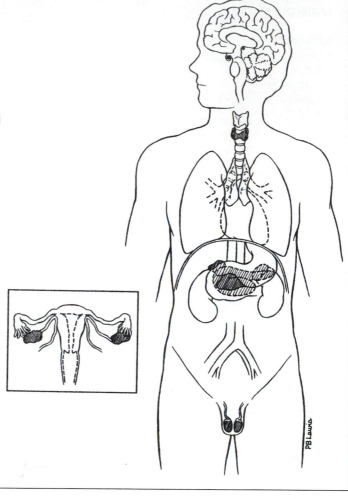

FIGURE 1–10
RESPIRATORY SYSTEM

Components:
- Nasal cavity
- Pharynx
- Larynx
- Trachea
- Bronchi
- Lungs

Functions:
- Supplies oxygen and removes carbon dioxide.
- Helps regulate acid–base balance.

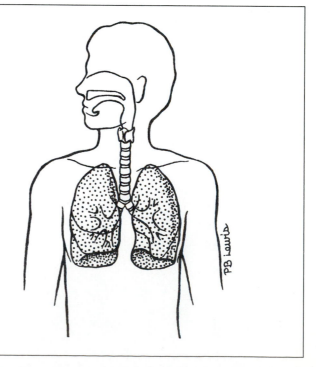

FIGURE 1–11
DIGESTIVE SYSTEM

Components:
- Mouth
- Salivary glands
- Digestive tube
- Liver and gall bladder
- Pancreas

Functions:
- Physical and chemical breakdown of food into nutrients for use by the cells of the body.
- Removes solid waste.

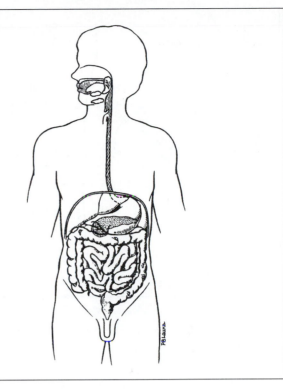

FIGURE 1–12
URINARY SYSTEM

Components:
- Kidneys
- Ureters
- Urinary bladder
- Urethra

Functions:
- Filters blood to eliminate waste and excess fluid.
- Helps maintain acid–base balance in the body.

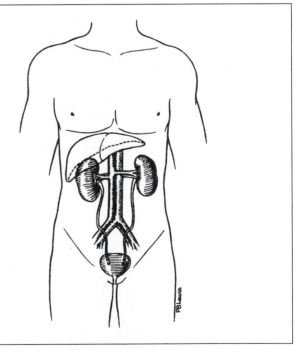

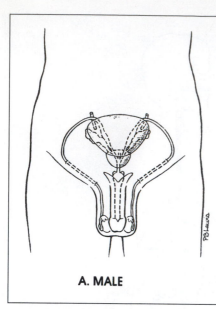

FIGURE 1–13
REPRODUCTIVE SYSTEM

Components:
- **Male:** testes, penis, duct system, glands
- **Female:** ovaries, uterine tubes, uterus, vagina, external genitalia. Accessory organs: mammary gland

Functions:
- Hormone production
- Production of germ cells for reproduction of the organism
- Houses developing fetus

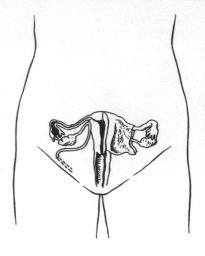

A. MALE

B. FEMALE

INTEGUMENTARY SYSTEM

Components:
- Skin, sweat, and oil glands
- Hair
- Nails
- Teeth

Functions:
- Protects deeper structures from foreign elements and from drying.
- Helps regulate body temperature.
- Eliminates some wastes.
- Receives some sensory stimuli.

Note: This is the only body system we will not include in this guide. It is the protective layer over all the body, and the omission is due to the histological nature of its anatomy. For an understanding of this system, please refer to an anatomy textbook.

Exercise One

Name _____

1. Label each figure with the appropriate letter from the following list:

   a. Anterior view

   b. Medial side of left lower limb

   c. Proximal upper limb (right)

   d. Superficial chest

   e. Deep abdomen

   f. Lateral view

   g. Distal lower limb (left)

   h. Lateral side of left thigh

   a. _____

   b. _____

2. Write a sentence to demonstrate an understanding of each of the relative pairs.
   (Example: The knee is *distal* to the hip.)

   a. *(superior, inferior)* _____

   _____

   b. *(superficial, deep)* _____

   _____

   c. *(medial, lateral)* _____

   _____

   d. *(proximal, distal)* _____

   _____

3. Complete the following sentences with the correct directional term.

   a. The wrist is _____ to the elbow.

   b. The neck is _____ to the abdomen.

   c. To separate the thorax from the abdomen, a cut in the _____
      plane would be the most appropriate.

   d. The skin is _____ to bone.

11

Osteology: The Study of Bone

The bones of the body provide a vertical axis, *axial skeleton,* from which the bones of the upper and lower limbs, *appendicular skeleton,* extend. We will study each bone of the skeleton and its major markings. There are some general terms and functions that should be understood before specific bones are introduced.

■ OBJECTIVES

1. List the functions of the skeleton.
2. Recognize different types of bones.
3. Identify the regions of a long bone and the kinds of bony material of which it is composed.
4. Define the microscopic unit, *osteon,* of compact bone.
5. Identify all the bones of the axial and appendicular skeleton.
6. List and define the articular and non-articular bone markings.

■ METHODS

1. Observe examples of cut and broken bones.
2. Using the long bone x-rays provided, identify both developing bone and adult bone.
3. Follow the directions as you study this lesson.

A. FUNCTIONS OF THE SKELETON

1. *support*—for the soft tissues of the body.
2. *movement*—bones serve as levers and joints as fulcra.
3. *protection*—to vital organs.
4. *storage of minerals*—calcium and phosphorus.
5. *production of blood cells* (hemopoiesis).

B. TYPES OF BONES

	Examples
1. long bones	femur, tibia, metatarsals
2. short bones	carpals and tarsals
3. flat bones (thin)	ribs, bones of skull, sternum
4. irregular bones	vertebrae, os coxae
5. sesamoid bones ("seed-like" bones that develop in certain tendons).	patella

C. GROSS ANATOMY OF A LONG BONE

The bones you study in the laboratory are hard and dry, but remember, in the living body they contain living cells and require blood and nerves. While the inorganic salts (of calcium and phosphorus) are hard, the organic material (collagen fibers) allows some flexibility, and the living cells are actively remodeling. **Osteocytes** are mature bone cells, **osteoclasts** are cells that tear down bone, and **osteoblasts** build new bone.

The strength of bone, as well as sites of certain bone functions, remain apparent in the material available in the lab. Using these bones, find each of the parts labeled in Figure 2–1. The marrow and arteries will not be seen.

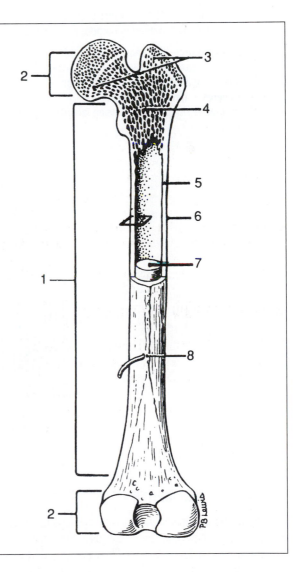

FIGURE 2–1
LONG BONE

In this illustration, a posterior section of the proximal end of the bone has been removed.

1. **Diaphysis** or shaft.

2. **Epiphysis**—found at both proximal and distal ends of long bones.

3. **Epiphyseal line**—where the epiphysis and the diaphysis fuse after the cartilaginous epiphyseal plate is no longer needed to increase bone length.

4. **Spongy (cancellous) bone (also in distal epiphysis)**—contains red marrow in the proximal epiphysis; the blood cell producing red marrow is also found in spongy bone of flat bones.

5. **Compact bone**—the external coat of solid bone.

6. **Periosteum**—fascial covering found on all bones.

7. **Yellow marrow**—mostly fat. It is seen here in the medullary cavity, a space lined with endosteum; some osteoclasts are found here.

8. **Nutrient artery** entering nutrient foramen.

D. MICROSCOPIC ANATOMY OF COMPACT BONE

Microscopic structures will not be seen in the gross bone, but you should be familiar with the terminology. (See Figure 2–2.)

FIGURE 2–2
COMPACT BONE

Diagram of a small section of bone (see inset from Figure 2–1) magnified to show osteons. Trabeculae of the spongy bone are shown toward the medullary cavity.

The osteon (Haversian system) is the structural unit of most compact bone. Each osteon is composed of the following:

- **Haversian canal**—for passage of blood vessel.
- **Lamellae**—concentric layers of bony tissue.
- **Lacunae**—spaces containing osteocytes.
- **Osteocytes**—mature bone cells.
- **Canaliculi**—connections between lacunae.

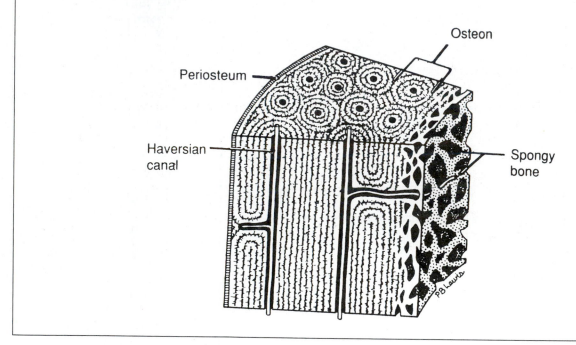

■ CLINICAL COMMENTS

Osteoporosis is a condition in which bone resorption occurs faster than bone deposition. This results in thinner compact bone and fewer trabeculae (interconnecting pieces of bone) in spongy bone. Because the bone is weaker, fractures are more likely to occur. Compression fractures of the spine and fractures of the neck of the femur are most frequent. Postmenopausal women and anyone who is immobile are at risk. Exercise and calcium are needed to keep bones strong.

Figure 2–3 can be used as a reference in each section of the book. It is a good illustration to photocopy and use to draw muscles, vessels, and nerves as you learn both the lower and the upper limbs. You may want to enlarge upper and lower limbs when appropriate.

The articulated skeleton is shown in both anterior and posterior views. *Use a light color to shade the bones of the axial skeleton.* These include: skull, vertebral column, sternum, and ribs.

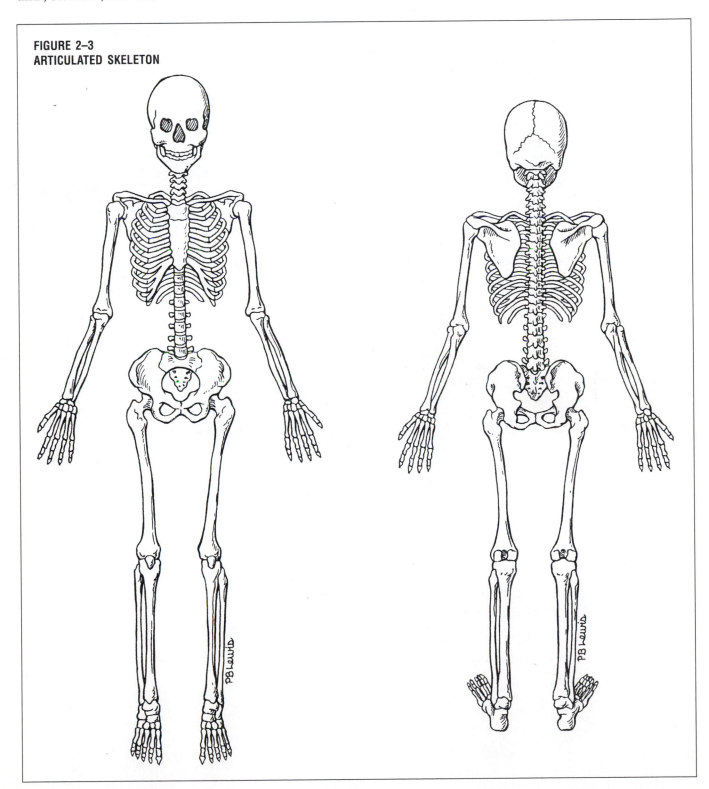

**FIGURE 2–3
ARTICULATED SKELETON**

Exercise Two

1. Using the skeleton at the right, follow the directions below:

   a. The skeleton pictured is a (an) _____ view.
   b. Color the most proximal long bone of the right lower limb.
   c. On the left lower limb, color the leg bone, which is seen in the lateral position between the knee and the ankle. **Remember:** When describing anatomical material we use left and right according to the position on the body being studied. So, it may be on the right side or the left side of the picture.

2. List the structures of the diaphysis (on the right) in the correct order from superficial to deep.

   a. _____   Endosteum (of medullary cavity)

   b. _____   Compact bone

   c. _____   Periosteum

   d. _____   Yellow marrow

   e. _____   Spongy bone

3. Choose the appropriate word from the group below and write it beside its definition.

Diaphysis	Osteon	Epiphyseal plate
Osteoblast	Yellow marrow	Periosteum
Red marrow		

   _____ a. A structure not found in an adult.

   _____ b. Covering found on all bones.

   _____ c. Another name for the shaft of a long bone.

   _____ d. Name of a bone-forming cell.

   _____ e. Major unit of compact bone.

   _____ f. Site of blood-cell formation.

   _____ g. Found in the cavity of the diaphysis.

Bones of the Pelvic Girdle and Lower Limb

As you begin to learn the details of the bones, you will find that some terms are used repeatedly. If you understand this terminology, the names of the bone markings will be easier to learn and more meaningful to you. Many bone markings are sites of attachment for muscles; thus understanding their position on the bones will help you understand muscle actions in the following lab sessions.

■ OBJECTIVES

1. Recognize both articular and non-articular bone markings.
2. Identify specific bone markings where *numbered* on the illustrations.
3. Determine whether the following bones are from the right or the left side of the body: os coxae, femur, tibia, foot (whole).
4. Use directional terminology to describe structures of the skeleton.

■ METHODS

1. Compare the markings in the lab guide illustrations with those on the bones in the lab.
2. Study skeletons and x-rays to see how the individual bones articulate with each other.
3. Observe on the skeleton the correct orientation of the bones, particularly the os coxae.
4. Cover the key to each illustration and see if you can identify each marking. Leave the leader lines unlabeled throughout this book so they can be used this way for repeated review.
5. On your own body, feel the bone markings indicated by an asterisk (*).

BONE MARKINGS

These are characteristics of bone that indicate the following: weight-bearing functions, passage of blood vessels and nerves, muscle attachments, and joints. Study this list to help you understand the specific markings on each of the bones.

1. **process:** a roughened bony prominence usually serving as the site of attachment for muscles or connective tissue structures.
2. **trochanter:** relatively large, blunt type of process found only on the femur.
3. **tuberosity:** a large, blunt or rounded process.
4. **tubercle:** a small, blunt or rounded process.
5. **spine:** a pointed projection of bone.

6. **crest:** a prominent border that may be rough.
7. **fossa:** a saucer-like depression.
8. **foramen:** a hole in a bone: size is extremely variable.
9. **head:** a rounded articular surface joined to the shaft of the bone by a constriction, the neck.
10. **condyle:** a smooth structure, either concave or convex, joined directly to the shaft of a long bone.
11. **facet:** a smooth surface for articulation.

Note: Items 9–11 are *articular* markings. Articular refers to a joint, so these indicate where bones are joined.

A. BONES OF THE LOWER LIMB

PELVIC GIRDLE

The pelvic girdle is made up of two ossa coxae, *appendicular skeleton* bones, that join anteriorly at the symphysis pubis and posteriorly to the sacrum, an *axial skeleton* bone. The pelvis is held together by strong ligaments to provide a sturdy structure to support the body weight in mobility.

When in the correct anatomical position, the anterior superior iliac spine and the pubic tubercle are in a vertical plane.

FIGURE 3–1
PELVIC GIRDLE (ANTERIOR VIEW OF FEMALE)

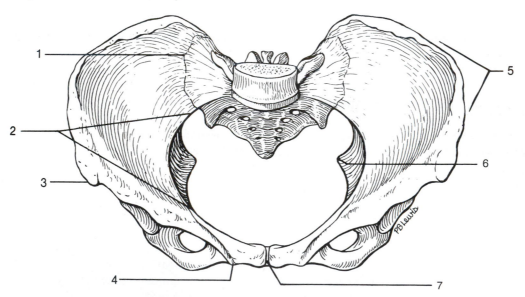

1. **Sacroiliac joint**—the attachment of the lower limb with the axial skeleton.

2. **Pelvic brim**—Inferior to the pelvic brim, the *true pelvis* is located between the pelvic bones. The *false pelvis* is the space above the pelvic brim and between the iliac bones.

3. **Anterior superior iliac spine**

4. **Pubic tubercle**

5. **Iliac crest**

6. **Ischial spine**

7. **Symphysis pubis**—the joining of the two ossa coxae anteriorly.

Note: The pelvic inlet (entrance to true pelvis) in the male is smaller and more oval. The male pelvis is deeper, the ilia less flared, and the bones are heavier and thicker.

SACRUM

This *axial skeleton* bone will be described here because it is a part of the pelvic girdle. The sacrum is formed from a fusion of five sacral vertebrae. (See Figure 3–2.)

FIGURE 3–2

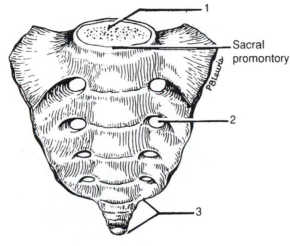

A. ANTERIOR VIEW

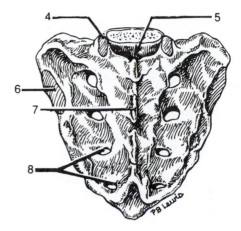

B. POSTERIOR VIEW

1. **Body** of first sacral vertebra
2. **Ventral (anterior) sacral foramen**—ventral rami of sacral spinal nerves emerge here.
3. **Coccyx**—the fusion of four or five small vertebrae.
4. **Superior articular surface**—for articulation with the fifth lumbar vertebra

5. **Sacral canal**—for passage of nerves.
6. **Auricular (ear-like) surface**—for articulation with the ilium
7. **Spinous tubercles**
8. **Posterior sacral foramina**—dorsal rami of sacral spinal nerves emerge here.

OS COXAE (INNOMINATE OR HIP BONE)

This is actually a fusion of three bones. Figure 3–3 shows the lines of fusion. As you learn the markings in Figures 3–4 and 3–5, notice that most marking names refer to the individual bone.

FIGURE 3–3
OS COXAE

a. ilium

b. Ischium

c. Pubis

Note: Because the pubis is an anterior structure, it can help you decide whether the os coxae is a right or left bone. Recognizing one anterior structure, you need to identify a marking from either the lateral or medial aspect so you can distinguish right from left. The bowl-shaped fossa, acetabulum, is a good choice for that purpose. Since the head of the femur fits into it, it must be lateral.

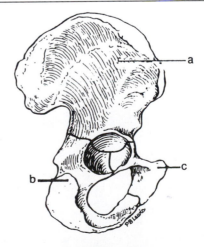

LATERAL VIEW

FIGURE 3–4
RIGHT OS COXAE (LATERAL VIEW)

1. **Greater sciatic notch**—this becomes a foramen when closed by the *sacrospinous ligament,* which extends from the sacrum to the ischial spine

2. **Ischial spine**

3. **Ischial tuberosity**

4. **Iliac crest**

5. **Anterior superior iliac spine**

6. **Acetabulum**—a bowl-shaped articular cavity formed from all three bones

7. **Obturator foramen**

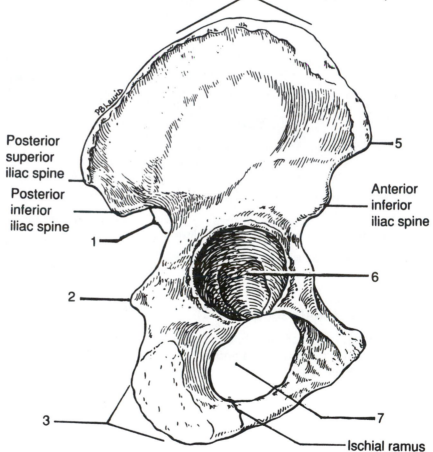

Posterior superior iliac spine

Posterior inferior iliac spine

Anterior inferior iliac spine

Ischial ramus

FIGURE 3–5
RIGHT OS COXAE (MEDIAL VIEW)

Remember: If it has an asterisk, feel it on your own body.

1. **Iliac crest***
2. **Iliac fossa**
3. **Anterior superior iliac spine***
4. **Superior pubic ramus**
5. **Pubic tubercle**
6. **Symphysis pubis***—where bodies of two pubic bones join
7. **Inferior pubic ramus**
8. **Articular surface**—for the sacrum
9. **Ischial spine**
10. **Obturator foramen**—formed by ischium and pubis

Note: A ramus is an arm or a branch. The superior and inferior rami of the pubic bone extend posteriorly from the anteriorly positioned body.

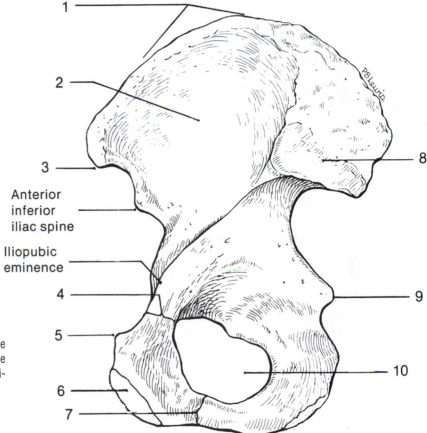

Anterior inferior iliac spine

Iliopubic eminence

■ **Student Activities**

1. In Figure 3–1, label the obturator foramen and the acetabulum. Draw, with yellow, a sacrospinous ligament from the sacrum to the ischial spine. This creates the greater sciatic foramen.
2. In Figure 3–3, color each bone a different color.

THE THIGH

The femur is the only bone of the thigh (hip to knee) and is the largest bone in the body. It articulates with the acetabulum proximally and the tibia and patella distally.

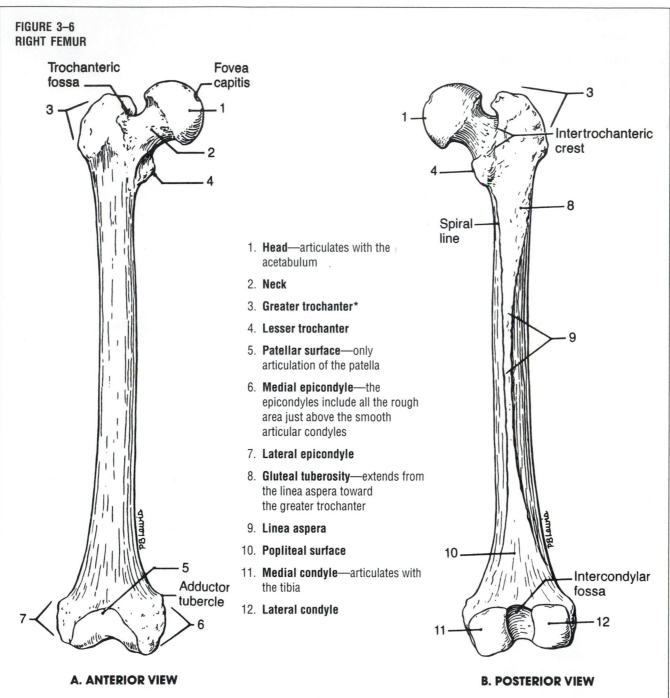

FIGURE 3–6
RIGHT FEMUR

Trochanteric fossa

Fovea capitis

Intertrochanteric crest

Spiral line

1. **Head**—articulates with the acetabulum

2. **Neck**

3. **Greater trochanter***

4. **Lesser trochanter**

5. **Patellar surface**—only articulation of the patella

6. **Medial epicondyle**—the epicondyles include all the rough area just above the smooth articular condyles

7. **Lateral epicondyle**

8. **Gluteal tuberosity**—extends from the linea aspera toward the greater trochanter

9. **Linea aspera**

10. **Popliteal surface**

11. **Medial condyle**—articulates with the tibia

12. **Lateral condyle**

Adductor tubercle

Intercondylar fossa

A. ANTERIOR VIEW

B. POSTERIOR VIEW

Remember: If there is an asterisk, you can feel this marking on your body.
Note: To distinguish left from right, the head must be a medial structure to articulate with the acetabulum. The linea aspera is on the posterior shaft and is rough.

FIGURE 3–7
THE RIGHT KNEE (ANTERIOR VIEW)

Patella*
A sesamoid bone that forms in the tendon of the quadriceps femoris muscle. It serves as a fulcrum, the support or point around which the action occurs, and it helps protect the knee joint.

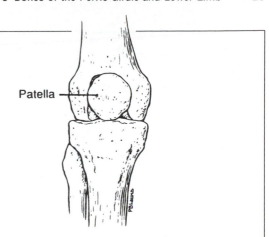

Patella

BONES OF THE LEG

The tibia and fibula are the two bones of the leg (knee to ankle). The tibia is the medial bone and is the weight-bearing bone. The fibula is thin and found in the lateral position. It is primarily for muscle attachment.

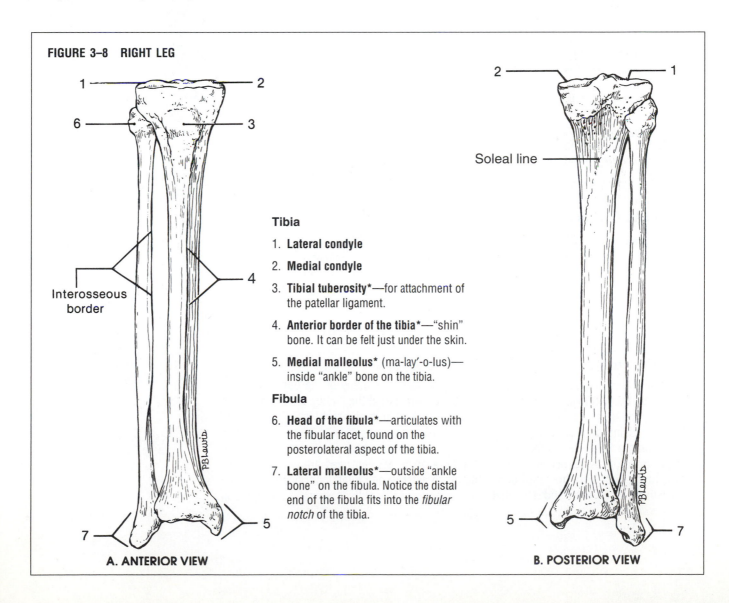

FIGURE 3–8   RIGHT LEG

Interosseous border

Soleal line

Tibia

1. **Lateral condyle**

2. **Medial condyle**

3. **Tibial tuberosity***—for attachment of the patellar ligament.

4. **Anterior border of the tibia***—"shin" bone. It can be felt just under the skin.

5. **Medial malleolus*** (ma-lay'-o-lus)— inside "ankle" bone on the tibia.

Fibula

6. **Head of the fibula***—articulates with the fibular facet, found on the posterolateral aspect of the tibia.

7. **Lateral malleolus***—outside "ankle bone" on the fibula. Notice the distal end of the fibula fits into the *fibular notch* of the tibia.

A. ANTERIOR VIEW

B. POSTERIOR VIEW

BONES OF THE FOOT

FIGURE 3–9
RIGHT FOOT (SUPERIOR VIEW)

Tarsal Bones (7)
a. Talus—articulates with both the tibia and the fibula

b. Calcaneus—the heel bone

c. Navicular

d. Cuboid

e–g. Cuneiforms (3)
Named from medial to lateral: medial, intermediate, and lateral, or, first, second, and third.

Metatarsals (5)
Numbered one (1) through five (5) from medial to lateral.

h. Second metatarsal
i. First metatarsal, etc.

Phalanges (14 bones)—a single bone is called a *phalanx*.
Hallux—first or great toe has two phalanges:

j. Proximal phalanx of hallux
k. Distal phalanx of hallux

Digits two (2) through five (5) have three phalanges each.

l. Proximal phalanx of fifth digit
m. Middle phalanx of fifth digit
n. Distal phalanx of fifth digit

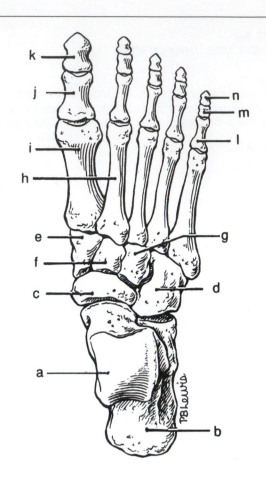

■ CLINICAL COMMENTS:

Ankle sprains, injuries in which ligaments are stretched or some of the collagen fibers are torn, are more common on the lateral side. These occur when the foot is inverted with weight on the ankle. Medial injuries are less frequent because there are more ligaments on the medial side and the fibula helps to splint the ankle to prevent eversion.

■ Student Activities

With your books closed, sketch each bone and include as many of the bone markings as you can remember. You do not need to be concerned that the pictures look good; just be sure the structures are in the right relationship and in the correct view.

 Using the bones on the lab tables, pick up several examples of an os coxae, a femur, and a tibia. Determine if each is left or right. **Remember:** This means from the left or right of the person from which the bone came. All you need are two directional structures, such as a posterior and a lateral; an anterior and a lateral; a posterior and a medial; or an anterior and a medial. As you perform this activity, imagine the bone in your own body.

Exercise Three

Name_____

1. Fill in the blanks with the name of the appropriate lower extremity bone.

   a. The most inferior bone of the os coxae is the _____ .
   b. The bone involved in formation of the acetabulum but not the obturator fora-

      men is the _____ .

   c. The major weight-bearing bone of the leg is the _____ . It

      is on the _____ side of the leg.

   d. Name all the bones of the thigh. _____

2. On the pelvis at the right:

   a. Draw a red line to indicate the pelvic brim.
   b. Outline the sacroiliac joint in green.
   c. Place the following labels on the illustration:
      1. pubic tubercle
      2. anterior superior iliac spine
      3. ischial spine
      4. obturator foramen
      5. iliac fossa

3. On the illustration at the right, label all visible bones. Color the sesamoid bone.
   Is the picture a right or left knee? _____

4. In the space provided, write the name of the bone on which you would find the
   marking. In the first column use the appropriate letter to indicate whether the
   marking is anterior (A), posterior (P), lateral (L), or medial (M). These words are
   defined with reference to the anatomical position.

A, P, L, or M	Name of Bone	Marking
_____	_____	a. linea aspera
_____	_____	b. soleal line
_____	_____	c. medial malleolus
_____	_____	d. popliteal surface
_____	_____	e. gluteal tuberosity
_____	_____	f. lateral malleolus
_____	_____	g. patellar surface
_____	_____	h. tibial tuberosity

5. In Figure 2–3 (you might want to use a photocopy), label all the lower limb bones
   with the correct name.

Lesson 4

Arthrology: The Study of Joints

This brief section on joints should familiarize you with joint terminology and introduce you to the articulations—places where bones attach to bone—of the lower limb. The detailed anatomy of specific joints is not included in this text.

■ OBJECTIVES

1. List and define the major classifications of joints.
2. Describe a synovial joint and list the types.
3. Classify each joint of the lower limb.

■ METHODS

1. Observe joint models on display.
2. Find each joint of the lower-limb on both the skeleton and the x-rays. Where possible, move or feel each joint on your own body.

A. CLASSIFICATION OF JOINTS

The classification of a joint depends on the tissue between the bones and on the freedom of movement allowed at the joint. Table 4–1 summarizes the major types of joints and gives examples of each. Figures 4–1 through 4–3 illustrate them.

TABLE 4–1. MAJOR TYPES OF JOINTS

Type of Joint	Movement	Examples
Synarthroses (fibrous) Suture—held tightly with little fiber	Immovable	Sutures of skull
Syndesmosis—slightly longer fibers	Slight "give"	Tibia to fibula (distal articulation)
Amphiarthroses (cartilaginous) Synchondroses—hyaline cartilage between bone	None	1st costal cartilage to sternum
Symphyses—fibrous cartilage between bone	Slight movement	Pubic bones and intervertebral discs
Diarthroses (synovial) Named on basis of movement	Free movement	Most extremity joints
Plane	Small surfaces slide/glide on each other	Facets of vertebrae

TABLE 4–1. (CONT.)

Type of Joint	Movement	Examples
Hinge	Movement in one plane	Knee
Pivot	Movement around a single axis	First cervical vertebra on 2nd
Condyloid	Two directions of movement	Wrist
Ball and socket	Move in many axes with common center	Hip, shoulder
Saddle	Movement in two planes	Carpometacarpal joint of thumb

B. ILLUSTRATIONS TO DESCRIBE EACH TYPE OF JOINT

FIGURE 4–1
SYNARTHROSIS

Fibrous connective tissue (ligaments) holds two bones together.
This example is a joint with slight give.

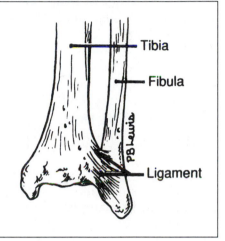

FIGURE 4–2
AMPHIARTHROSIS

A cartilaginous disc connects the two bones anteriorly. This
example is a joint with slight give.

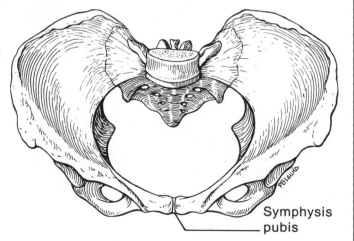

FIGURE 4–3
DIARTHROSIS (SYNOVIAL JOINT)

This is the most complicated and most common type of joint. Hyaline cartilage covers the ends of the bones, which are separated by an articular cavity. Synovial joints are involved in muscle actions throughout this course. Descriptions of the important parts of these joints are described here and illustrated in Figure 4–3.

- **Synovial cavity**—contains synovial fluid that reduces the friction of movement.
- **Articular cartilage (a form of hyaline cartilage)**—provides protection for the ends of bones during movement. Color it yellow.
- **Synovial membrane**—lines the cavity and produces the synovial fluid. Color it pink.
- **Articular capsule**—greatly thickened continuation of periosteum surrounding the joint. In a few joints the articular capsule extends between the bones as an articular disc dividing the cavity in two.

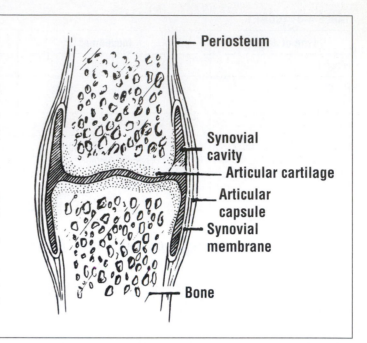

FIGURE 4-4
LIGAMENTS OF THE KNEE

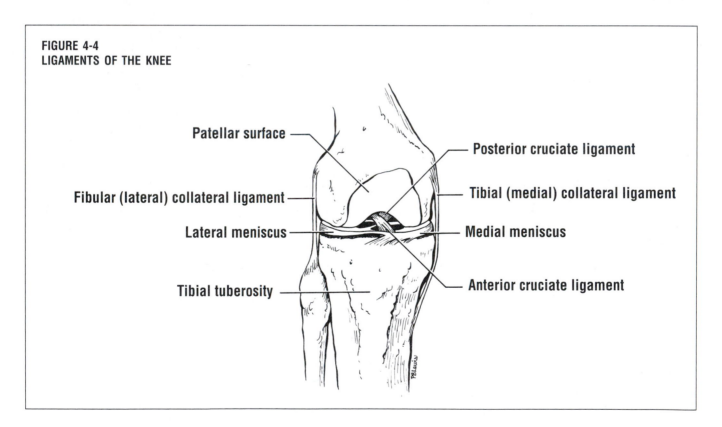

■ CLINICAL COMMENTS

The knee, the most complicated joint, is frequently injured, especially during contact sports. The anterior cruciate and tibial (medial) collateral ligaments are commonly torn in football accidents if a player is hit from the anterolateral aspect when his or her foot is planted. Another common knee injury occurs when the body suddenly changes direction. Because the menisci are not firmly attached, they may tear. The *arthroscope,* a very small viewing instrument with a fiberoptic light source, can be inserted through a tiny incision and allow the joint to be viewed and surgically repaired.

C. JOINTS OF THE LOWER LIMB

Table 4–2 organizes the joints we are studying in this unit. The movements are listed here, but definitions and illustrations of the major diarthrotic movements are included in Lesson 5.

TABLE 4–2. JOINTS OF THE LOWER LIMB

Joint	Type	Movements
Pubic symphysis	Symphysis	Slight "give"
Sacroiliac	Part synchondrosis part diarthrosis	No movement in part; slight gliding movement
Hip	Diarthrosis (ball and socket)	Flexion, extension, abduction, adduction, circumduction, and rotation
Knee (between the femur and tibia)	Diarthrosis (hinge)	Flexion, extension, slight rotation
Proximal ends of tibia and fibula	Diarthrosis (gliding)	Gliding
Distal ends of tibia and fibula	Synarthrosis (syndesmosis)	Slight "give"
Ankle (between distal tibia and fibula, and the talus)	Diarthrosis (hinge)	Dorsiflexion, plantar flexion
Ankle (between the calcaneus and talus)	Diarthrosis (gliding)	Inversion, eversion
Between the tarsals and metatarsals	Diarthrosis (gliding)	Gliding
Metatarsophalangeal (MP)	Diarthrosis (condyloid)	Flexion, extension, abduction, adduction
Interphalangeal (IP)	Diarthrosis (hinge)	Flexion, extension

■ CLINICAL COMMENTS

Arthritis is an inflammation of the joints and exists in many forms. The most common form, osteoarthritis, causes pain, swelling, and stiffness as the articular cartilage degenerates. The cause is not always known. Another type, rheumatoid arthritis, is thought to be caused by an immune response to inflammation of the synovial membrane.

■ Student Activities
Using the skeletons and x-rays, find each joint listed in Table 4–2. Be sure you understand the classification.

As you read each joint classification, move the joint on your own body.

Lesson 5

Myology: The Study of Muscles

Before you begin to learn specific muscles of the muscular system, a brief introduction to muscle tissue and body movements is important. Our major emphasis will be on skeletal muscle.

■ OBJECTIVES

1. State the general functions of muscle tissue.
2. Describe the connective tissue elements that connect muscle cells to other body structures.
3. List the types of muscle tissue.
4. List the actions and possible roles skeletal muscles can assume in movement.

■ METHODS

1. Study the text and illustrations included in this section.
2. Use the skeletons to see how the bones relate to each other when performing the actions described.
3. Complete the student activities.

A. MUSCLE FUNCTION

Muscle tissue, which makes up almost half the total body weight, has the unique ability to contract or become shorter. This characteristic allows muscle tissue to serve three major functions:

1. **Production of movement** such as the large muscle action required in walking, as well as less obvious motion such as that involved in changing the size of blood vessels or the pupil of the eye.
2. **Production of heat** as the result of the mechanical contraction. This heat is necessary in the maintenance of the body temperature.
3. **Maintenance of posture** or ability to hold the body in stationary positions. This is possible because skeletal muscles are always in a state of partial contraction, called *tonus* (muscle tone).

B. TYPES OF MUSCLE

1. **Cardiac muscle** is found exclusively in the heart. This tissue is characterized by its involuntary action and striated appearance when seen under a microscope.
2. **Visceral (smooth) muscle** is associated with internal structures such as blood vessels and the digestive tube. It is also involuntary, but it does not have the striated appearance.
3. **Skeletal muscle** is the muscle type that attaches to the bones of the skeleton. It is usually voluntary and is striated.

C. SKELETAL MUSCLE

Because this is the muscle type encountered in the study of the gross anatomy of the lower and upper limbs, it is described in some detail here.

1. **Parts of a muscle**
   a. **Muscle belly**—this is the fleshy or contracting part of the muscle located between the tendons of origin and insertion.
   b. **Origin** (usually more proximal)—the tendon or muscle attachment that is located on the body part that is less movable.
   c. **Insertion** (usually more distal)—the tendon or muscle attachment that is located on the body part that is more movable.

   Note: The general terms **proximal attachment** and **distal attachment** are often preferable to origin and insertion, because the movable part and the stationary part are interchangeable in some cases.

2. **Connective tissue elements**
   The connective tissue fibers (collagen) are continuous from the **endomysium,** which surrounds the individual muscle fiber (cell), through the **perimysium,** which packages the cells into fascicles, and the **epimysium,** which is the fascia surrounding the entire muscle. The fibers are then continuous with those of the tendon holding the muscle to bone. It is this continuity of fibers that lends great strength to muscle attachments, since the connective tissue elements continue into the bone itself. (See Figures 5–1 and 5–2.)

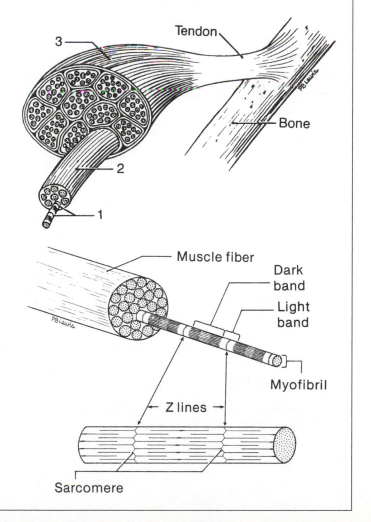

FIGURE 5–1
CONNECTIVE TISSUE COVERINGS OF A SKELETAL MUSCLE

1. **Endomysium**—surrounds an individual fiber

2. **Perimysium**—surrounds a bundle of fibers called a *fascicle*

3. **Epimysium**—surrounds the whole muscle belly

FIGURE 5–2
MICROSCOPIC ANATOMY

The striated appearance of a skeletal muscle is due to the arrangement of thick and thin myofilaments (protein structures) within the cells. These can be seen as darker and lighter bands because of their organized arrangement. This arrangement divides muscle fibers into units called *sarcomeres.* When the biochemistry of the cell causes the myofilaments within a sarcomere to slide over each other, the fiber and thus the muscle shortens or contracts.

3. **Roles of skeletal muscle in action**

During any activity many muscles are involved in production of smooth movements. Although we will learn the major actions a muscle or muscle group can perform, that muscle or group may also be involved in many movements in which it is not producing the major activity. Under different conditions it may assume any of the following roles:

a. **Prime mover (agonist)**—major agent that initiates and maintains a particular action.

b. **Antagonist**—opposes the movement of the prime mover or initiates and maintains the converse of the prime movement.

c. **Synergist**—steadies or eliminates unwanted movement when a muscle crosses two joints. Example: When you make a fist, flexors bend the fingers. But to keep the fist from flexing toward the forearm, extensors (synergists) on the posterior forearm contract to stabilize wrist position.

d. **Fixator**—maintains the position of a body part not actually involved in movement. Example: Certain upper limb muscles hold your arms and forearm steady while your fingers type.

4. **Actions produced by skeletal muscle**

The lower limb will be used to illustrate these actions. Refer to Figure 5–3 when studying Lesson 6.

a. **Flexion**—decrease in angle between two body parts.

b. **Extension**—increase in angle between two parts (opposite of flexion).

c. **Abduction**—moving laterally or away from the midline of the body.

d. **Adduction**—moving medially or toward the midline.

e. **Rotation**—movement around the long axis of the bone.

f. **Circumduction**—circumscribing a cone with the joint as its apex. It is a combination of flexion, abduction, extension, and adduction at the hip.

■ **Student Activities**

Fill in the blanks in Figure 5–3 identifying the illustrated action.

FIGURE 5–3

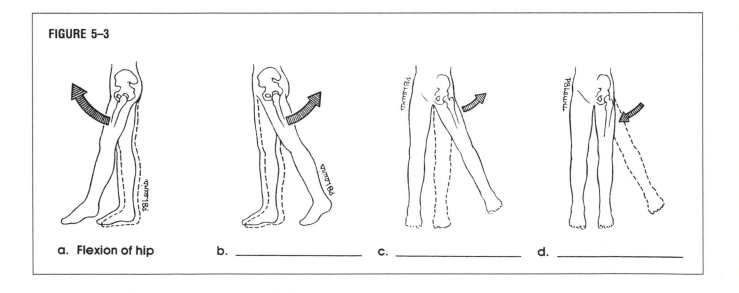

a. **Flexion of hip**   b. _____   c. _____   d. _____

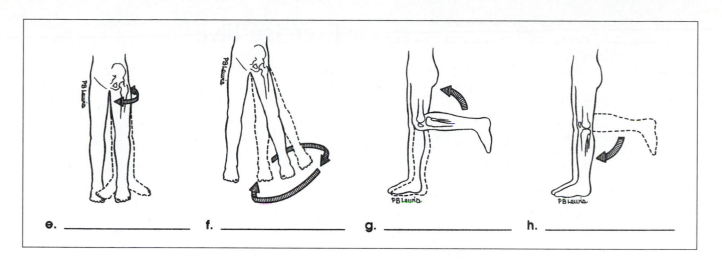

e. _____   f. _____   g. _____   h. _____

■ CLINICAL COMMENTS

Several muscular diseases cause a weakening of muscles. **Myasthenia gravis,** an immune disease, usually starts with a weakness of the muscles of the eye and then moves down the body. **Muscular dystro-
phy** is a genetic disease in which muscle tissue does not develop normally.

Muscle testing is important in understanding the site of muscular problems, and knowing the muscles and
their actions is an important part of testing. An electromyogram (EMG) is a recording of the electrical activity in skeletal muscle and can be used to help determine the cause of muscular weakness.

Name _____

1. Perform with your own lower limb all actions illustrated in this lesson.

2. Answer the following questions:

_____ a. What is the term for the state of partial contraction of a muscle?

_____ b. What muscle type is voluntary and striated?

_____ c. Give the name of a bundle of muscle fibers.

_____ d. What connective tissue element surrounds the whole muscle belly?

_____ e. Name the connective tissue structure that attaches muscle to bone.

_____ f. If you dissect a muscle, which connective tissue would you find as the deepest layer?

_____ g. Which muscle type moves your leg?

_____ h. Would you expect any muscle type other than skeletal to be found in the lower limb?

3. Referring to the illustration below, complete the following:

_____ a. Label all structures indicated.

_____ b. How many fibers are in the fascicle that you just labeled?

_____ c. Can you tell if the tendon shown is of the origin or the insertion?

_____ d. What is the outer covering of bone with which the fibers of the tendon are continuous?

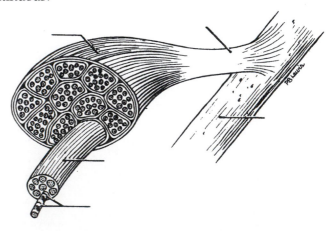

Muscles of the Hip and Thigh

To study the muscles it is helpful to group them according to region and action. Try to avoid memorizing by really understanding each muscle in its position. If you can picture, both mentally and by drawing (use your photocopied skeletons, Figure 2–3), each muscle and its attachments, you can figure out the action. Recognition of the muscle will be easier if you consider its relationship to the structures around it.

You will notice that many of the facts in the muscle charts are not in bold type. For most students, these indicate details that may help in understanding muscles but need not be committed to memory.

■ OBJECTIVES

1. Recognize hip and thigh muscles as indicated in the text.
2. Describe the attachments and/or position of muscles and muscle groups as indicated.
3. Define the actions of each muscle or its group. Refer to Lesson 5 if needed.

■ METHODS

1. Observe the demonstration of each muscle.
2. Identify each of the assigned lower-limb muscles until you can easily name each one.
3. Look at the lower-limb bones and the skeletons, imagining each muscle on the bone markings you studied earlier.

A. MUSCLES OF THE POSTERIOR GLUTEAL (HIP) REGION

These muscles form the buttocks. The large, coarse fibers, especially of gluteus maximus, are important in maintaining the upright posture in the human.

[**Note:** The description of a muscle action requires both the action produced and the joint or body part moved. The action occurs at the joint; the body part that moves is often used in action description. You should recognize it either way. Example: flex knee = flex leg.]

TABLE 6-1. POSTERIOR GLUTEAL MUSCLES

Name	Origin	Insertion	Action	Innervation
Gluteus maximus	**Posterior portion of ilium; post. lower part of sacrum and coccyx,** sacrotuberous ligament	**Gluteal tuberosity and iliotibial tract of fascia lata**	**Extension and lateral rotation of hip (thigh)**	**Inferior gluteal nerve**
Gluteus medius	**Outer surface and crest of ilium** between posterior and anterior gluteal lines	Lateral surface of **greater trochanter of femur**	**Abducts hip (thigh);** anterior fibers med. rotate and flex; post. fibers lat. rot. and extend	**Superior gluteal nerve**
Gluteus minimus	**Outer surface of ilium** between anterior and inferior gluteal lines	Anterior surface of **greater trochanter of femur**	**Abducts thigh;** medially rotates hip (thigh)	**Superior gluteal nerve**
Tensor fasciae latae	**Anterior portion of crest of ilium;** anterior sup. iliac spine	**Iliotibial tract of fascia lata**	**Flex, abduct,** and medially rotate **hip (thigh)**	**Superior gluteal nerve**

FIGURE 6–1
SUPERFICIAL POSTERIOR GLUTEAL AND THIGH MUSCLES

1. **Gluteus medius.** Fibers of this muscle can be seen passing under the larger gluteus maximus muscle. This is a very important muscle in walking. It works with gluteus minimus to stabilize the pelvis. The contracted fibers on the weight-bearing side keep the pelvis from dropping on the side with the lifted foot.

2. **Gluteus maximus.** This large, powerful extensor of the hip is needed for strength when climbing stairs and running. *Color the muscle pink . . . be sure to stop at the fascia!*

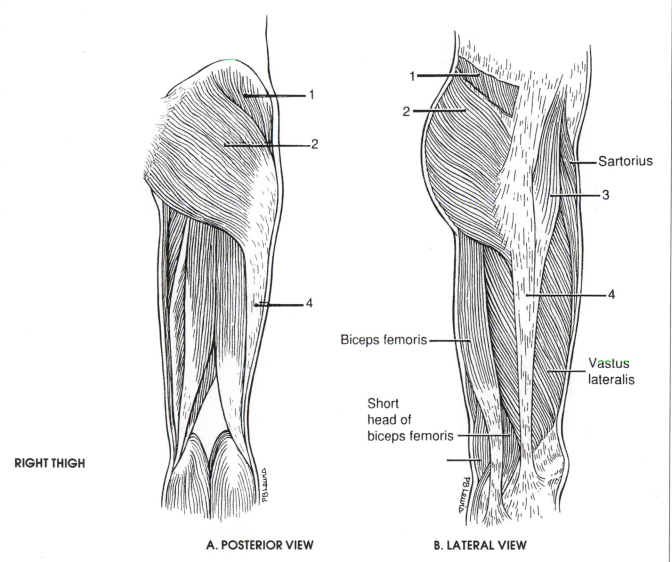

RIGHT THIGH

A. POSTERIOR VIEW   **B. LATERAL VIEW**

Sartorius

Biceps femoris

Short
head of
biceps femoris

Vastus
lateralis

3. **Tensor fasciae latae.** Because this muscle tenses a part of the fascia lata, it helps stabilize the knee. *Color it pink . . . be careful to color only muscle fibers!*

4. **Iliotibial tract.** This is a thickened (more connective tissue fibers) strip of *fascia lata,* the name of the deep fascia that invests the entire thigh. From the fascia lata, sheets of connective tissue extend between muscle groups. *Color it yellow.*

B. DEEP MUSCLES OF THE POSTERIOR GLUTEAL REGION

The deep lateral rotators are more important as postural muscles (synergistic) than as prime movers. Except for piriformis, you should learn the origins and insertions simply as having origin on the ilium and ischium and insertion on the greater trochanter. Table 6–2 is to be used if you are interested.

TABLE 6–2. DEEP LATERAL ROTATORS

Name	Origin	Insertion	Action	Innervation
Piriformis	**Anterior sacrum**	**Greater trochanter of femur**	**Lateral rotation of hip (thigh);** some abduction	**N. to piriformis**
Obturator internus	Bony inner margin of obturator foramen and inner obturator membrane	Greater trochanter of femur	Lateral rotation of hip or thigh; some abduction	N. to obturator internus
Gemellus superior	Ischial spine	Greater trochanter of femur	Lateral rotation of hip or thigh; some abduction	N. to obturator internus
Gemellus inferior	Ischial tuberosity	Greater trochanter of femur	Lateral rotation of hip (thigh); some abduction	N. to quadratus femoris
Quadratus femoris	Ischial tuberosity	Lower posterior greater trochanter	Lateral rotation of thigh	N. to quadratus femoris
Obturator externus	Bony outer margin of obturator foramen and outer obturator membrane	Trochanteric fossa	Lateral rotation of thigh	Obturator n.

FIGURE 6-2
DEEP MUSCLES OF THE POSTERIOR HIP

1. _____

2. _____

3. **Gluteus minimus.** With gluteus medius, it is important in stabilizing the pelvic girdle in walking.

4. **Piriformis.** A pear-shaped muscle that passes from the true pelvis via the greater sciatic foramen. It is an important landmark muscle; the superior gluteal n. emerges superior to pirifomis and the sciatic n. and inferior gluteal n. emerge inferior to it.

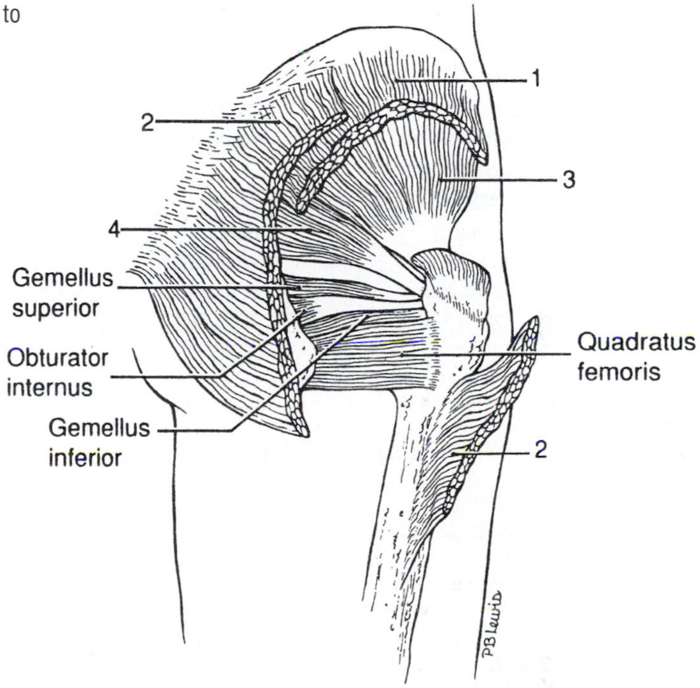

Gemellus superior

Obturator internus

Gemellus inferior

Quadratus femoris

■ **CLINICAL COMMENTS**

Because of the position of the nerves relative to the piriformis muscle, it is important to avoid that area when you give an injection in the gluteal region. The safe place to insert the needle is in the upper outer quadrant.

C. MUSCLES OF THE ANTERIOR HIP (ILIAC REGION)

These muscles lie over the anterior hip joint and can pull the trunk down (flexion of trunk) or raise the thigh (flexion of the thigh) but flex the hip joint in either action.

TABLE 6–3. MUSCLES OF THE ANTERIOR HIP

Name	Origin	Insertion	Action	Innervation
Psoas major	All lumbar vertebrae, transverse processes and bodies	Lesser trochanter of femur	Flexes thigh; flexes trunk (or flexes hip)	Lumbar nerves L1–L3
Psoas minor	Bodies of last thoracic and first lumbar vertebrae	Iliopubic eminence	Flexes pelvis or lumbar spine	Lumbar nerve L1
Iliacus	Iliac fossa	Lesser trochanter of femur	Flexes hip	Femoral n.

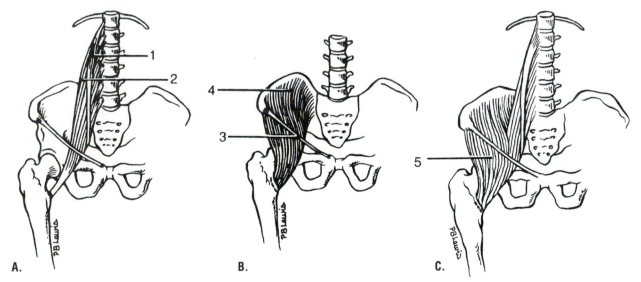

FIGURE 6–3
MUSCLES OF THE ANTERIOR ILIAC REGION

A.   B.   C.

1. **Psoas minor** only exists about 60% of the time. Because it does not cross the hip joint, it can only perform minor flexion of the trunk.

2. **Psoas major.**

3. **Inguinal ligament.** This very important landmark structure extends from the anterior superior iliac spine to the pubic tubercle. It marks the division between the trunk and the thigh.

4. **Iliacus** fills the iliac fossa.

5. **Iliopsoas** is formed where the psoas major and iliacus muscles join after passing under the inguinal ligament.

D. MUSCLES OF THE THIGH

Three groups of muscles surround the femur. The muscles are separated into anterior, medial, and posterior groups by connective tissue sheets. If considered as a group, each has its own major action and innervation. Exceptions will be seen with individual muscles.

FIGURE 6–4
MUSCLES OF THE THIGH

The thigh is shown in cross section, a transverse plane through the mid-thigh, to demonstrate the three groups with the major action of each group.

a. Anterior femoral muscles

  Major action _____

  Innervation _____

b. Medial femoral muscles

  Major action _____

  Innervation _____

c. Posterior femoral muscles

  Major actions _____

  Innervation _____

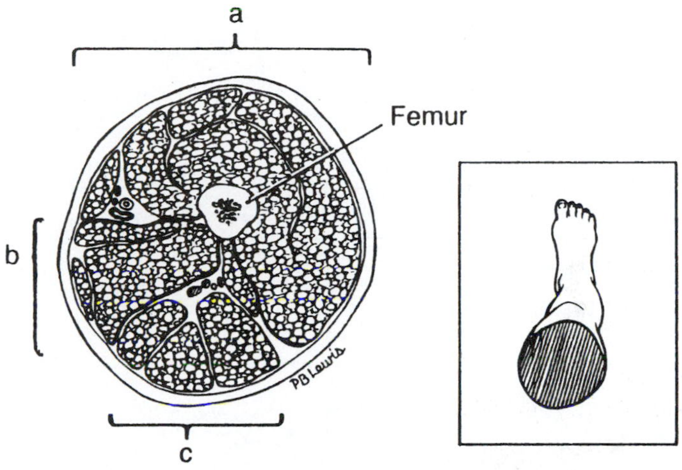

ANTERIOR FEMORAL MUSCLES

These muscles cover the entire anterior portion of the thigh, and, as a group, they are *the* extensors of the leg.

TABLE 6–4. ANTERIOR FEMORAL MUSCLES[a]

Name	Origin	Insertion	Action	Innervation
1. **Sartorius** (Figure 6–5)	**Anterior superior iliac spine**	**Upper part of medial surface of tibia**	**Flexes leg and thigh**	
2. **Rectus femoris** (Figure 6–6A)	**Anterior inferior iliac spine; superior margin of acetabulum**		**Extension of leg;** some flexion of thigh	
3. **Vastus lateralis** (Figure 6–6B)	**Lateral lip of linea aspera;** lower part of greater trochanter	**Tibial tuberosity** (by way of patella and patellar ligament)		**Femoral n.**
4. **Vastus medialis** (Figure 6–6C)	**Medial lip of linea aspera;** intertrochanteric line		**Extension of leg or knee**	
5. **Vastus intermedius** (Figure 6–6D)	**Anterior shaft of upper femur**			

[a]The anterior femoral muscles are illustrated in Figures 6–5 and 6–6.

FIGURE 6–5
SARTORIUS MUSCLE

This is a narrow strap and is the longest muscle in the body. (In addition to actions listed in Table 6–4, it helps abduct the thigh and laterally rotate the thigh.)

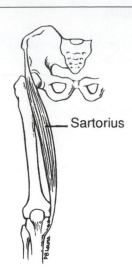

— Sartorius

FIGURE 6–6
QUADRICEPS FEMORIS

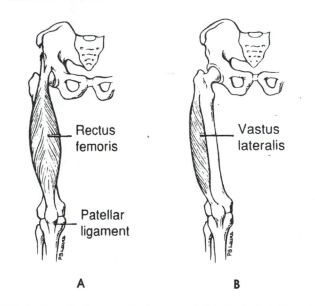

Rectus femoris

Patellar ligament

A

Vastus lateralis

B

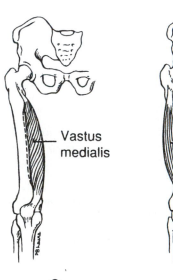

Vastus medialis

C

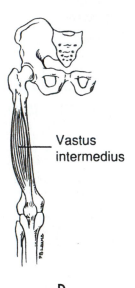

Vastus intermedius

D

This is the collective name for muscles 2–5 in Table 6–4. The common tendon of these four muscles, the quadriceps tendon, encases the patella; the patellar ligament then attaches to the tibial tuberosity, and so the quadriceps femoris is the great extensor of the leg at the knee.

MEDIAL FEMORAL MUSCLES

As a group, these are the adductors of the thigh; they originate from the medial pelvis (largely pubis) and insert on the posterior femur. They serve primarily as synergists. (See Table 6–5.)

TABLE 6–5. MEDIAL FEMORAL MUSCLES

Name	Origin	Insertion	Action	Innervation
Gracilis	**Pubic bone;** medial surface of body and inferior ramus	**Upper part of medial surface of tibia**	Flexes knee (leg); some **adduction of hip (thigh)**	**Obturator n.**
Pectineus	Pectin of **Pubis**	Upper part of posterior femur	**Adducts, flexes hip (thigh)**	**Femoral n.** and some obturator n.
Adductor longus	**Pubic bone,** between crest and symphysis	Linea aspera	**Adducts,** flexes hip (thigh); some lateral rotation	**Obturator n.**
Adductor brevis	Inferior **pubic** ramus	Upper part of posterior femur	**Adducts hip;** some lateral rotation	
Adductor magnus	Rami of pubis and **ischium**	Linea aspera; adductor tubercle	**Adducts hip;** lateral and possibly medial rotation	**Obturator n.** and some tibial n.

FIGURE 6–7   MEDIAL FEMORAL MUSCLES

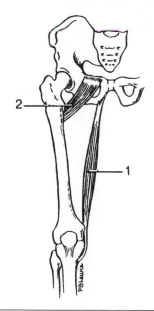

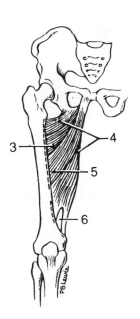

1. **Gracilis** inserts very close to sartorius.

2. **Pectineus** is beside, and in the same plane as, iliopsoas.

3. **Adductor brevis** is the smallest of the three adductors and is sandwiched between the other two.

4. **Adductor magnus** is very large and can be seen as easily from the posterior aspect of the thigh.

5. **Adductor longus** is the most superficial adductor muscle.

6. **Adductor hiatus** is an opening in the tendon of insertion of the adductor magnus.

■ **Student Activities**

In Figure 6–7, color adductor magnus pink. Magnus means large . . . you can see it in two places because of its size.

FIGURE 6–8
ANTERIOR VIEW OF THE ILIAC REGION AND THIGH

Now that you have seen each of these structures, cover the key and identify each one.

1. Psoas major m.
2. Iliacus m.
3. Iliopsoas m.
4. Pectineus m.
5. Adductor longus m.
6. Sartorius m.
7. Adductor magnus m.
8. Gracilis m.
9. Rectus femoris m.
10. Vastus medialis m.
11. Vastus lateralis m.
12. Quadriceps tendon
13. Patella
14. Patellar ligament

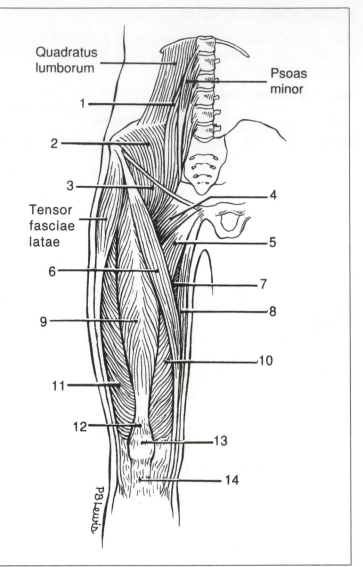

■ **CLINICAL COMMENTS**

Muscle injuries are quite common. Forceful contraction of a muscle, particularly if it has not been warmed up, can cause tearing and bleeding of muscle tissue and results in pain, often severe. This is particularly common with the hamstrings.

POSTERIOR FEMORAL MUSCLES

This muscle group is composed of only three muscles, but its actions are very important at both the hip and knee joints. These muscles are commonly called the hamstring muscles.

TABLE 6–6. POSTERIOR FEMORAL MUSCLES

Name	Origin	Insertion	Action	Innervation
Biceps femoris a. long head	Ischial tuberosity	Head of fibula; lateral condyle of tibia	Flexes leg; extends thigh	Tibial n. (div. of sciatic)
b. short head	Linea aspera of shaft of femur	With the long head—they share a common tendon	Flexes leg	Common fibular (peroneal) n.
Semitendinosus	Ischial tuberosity	Upper part of medial tibia	Flexes leg; extends thigh	Tibial n.
Semimembranosus	Ischial tuberosity	Posterior upper tibia; medial condyle	Flexes leg and extends thigh	Tibial n.

FIGURE 6–9
POSTERIOR VIEW OF GLUTEAL REGION AND THIGH

1. _____

2. _____

3. _____

4. **Semitendinosus** inserts on the tibia with the sartorius and gracilis muscles. It attaches distally as a long tendon.

5. **Biceps femoris.** This muscle is easily identified as the only muscle of the thigh that inserts on the lateral aspect of the leg. The long head hides most of the short head; the two heads join to form a common belly and common distal attachment.

6. **Semimembranosus** muscle is so named because its proximal attachment is a flattened, wide aponeurosis (tendon) in the upper thigh.

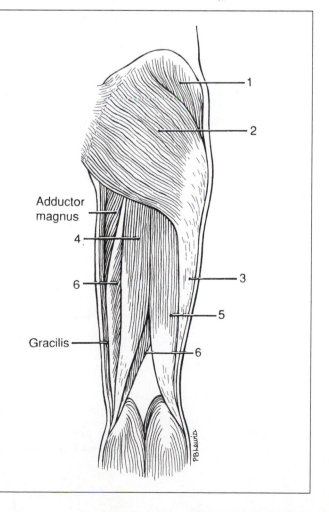

Exercise Six

Name _____

1. In Figure 6–9, underline the name of each hamstring muscle with a different color; color the named muscle with the corresponding color. To the right of each muscle that is *not* a posterior femoral group muscle, write the name of the compartment to which it does belong.

2. In Figure 6–4 and Figure 6–8, use a different color for each group of muscles. (Ant. = pink; med. = blue; post. = yellow.)

3. Fill in the blanks in Figures 6–4 and 6–9.

4. Use a copy of the skeleton in Figure 2–3 to draw each muscle on its attachments.

5. Matching—each letter may be used more than once, and more than one letter may be used to define the numbered terms.

_____ 1. Iliac fossa	a. Adducts hip
_____ 2. Tonus	b. Includes biceps femoris m.
_____ 3. Gluteus maximus m.	c. Covering of the thigh muscles
_____ 4. Posterior femoral m.	d. Attachment for extensors of the leg (knee)
_____ 5. Abduction	e. Study of muscles
_____ 6. Tibial tuberosity	f. Attachment for iliacus m.
_____ 7. Quadriceps femoris m.	g. Includes rectus femoris m.
_____ 8. Adductor magnus m.	h. Major extensor of the thigh
_____ 9. Myology	i. Moving away from the midline
_____ 10. Fascia lata	j. Partial contraction

6. Write the answers to the following questions.

_____ a. If looking at a posterior view of the thigh, what muscle would be seen medial to the semitendinosus and semimembranosus?

_____ b. Name the muscle that is a combination of two muscles.

_____ c. Name the only thigh muscle that attaches on the lateral side of the leg.

_____ d. If you have your left foot on the ground and your right foot on a step, is your right knee flexed or extended?

_____ e. Refer to question 6d. To lift your body onto the step, which group of thigh muscles would act at the knee?

_____ f. A muscle which would act as an antagonist to the iliopsoas muscle would be the _____ .

_____ g. The action gluteus maximus has in common with biceps femoris is _____ .

46

Muscles of the Leg and Foot

Deep to the skin there is a layer of fascia that covers all muscles. You learned that this fascia is called *fascia lata* on the thigh. Fibers of this connective tissue are continuous onto the leg, but the name changes to **crural fascia.** Crural fascia covers the muscles that surround the tibia and fibula. Connective tissue sheets from this fascia separate the muscles into compartments. The muscles of the leg should be studied in the same manner as those of the thigh.

■ OBJECTIVES

1. Recognize all groups of leg and foot muscles.
2. Describe the position of the major muscles as indicated.
3. Define the action of each muscle or muscle group.

■ METHODS

1. Observe the demonstration of each muscle.
2. Identify each indicated leg and foot muscle until you can name each muscle.
3. Using the bones of the lower limb and the skeletons, imagine each muscle in its position. Move the bones to simulate the action that would be created by each muscle.

A. MUSCLES OF THE LEG

FIGURE 7–1
SUPERIOR VIEW OF TRANSVERSE SECTION OF RIGHT LEG

a. Anterior crural muscles

    Color all three muscles pink.

b. Lateral crural muscles

    Color both muscles blue.

c. Posterior crural muscles

    Color the three deep muscles yellow.

d. Crural fascia

    Notice the transverse intermuscular septum separating the posterior crural muscles into a deep and a superficial group.

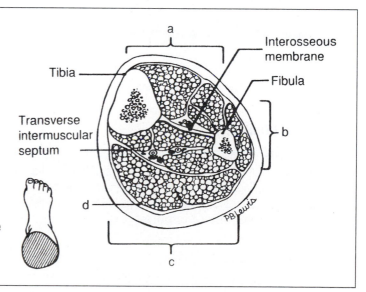

TERMS OF MOVEMENT

The muscles of the leg and foot will produce actions across the knee joint (illustrated in Lesson 5) as well as across the ankle, metatarsophalangeal, and interphalangeal joints. Remember, even if you do not learn exact attachments of a specific muscle, it is necessary to know which joints are crossed because some movement will occur if the muscle crosses the joint.

The following actions and action terminology are added here and illustrated in Figure 7–2 to help you understand movements at the ankle and digits.

(a) **Dorsiflexion:** brings the dorsum of the foot toward the anterior leg. (Lifts ball of foot off the ground.)
(b) **Extension** of the toes.
(c) **Plantar flexion:** the plantar aspect (sole) of the foot approaches the posterior leg. (Lifts heel of foot off the ground.)
(d) **Flexion** of the toes.
(e) **Inversion** (supination): turns the plantar surface inward parallel to the median plane.
(f) **Eversion** (pronation): opposite of inversion—turns the plantar surface to the outside.

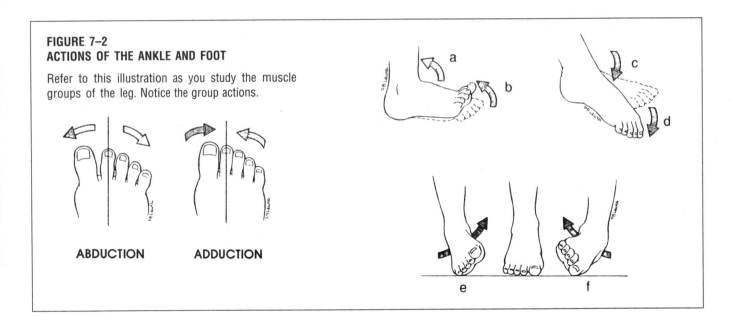

FIGURE 7–2
ACTIONS OF THE ANKLE AND FOOT

Refer to this illustration as you study the muscle groups of the leg. Notice the group actions.

ABDUCTION   ADDUCTION

■ CLINICAL COMMENT

A **sprained ankle** is most commonly caused when the foot is forcefully inverted. This stretches the lateral ligaments causing some of the collagen fibers to tear. The ligament is still functional, but there is pain and usually swelling. A more serious accident can result in a completely separated or *torn ligament*. A sprain rarely occurs on the medial side of the ankle because the stronger medial ligaments and the laterally positioned fibula prevent excessive eversion.

ANTERIOR CRURAL MUSCLES

To appreciate the position of these muscles you can feel them on your own leg. They are just lateral to the anterior border (shin) of the tibia. As a group, they are the major dorsiflexors of the foot and extensors of the toes. See Figure 7–2. Specific attachments are included for information only. You do not need to memorize them. (See Table 7–1.)

TABLE 7–1. ANTERIOR CRURAL MUSCLES

Name	Origin	Insertion	Action	Innervation
Tibialis anterior	Lateral condyle and upper tibia; interosseous membrane	Medial surface of 1st cuneiform and 1st metatarsal	**Dorsiflexes and inverts foot**	
Extensor digitorum longus	Lateral condyle of tibia; upper 3/4 anterior fibula; interosseous membrane	Dorsal surface, middle and distal phalanges of digits 2–5	**Extends digits 2–5; dorsiflexes foot**	**Deep fibular (peroneal) n.**
Extensor hallucis longus	Anterior middle fibula; interosseous membrane	Dorsal surface, base of distal phalanx of hallux	**Extends hallux; dorsiflexes and inverts foot**	
Fibularis (peroneus) tertius	Lower third of medial fibula; interosseous membrane	Base, fifth metatarsal	**Dorsiflexes and everts foot**	

■ CLINICAL COMMENTS

Shin-splints are small tears in the periosteum where the tibialis anterior muscle attaches to the tibia. This is a painful condition and is most likely to occur if the muscle has not been warmed up.

FIGURE 7–3
ANTERIOR CRURAL MUSCLES

1. **Tibialis anterior.** The large belly ends as a long tendon. This muscle is very active in walking and running where a combination of dorsiflexion and inversion of the ankle are important.

2. **Extensor digitorum longus.** The belly ends in a tendon that divides into four slips, one for each of the four lateral digits.

3. **Extensor hallucis longus.** The belly of this muscle is almost hidden between tibialis anterior and extensor digitorum longus.

4. **Fibularis (peroneus) tertius.** The tendon of this muscle is actually a part of extensor digitorum longus tendon.

5. **Superior extensor retinaculum.** To keep the tendons from "bow-stringing" at the ankle, the crural fascia thickens to form bands called retinacula.

In the illustrations of the individual muscles, part **B,** you can see the origins and insertions of the three large anterior crural muscles.

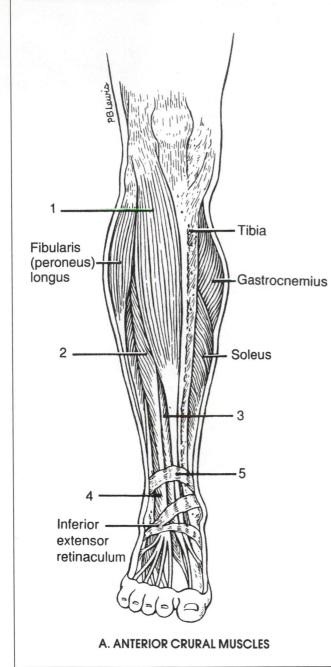

A. ANTERIOR CRURAL MUSCLES

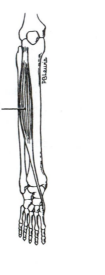
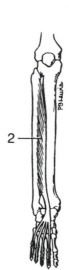
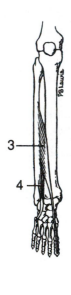

B. INDIVIDUAL MUSCLES

LATERAL CRURAL MUSCLES

This group consists of only two muscles, the evertors of the foot. Notice the use of the term *fibular* when referring to many of the structures on the fibular or lateral side of the leg. New anatomical terminology has replaced the word peroneal with fibular. The muscles are now called fibularis tertius, fibularis longus and fibularis brevis. The retinaculum is the fibular retinaculum. (See Table 7–2.)

TABLE 7–2. LATERAL CRURAL MUSCLES

Name	Origin	Insertion	Action	Innervation
Fibularis (peroneus) longus	Head and upper 2/3 of lateral fibula	Base of first metatarsal; first cuneiform	**Plantar flexes and everts foot**	**Superficial fibular (peroneal) n.**
Fibularis (peroneus) brevis	Lower 2/3 of lateral fibula	Base of fifth metatarsal		

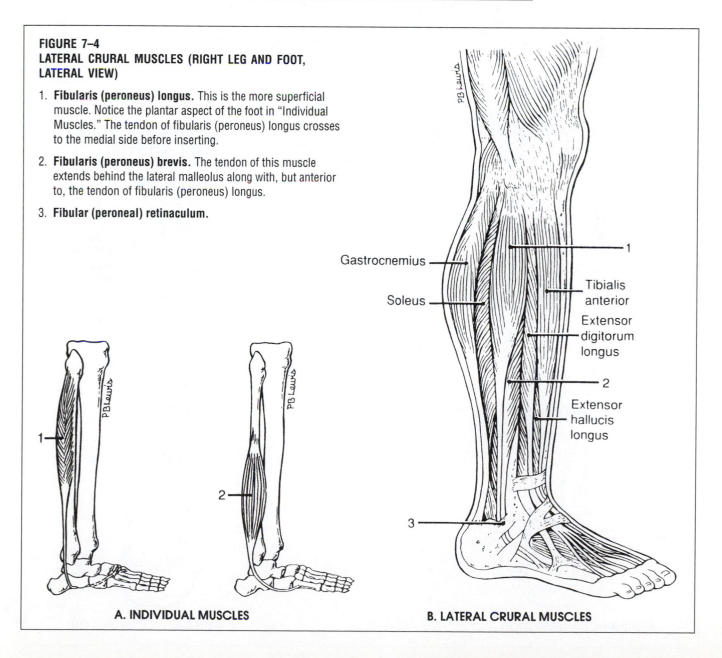

FIGURE 7–4
LATERAL CRURAL MUSCLES (RIGHT LEG AND FOOT, LATERAL VIEW)

1. **Fibularis (peroneus) longus.** This is the more superficial muscle. Notice the plantar aspect of the foot in "Individual Muscles." The tendon of fibularis (peroneus) longus crosses to the medial side before inserting.

2. **Fibularis (peroneus) brevis.** The tendon of this muscle extends behind the lateral malleolus along with, but anterior to, the tendon of fibularis (peroneus) longus.

3. **Fibular (peroneal) retinaculum.**

Gastrocnemius

Soleus

Tibialis anterior

Extensor digitorum longus

Extensor hallucis longus

A. INDIVIDUAL MUSCLES

B. LATERAL CRURAL MUSCLES

POSTERIOR CRURAL MUSCLES

Partially separated from the anterior muscles by the interosseous membrane, the posterior muscles can be regarded as two groups. The **superficial group** and **deep group** are separated by a fascial sheet. Learning specific attachments is unnecessary. You *do* need to know which joints are crossed. The muscles with asterisks (*) cross both knee and ankle joints.

TABLE 7–3. SUPERFICIAL GROUP: POSTERIOR CRURAL MUSCLES

Name	Origin	Insertion	Action	Innervation
Gastrocnemius*	Medial and lateral condyles of femur	Posterior calcaneus via calcaneal tendon	**Flexes leg; plantar flexes foot**	
Soleus	Upper fibula; soleal line and middle 1/3 of tibia	Posterior calcaneus via calcaneal tendon	**Plantar flexes foot**	**Tibial n.**
Plantaris*	Posterior femur above lateral condyle	Posterior calcaneus	**Flexes leg; plantar flexes foot**	

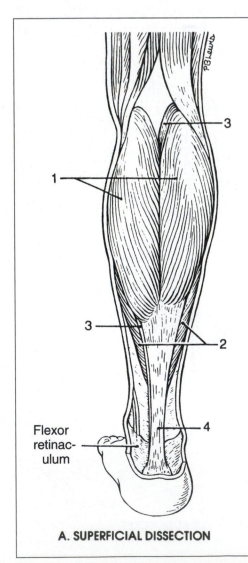

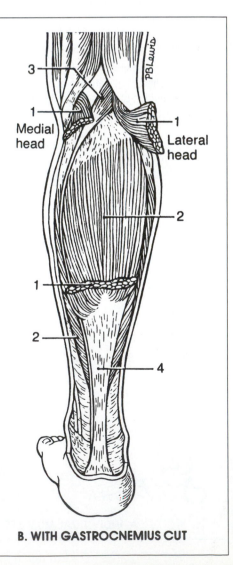

FIGURE 7–5
POSTERIOR CRURAL MUSCLES: SUPERFICIAL GROUP (RIGHT LEG, POSTERIOR VIEW)

1. **Gastrocnemius.** Both heads of this muscle can be seen attaching into the calcaneal (Achilles) tendon.

2. **Soleus.** With gastrocnemius, this muscle makes up the large fleshy part of the calf of the leg. The two muscles share the calcaneal tendon.

3. **Plantaris.** The small belly terminates in a very long tendon.

4. **Calcaneal tendon.** This is the largest tendon in the body; attaches to the calcaneus.

Flexor retinaculum

Medial head

Lateral head

A. SUPERFICIAL DISSECTION

B. WITH GASTROCNEMIUS CUT

DEEP GROUP: POSTERIOR CRURAL MUSCLES

The tendons of the last three muscles in the chart pass behind the medial malleolus. In this position they are all plantar flexors and invertors of the foot. Details are in Table 7–4.

TABLE 7–4. DEEP GROUP: POSTERIOR CRURAL MUSCLES

Name	Origin	Insertion	Action	Innervation
Popliteus	Lateral condyle of femur	Posterior tibia above soleal line	**Flexes leg; rotates tibia medially**	
Flexor hallucis longus	Lower 2/3 fibula; interosseous membrane	Base of distal phalanx of hallux	**Flexes hallux; plantar flexes foot**	
Flexor digitorum longus	Posterior tibia	Base of distal phalanx of digits 2–5	**Flexes digits 2–5; plantar flexes and inverts foot**	**Tibial n.**
Tibialis posterior	Posterior interosseous membrane; tibia and fibula	Navicular, cuneiforms, cuboid; metatarsals 2–4	**Plantar flexes and inverts foot**	

FIGURE 7–6A
POSTERIOR CRURAL MUSCLES: DEEP GROUP (RIGHT LEG, POSTERIOR VIEW)

1. **Popliteus.** This flat muscle forms part of the floor of the popliteal fossa. It is considered the muscle that "unlocks" the fully extended knee so flexion can begin.

2. **Flexor hallucis longus.** Although in the most lateral position, this muscle flexes the most medial digit, the hallux.

3. **Flexor digitorum longus.** The tendons of this muscle pass through openings in the tendons of flexor digitorum brevis to reach the distal phalanges of the lateral four digits.

4. **Tibialis posterior.** The belly of this muscle is overlapped by those of flexor hallucis longus and flexor digitorum longus, and it can be seen by looking between them.

5. **Tendon of tibialis posterior**

6. **Flexor retinaculum**

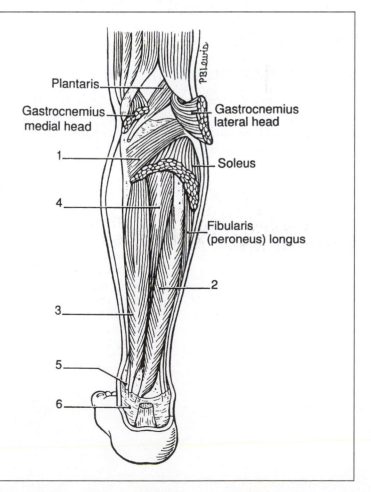

FIGURE 7–6B
INDIVIDUAL MUSCLES OF THE POSTERIOR DEEP CRURAL GROUP

In this posterior view of the right leg, notice the three tendons of the long muscles passing behind the medial malleolus. They can easily be identified in the lab by locating the medial malleolus. The tendon just posterior is *t*ibialis posterior, next is flexor *d*igitorum longus, and then, flexor *h*allucis longus—or, *Tom, Dick,* and *H*arry.

Figure 7–6A illustrates the bellies of these muscles; notice that they are *not* in the same order as the tendons. The numbers correspond with those in Figure 7–6A.

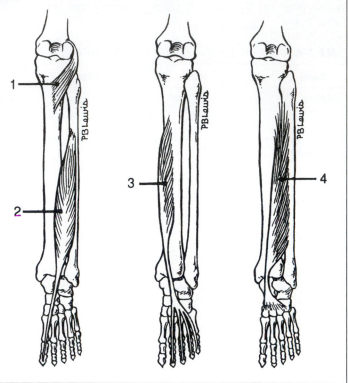

B. MUSCLES OF THE FOOT

MUSCLE OF THE DORSUM OF THE FOOT

There is only one intrinsic muscle of the dorsum of the foot. An intrinsic muscle is one that has both attachments within the same body part. You will notice that all other tendons on the dorsum of the foot are from muscles that originate on another body part, the leg. Therefore, they are extrinsic muscles.

TABLE 7–5. MUSCLE OF THE DORSUM OF THE FOOT

Name	Origin	Insertion	Action	Innervation
Extensor digitorum brevis	Lateral calcaneus	Base of proximal phalanx of hallux; into ext. digitorum longus tendons of digits 1–4	**Extends digits 1–4**	**Deep fibular (peroneal) n.**

FIGURE 7–7
RIGHT LEG AND FOOT (ANTERIOR VIEW)

1. **Extensor digitorum brevis.** Color the belly and tendons of this muscle. Use a pale red color.

      Note: Some textbooks refer to the medial part of this muscle as *extensor hallucis brevis.*

      Color all the anterior crural muscles with a yellow pencil, the lateral crural muscles blue, and the posterior crural muscles green.

      Label the remaining structures of Figure 7–7. Try to do it without referring to the other illustrations.

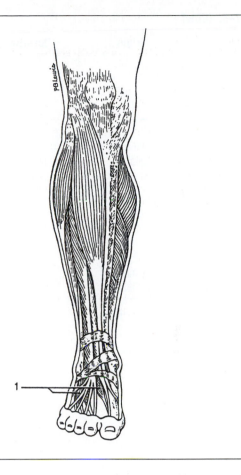

MUSCLES OF THE PLANTAR ASPECT OF THE FOOT

These muscles are arranged in four layers and are covered by a thick fascial structure called the **plantar aponeurosis.** Most students will not need to know the details of these muscles; however, they are included here for your reference. For general understanding, learn the first layer; read about the others.

TABLE 7–6. MUSCLES OF THE PLANTAR ASPECT OF THE FOOT

Name	Origin	Insertion	Action	Innervation
First layer Abductor hallucis	Calcaneus and flexor retinaculum	Proximal phalanx of hallux	Abducts hallux	Medial plantar n.
Flexor digitorum brevis	Calcaneus and plantar aponeurosis	Middle phalanx of digits 2–5	Flexes digits 2–5	
Abductor digiti minimi	Calcaneus and plantar aponeurosis	Base of proximal phalanx of fifth digit	Abducts fifth digit	Lateral plantar n.
Second layer Quadratus plantae	Calcaneus	Tendon of flexor digitorum longus	Flexes digits 2–5	Lateral plantar n.

TABLE 7–6. (CONT.)

Name	Origin	Insertion	Action	Innervation
Lumbricals (4)	Tendons of flexor digitorum longus	Tendons of extensor digitorum longus	Flex MP joints 2–5; extend IP 2–5	Medial (first) and lat. plantar n.
Third layer Flexor hallucis brevis	Cuboid and lateral cuneiform	Proximal phalanx of hallux	Flexes hallux	Medial plantar n.
Adductor hallucis	Oblique head; metatarsals 2–4 Transverse head: ligaments of MP joints	Proximal phalanx of hallux	Adducts hallux	Lateral plantar n.
Flexor digiti minimi brevis	Fifth metatarsal	Proximal phalanx of fifth digit	Flexes fifth digit	Lateral plantar n.
Fourth layer Dorsal interossei (4)	Bases metatarsals 3–5	Proximal phalanx of same digit	Abduct digits; flexes MP joints	Lateral plantar n.
Plantar interossei (3)	Bases of adjacent metatarsals	Proximal phalanges of digits 2–4	Adduct digits; flexes MP joints	Lateral plantar n.

FIGURE 7–8
PLANTAR MUSCLES

Plantar view of the right foot, first layer. The plantar aponeurosis has been removed.

1. Abductor hallucis
2. Flexor digitorum brevis
3. Abductor digiti minimi

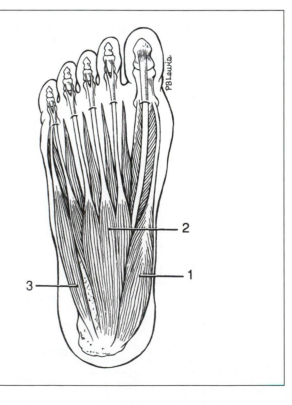

Name _____

1. In Figure 7–3, color each of the anterior crural muscles with a different color. Be sure you color the tendon as far as it is visible. **Note:** The most lateral tendon is that of fibularis (peroneus) tertius!

2. In Figure 7–4, color the lateral crural muscles with different colors. Choose a third color for the fibular (peroneal) retinaculum.

3. In Figure 7–5A,B, color each of the superficial posterior crural muscles a different color.

4. In Figure 7–6A, color the four deep posterior muscles in different colors. Be careful to have the tendons in the correct order (remember *Tom*, *Dick*, and *Harry*). Notice that the bellies are not in the same order as the tendons.

    Color the fibular (peroneal) retinaculum and the flexor retinaculum with different colors.

5. In Figure 7–8, color the superficial layer of plantar muscles.

6. Answer the following:

   a. A muscle that has both its origin and insertion within an anatomical part is a

      (an) _____ muscle.

   b. Another term for Achilles tendon is _____ .

   c. The lateral crural muscles are most important in what

      action? _____ .

   d. Tibialis anterior is found just _____ to the crest of the tibia.

   e. The hamstrings share an action with gastrocnemius. It

      is _____ .

7. Using the illustrations on the right, list the correct names for the labeled structures.
   1. _____
   2. _____
   3. _____
   4. _____
   5. _____
   6. _____
   7. _____
   8. _____
   9. _____
   10. _____

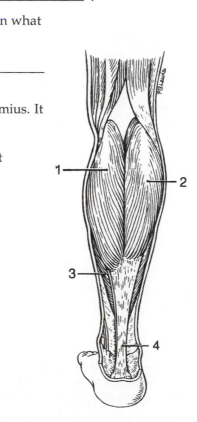
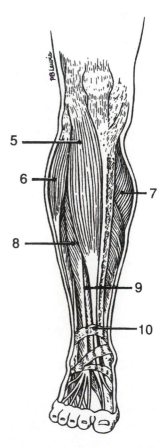

Introduction to the Nervous System

The nervous system, the major communication system of the body, will be studied in great detail later in this course. However, it is important that you have a basic understanding of what the nerve cell processes are and where they originate before we discuss the nerves of the lower limb. Because the nerve cells are microscopic, they will be represented schematically.

■ OBJECTIVES

1. Define general terms related to the nervous system.
2. List the structures of the central nervous system and those of the peripheral nervous system.
3. Describe the principal parts of a neuron.
4. State the locations of both motor and sensory nerve cell bodies that are involved in the innervation of the limbs.

■ METHODS

1. Study the information presented, then complete *Student Activities.*

A. THE NERVOUS SYSTEM DIVISIONS

These divisions are the **central nervous system (CNS)** composed only of the brain and spinal cord, and the **peripheral nervous system (PNS),** which includes all other nervous structures.

CNS Structures

Brain—the major control structure. It is contained in, and protected by, the skull.

Spinal cord—a direct extension of the brain. It is contained in, and protected by, the bones of the spinal column.

PNS Structures

Cranial nerves—originate in brain structures; related to head and neck anatomy and to thoracic and abdominopelvic viscera.

Peripheral nerves—originate at the spinal cord; related to peripheral (limbs) and external structures.

Ganglia—groups of nerve cell bodies in the periphery.

Plexuses—intermingling of nerve cell processes.

B. HISTOLOGY OF THE NERVOUS SYSTEM

1. THE NEURON

The neuron is the **nerve cell,** the basic structural and *functional* unit of the nervous system. It is composed of a body, which is always found either in the central nervous system or in a ganglion, and of one or more nerve cell processes.

Structural Characteristics

The number of processes determine the following cell types:

a. Multipolar = many processes (motor cells, internuncial cells)
b. Bipolar = two processes (sensory cells for special senses)
c. Unipolar = one process (general sensory cells)

Illustrations of these microscopic cells are schematic.

Multipolar Neuron (Figure 8–1)

This is the most common type of neuron. It has many dendrites, short processes that extend from the nerve cell body and take information toward the cell body; it has only one axon, the process that takes information away from the nerve cell body.

Included among multipolar cells are those that carry motor information to the periphery. The cell bodies of the motor neurons for the skeletal muscles of the limbs are in the ventral horn of gray matter in the spinal cord. Because this information is on its way from the CNS to the periphery, these processes are *efferent*. It is interesting to note here that the nerve cell bodies are in the spinal cord, and, the nerve impulse must reach as far as the intrinsic foot muscles. That means some of the processes are several feet long.

If the information traveling in the processes of these motor neurons is interrupted proximal to the muscle, the muscle is paralyzed.

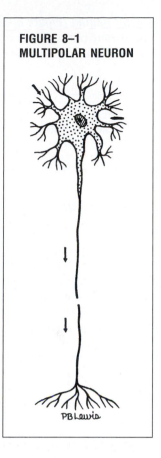

FIGURE 8–1
MULTIPOLAR NEURON

PB Lewis

Unipolar Neuron (Figure 8–2)

A sensory neuron with only one process; the process probably originated as one dendrite and one axon.

Sensory cells, *afferent* cells, bring information from the periphery into the central nervous system. If the afferent processes are interrupted, anesthesia, or absence of sensation, results.

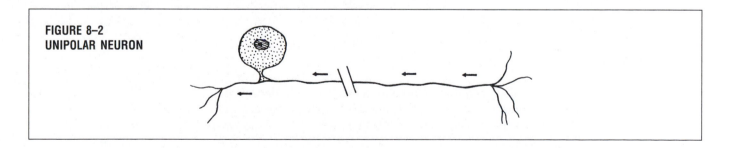

FIGURE 8–2
UNIPOLAR NEURON

The cell bodies of these sensory neurons are found in the dorsal root ganglia. (See Figure 8–5.)

Bipolar Neuron (Figure 8–3)

These neurons with one axon and one dendrite are found only in cranial nerves relating to the special senses and will be discussed later.

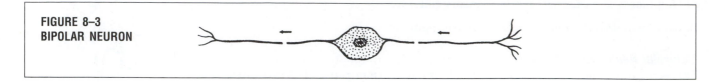

FIGURE 8–3
BIPOLAR NEURON

Functional Characteristics

Neurons are functional because of the following characteristics:

a. **Irritability:** The capacity to respond to a stimulation by changing cell activity.
b. **Conductivity:** The change in the cell activity is transmitted along the cell process as a nerve impulse. The impulse is conducted to the structure that is to receive the message, such as a muscle in the case of a motor neuron. Some "effect" will then result from the original stimulus. In the case of sensory information, the effect might be in the conscious awareness of the stimulus.

When a nerve impulse is transmitted from one nerve cell to another, the site of the membrane-to-membrane contact is called a **synapse.** A chemical *neurotransmitter* is usually involved in the transmission.

2. NEUROGLIA

Neuroglia, the supportive cells in the CNS, are necessary for the proper functioning of the neurons. Three kinds of neuroglia are:

a. **Microglia**—found throughout the gray and white matter; these small cells are phagocytic, and thus they serve to remove foreign material and dead cells.
b. **Oligodendroglia**—the cells that produce myelin, a fatty insulating material that aids in the conduction of impulses, the electrochemical changes that are transmitted along the membranes of nerve fibers.
c. **Astrocytes**—cells thought to help in the repair process and in transfer of nutrients from blood vessels to nerve cells. These cells are multipolar (many processes).

Neuroglial cells will not be studied in detail.

3. SCHWANN CELLS

These supportive cells of the PNS produce a myelin coating on the nerve fibers within peripheral nerves. In Figure 8–4, these cells can be seen wrapping around a nerve process. The space between adjacent Schwann cells is referred to as the *node of Ranvier.*

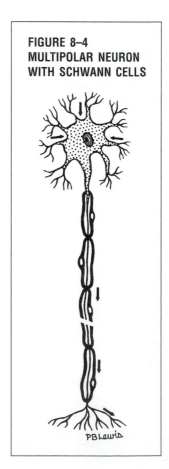

FIGURE 8–4
MULTIPOLAR NEURON
WITH SCHWANN CELLS

PBLewis

Each process is covered by a **neurilemmal sheath** composed of the Schwann cell and the myelin produced by it.

The neurilemma is necessary for repair of nerve fibers. If the nerve cell body is injured it cannot be repaired.

C. SPINAL CORD AND PERIPHERAL NERVES

These are the structures needed to understand the innervation of the upper and lower limbs. The brain and cranial nerves will be discussed in Unit III.

1. A NERVE

This is a bundle of many nerve cell processes enclosed in a fascial sheath called the **epineurium.** Spinal nerves are those that contain both afferent (sensory) and efferent (motor) processes, and that leave the region of the spinal cord at a specific level indicated by the number of the vertebra either above or below its exit. For instance, the third lumbar spinal nerve, L3, leaves the bony spinal column just below the third lumbar vertebra. (See Figure 9–1.)

The sensory (afferent) fibers that are a part of this nerve will bring peripheral information (e.g., touch, pressure, temperature, pain, position sense) from the limbs to the nerve cell bodies located in the dorsal root ganglion. The motor (efferent) fibers, whose cell bodies are located in the ventral horn of the spinal cord, will leave the cord as the ventral root. (See Figure 8–5.) Spinal nerves are **mixed nerves,** those that have both efferent (motor) and afferent (sensory) processes.

2. THE SPINAL CORD

The spinal cord contains the nerve cell processes that communicate information between the brain and the periphery. It is contained within the *vertebral canal* of the vertebral column; the spinal nerves leave this enclosure via the *intervertebral foramina*.

In order to understand the innervation of the upper and lower limbs, the parts of the spinal cord should be learned at this time.

■ CLINICAL COMMENTS

Most **brain tumors** develop from glial cells; usually they are astrocytomas. These tumors occur in different regions of the brain and may grow as large as 2 inches in diameter in a year. They are difficult to remove because they infiltrate the surrounding brain tissue.

FIGURE 8–5
SPINAL CORD SEGMENT (TRANSVERSE SECTION)

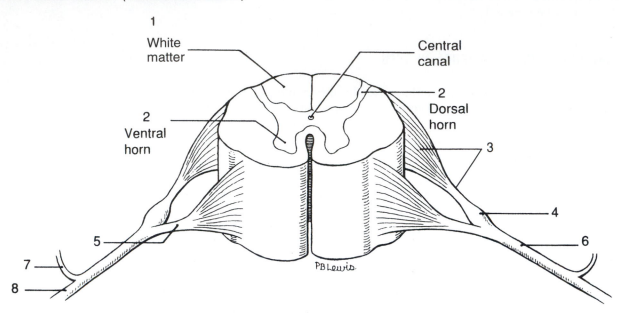

1. **White matter**—composed of nerve cell processes. They have a white appearance because of an insulating coat of a fatty substance called *myelin*.

2. **Gray matter**—composed of nerve cell bodies. Because they are without the myelin coating, the groups of cell bodies appear gray.

3. **Dorsal root**—sensory nerve processes bringing information into the dorsal horn of the spinal cord.

4. **Dorsal root ganglion**—the nerve cell bodies of the unipolar, sensory neurons form this enlarged structure.

5. **Ventral root**—nerve cell processes of efferent fibers on their way to muscles. The bodies of the motor neurons are located in the ventral horn of the gray matter.

6. **Spinal nerve**—a mixture of the incoming sensory processes and the outgoing motor processes. There are 31 pairs of these spinal nerves; they divide to form ventral and dorsal rami.

7. **Dorsal ramus**—the mixture of sensory and motor fibers that branch posteriorly.

8. **Ventral ramus**—the mixture of sensory and motor fibers that branch anteriorly. These are the processes that will be involved in the formation of nerve plexuses.

■ **Student Activities**

Using Figure 8–5, with a red pencil, put a nerve cell body in the ventral horn of gray matter and draw the efferent nerve cell process from that body out through the ventral root, the spinal nerve, and the ventral ramus.

   With a blue pencil, put a nerve cell body in the dorsal root ganglion. Draw its afferent process out through the spinal nerve and the ventral ramus. Now, extend its unipolar process into the dorsal horn of gray matter via the dorsal root.

   You can now see that spinal nerves are "mixed" nerves; they have both sensory and motor fibers. It is the mixed ventral rami that will intermingle to form the plexuses and the nerves of the limbs.

Nerves of the Lower Limb

In order for muscles to function, they must receive impulses from motor neuron processes. The nerve process releases a *neurotransmitter,* a chemical substance that causes a biochemical change in the muscle fiber. This change results in the contraction of the muscle fiber.

Within the nerves to each muscle there are also sensory fibers that are important in maintaining tonus in the muscle. These fibers will be discussed with reflexes in Unit III. The sensory fibers related to tonus are in addition to the fibers that carry conscious sensations from the skin and underlying tissue to the central nervous system.

Each nerve process can do only one thing; it is either a motor fiber going to a specific motor unit, or it is a sensory fiber carrying a specific sensation from a specific site.

■ OBJECTIVES

1. Describe the formation of a plexus of nerves.
2. Name the nerves (as listed in this exercise) of the lumbar and sacral plexuses, and list the muscles innervated by each.
3. List the cord levels of origin of each plexus and of the major nerves of the thigh and leg.
4. Describe the action(s) made possible by each nerve.

■ METHODS

1. Perform the indicated activities as you study the text; complete Exercise 9.
2. Observe the demonstration of the nerves; identify them on the materials available.

A. NERVE PLEXUS

This is an intermingling of nerve cell processes from ventral rami of different cord levels. The limbs are provided innervation (nerve supply) by plexuses. A plexus gives rise to peripheral nerves that provide innervation to the limbs.

**FIGURE 9–1
PELVIS (ANTERIOR VIEW)**

Lumbar Plexus formed by 12th thoracic (T12) and the first through the fourth lumbar (L1–4) spinal nerves.

1. Femoral n. _____

2. Obturator n. _____

Sacral Plexus formed of the fourth and fifth lumbar (L4, 5) and the first through the fourth (S1–4) sacral nerves (S4 not illustrated).

3. Superior gluteal n.

4. Inferior gluteal n.

5. Sciatic n. _____

6. Tibial division of sciatic n. = L4–S3

7. Common fibular (peroneal) division of sciatic n. = L4–S2

Note: Not all nerves formed by the sacral plexus are shown.

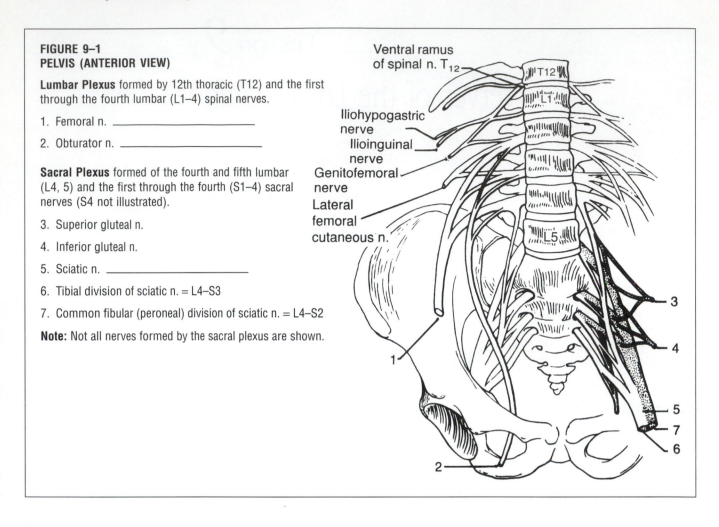

In Figure 9–1, ventral rami of spinal nerves T12–L5 emerge *below* the vertebra of the corresponding number. Ventral rami of S1–3 emerge from the *ventral sacral foramina.*

■ **Student Activities**

Use a different color for each nerve numbered in Figure 9–1; follow it back from its distal cut end to its origin. Fill in the blank with cord levels of origin where indicated.

B. DISTRIBUTION OF NERVES TO ANTERIOR AND POSTERIOR HIP MUSCLES

The innervations are included in the tables of Lessons 6 and 7 with the individual muscles. Some of the nerves are very small; they were not drawn on the illustration of the plexuses. Included in section B and C are the *nerves which should be seen.* The first two are nerves from the sacral plexus.

1. SUPERIOR GLUTEAL NERVE

This is the more superior of the two gluteal nerves and will be seen emerging superior to the piriformis muscle. It innervates:

a. Gluteus medius muscle
b. Gluteus minimus muscle
c. Tensor fasciae latae muscle

It can be seen between the gluteus medius and gluteus minimus muscles and entering the bellies of each.

2. INFERIOR GLUTEAL NERVE

This nerve emerges in the hip region below the piriformis muscle accompanied by the inferior gluteal vessels. Its fibers can be seen entering the large belly of the only muscle it innervates, the gluteus maximus muscle.

3. FEMORAL NERVE

(See Figures 9–3 and 12–1.) This is the largest nerve of the lumbar plexus. It passes through part of psoas major muscle and then descends between it and iliacus muscle. As it enters the thigh, the femoral n. passes under the inguinal ligament, which extends from the anterior superior iliac spine to the pubic tubercle. Along this course it innervates both

a. iliacus
b. anterior femoral muscles

FIGURE 9–2
RIGHT POSTERIOR GLUTEAL REGION

Using the information included in this text (or a reference book) draw the superior and inferior gluteal nerves and the large sciatic nerve at the appropriate location in the illustration.
    Write in the muscle names on the appropriate lines.

1. _____

2. _____

3. _____

4. _____

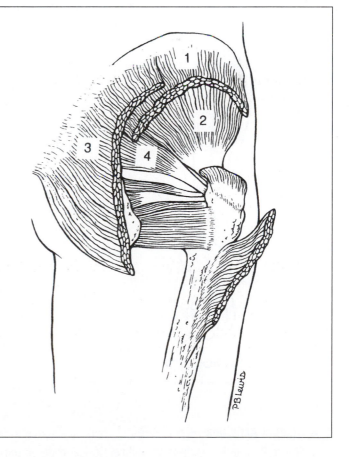

C. DISTRIBUTION OF NERVES TO THE THIGH, LEG, AND FOOT MUSCLES

FIGURE 9–3
NERVES OF THE RIGHT LOWER LIMB

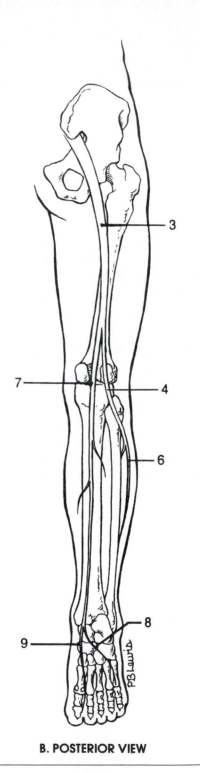

1. **Femoral n.:** This nerve innervates all the anterior femoral group of muscles, and part of pectineus.

2. **Obturator n.:** Passing through the obturator foramen, it leaves the pelvis to enter the medial thigh. It innervates most of the medial thigh muscles.

3. **Sciatic n.:** Its tibial division innervates the posterior femoral muscles.

4. **Common fibular (peroneal) n.:** The lateral division of the sciatic n. (Innervates short head of biceps femoris only.)

5. **Deep fibular (peroneal) n.:** Medial branch of the common peroneal n., it passes to the anterior compartment of the leg where it innervates all the muscles in that group. It then passes onto the dorsum of the foot.

6. **Superficial fibular (peroneal) n.:** The lateral branch of the common peroneal n., it innervates the lateral crural muscles.

7. **Tibial n.:** This nerve innervates all the posterior crural muscles as it continues toward the medial malleolus.

8. **Lateral plantar n.**

9. **Medial plantar n.:** The plantar nerves innervate all intrinsic muscles of the plantar aspect of the foot.

    Note: 4, 5, and 6 should now be called common fibular n., deep fibular n., and superficial fibular n.

A. ANTERIOR VIEW

B. POSTERIOR VIEW

■ **Student Activities**

In Figure 9–3, color each nerve yellow. Concentrate on the structures innervated by the nerve as you trace its distribution.

RELATIONSHIP OF NERVES WITH OTHER ANATOMICAL STRUCTURES

With minor exceptions, the lumbar plexus nerves, femoral n. and obturator n., provide innervation for the muscles of the anterior and medial thigh. The sacral plexus nerves, branches of tibial n. and common fibular (peroneal) n., supply the muscles of the posterior thigh and all the leg and foot.

In Figure 9–3, these nerves are illustrated with their relationships to the bones. Use Figure 9–3 and an atlas, a textbook, or the cadaver to sketch (lightly in pencil) the muscles that would surround or lie next to each of the nerves in the following list. Photocopy the illustrations if you prefer. The description of the location of each will help you find them in the body.

1. **Femoral n.:** After passing under the inguinal ligament, it lies in the femoral triangle (see Figure 12–1). Branches from this nerve can be seen entering the anterior femoral muscles. In this region the nerve is deep to the skin and underlying fascia only.
2. **Obturator n.:** The anterior division of this nerve can be seen deep to pectineus and between adductor longus and adductor brevis muscles.
3. **Sciatic n.:** The largest nerve in the body; it leaves the true pelvis by way of the greater sciatic foramen and normally emerges inferior to the piriformis muscle. This nerve passes between the greater trochanter and the ischial tuberosity. About two thirds of the way down the posterior thigh it divides into the tibial and common fibular (peroneal) nerves.
4. **Common fibular (peroneal) n.:** It can be palpated, felt with the fingers, as it passes against the neck of the fibula. It then immediately divides into the superficial fibular (peroneal) and the deep fibular (peroneal) nerves.
5. **Deep fibular (peroneal) n.:** This nerve can easily be found between the bellies of the tibialis anterior and the extensor digitorum longus muscles.
6. **Superficial fibular (peroneal) n.:** Lateral to the belly of extensor digitorum longus, this nerve can be seen sending fibers into the fibular (peroneal) muscles.
7. **Tibial n.:** This medial division of the sciatic n. enters the popliteal fossa (Figure 12–2), where it is lateral and superficial to the popliteal vessels. It passes down the posterior leg between the superficial and deep posterior crural muscles. It passes behind the medial malleolus and branches onto the plantar foot.

The tibial *n.* has a special position as it passes behind the medial malleolus. It is consistently located between the posterior tibial *a.* and the flexor hallucis longus m. tendon. Now we can complete the phrase "Tom, Dick, *a n*, Harry."

■ CLINICAL COMMENTS

Foot drop refers to the inability to dorsiflex and evert the foot. This is a result of injury to the common fibular (peroneal) nerve, the most easily injured branch of the sciatic nerve. A patient with foot drop drags his/her foot when walking.

■ **Student Activities**

Complete the following chart by listing muscles and filling in the second and third columns. This will be a useful study tool to help you understand innervations and actions as they relate to muscle groups.

Muscle Group (Position)	Major Group Action	Major Group Innervation
Anterior Hip Muscles 1. _____ 2. _____		
Anterior Femoral Muscles 1. _____ 2. Quadriceps Femoris a. _____ b. _____ c. _____ d. _____		
Medial Femoral Muscles 1. _____ 2. _____ 3. _____ 4. _____ 5. _____		
Posterior Femoral Muscles 1. _____ 2. _____ 3. _____		
Anterior Crural Muscles 1. _____ 2. _____ 3. _____ 4. _____		
Lateral Crural Muscles 1. _____ 2. _____		
Posterior Crural Muscles (Superficial) 1. _____ 2. _____ 3. _____		
Posterior Crural Muscles (Deep) 1. _____ 2. _____ 3. _____ 4. _____		

D. SENSORY INNERVATION OF THE LOWER LIMB

The sensory nerves will not be studied in great detail. In Figure 9–4, color only those regions from which sensations are carried by afferent processes within the named nerves that you have learned. You learned these as motor nerves to the skeletal muscle: numbers 9, 13, 14, and 15. *For students interested in the distribution of all sensory nerves, Figure 9–4 can be color-coded by underlining the name of the nerve and using the same color for the region from which sensations are carried by that nerve.*

FIGURE 9–4
DISTRIBUTION OF CUTANEOUS NERVES TO THE RIGHT LOWER LIMB

1. Iliohypogastric n.
2. Subcostal n.
3. Genitofemoral n.
4. Ilioinguinal n.
5. Dorsal rami $L_{1,2,3}$
6. Dorsal rami $S_{1,2,3}$
7. Lateral femoral cutaneous n.
8. Posterior femoral cutaneous n.
9. Obturator n.
10. Medial and intermediate femoral cutaneous n.
11. Lateral sural cutaneous n.
12. Saphenous n.
13. Superficial fibular (peroneal) n.
14. Deep fibular (peroneal) n.
15. Tibial n.
16. Sural n.
17. Medial plantar n.
18. Lateral plantar n.

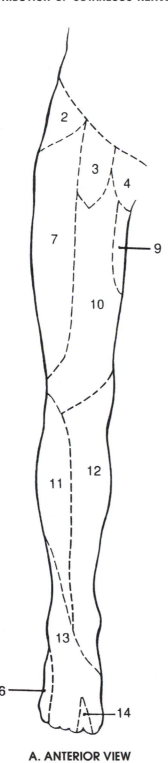

A. ANTERIOR VIEW

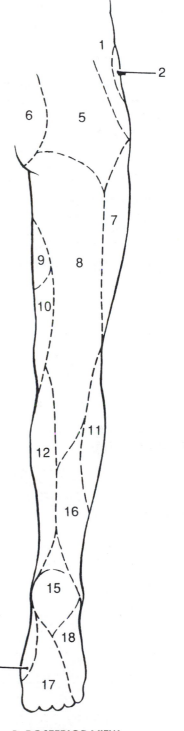

B. POSTERIOR VIEW

Exercise Nine

Name _____

1. Using the illustration below (and Lesson 8, if needed):
   a. Label all indicated structures on the corresponding label line.
   b. With a red pencil:
      1. Draw the nerve cell body of a motor neuron.
      2. Draw the path the process would take to become a part of a lower-limb nerve.
      3. Indicate with arrows the direction of the impulse.
   c. With a green pencil:
      1. Draw a lower limb sensory nerve cell body in its correct position.
      2. Draw the nerve cell process entering the appropriate ramus and continuing into the spinal cord.
      3. Use arrows to indicate the direction of the impulse.

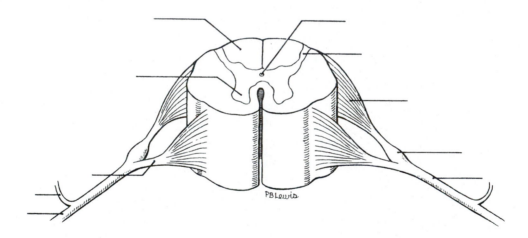

2. Match the muscle with its innervation.

   _____ 1. Fibularis (peroneus) longus   a. Obturator n.

   _____ 2. Adductor magnus   b. Tibial n.

   _____ 3. Gluteus maximus   c. Superior gluteal n.

   _____ 4. Semitendinosus   d. Superficial fibular (peroneal) n.

   _____ 5. Vastus medialis   e. Femoral n.

   _____ 6. Gluteus medius   f. Inferior gluteal n.

3. Name the one nerve that could be damaged to cause the following:

Nerve   Condition

_____ a. The patient can barely evert his foot.

_____ b. Each time the patient takes a step his pelvis drops.

_____ c. There is no muscular control of the foot.

_____ d. His toes drag when the patient walks.

_____ e. Can't get his legs together when doing "jumping jacks" in exercise class.

_____ f. He can't push the pedal down when riding his bike. (His hip works fine.)

4. Write the name of the nerve you would find in the position indicated.

_____ a. Between the bellies of tibialis anterior and extensor digitorum longus.

_____ b. Passing under the inguinal ligament.

_____ c. Deep to pectineus.

_____ d. Among the hamstrings near the pelvis.

_____ e. Between superficial and deep posterior crural muscles.

■ **Student Activities**

In Figure 7–6A (pg. 53), use a red line for the posterior tibial a. and a yellow line for the tibial n. and insert these structures in the correct relationship between "Dick" and "Harry."

Introduction to the Cardiovascular System

A distribution system is necessary to supply all body tissues with nutrients and oxygen and to take the waste products of cell metabolism from the cells to the excretory organs. The blood vessels and heart provide this service.

The heart, a thoracic structure to be studied in detail with that region, serves as a double pump to move the blood through the vessels. The right side of the heart receives blood that has been depleted of its oxygen supply. It pumps this blood, containing high levels of carbon dioxide, through the pulmonary arteries to the lungs. Here the carbon dioxide is exchanged for a new supply of oxygen. The blood returns to the left side of the heart by way of pulmonary veins and is distributed to the body systems by way of the large arterial structure, the aorta.

■ **OBJECTIVES**

1. State the purpose of the cardiovascular system.
2. Define the types of vascular structures through which blood travels.
3. Describe the basic histology of blood vessels.
4. List general characteristics of vessels.

■ **METHODS**

1. Study the following pages, completing activities described.

■ **CLINICAL COMMENTS**

Atherosclerosis is one of the most common conditions that threatens the blood supply to different areas of the body. Due to a variety of reasons (smoking, high-fat diet, excess weight, lack of exercise, high blood pressure), fatty plaque and hypertrophied smooth muscle build up in the lumen of the vessels. This leads to **arteriosclerosis,** occlusion and hardening of the vessels, which often results in death.

FIGURE 10–1
SCHEMATIC DIAGRAM OF THE ENCLOSED CIRCULATORY SYSTEM

Draw arrows beside each blood vessel to indicate the direction of blood flow:

(1) Into the right side of the heart and out to the lungs.

(2) Into the left side of the heart and out to the body systems.

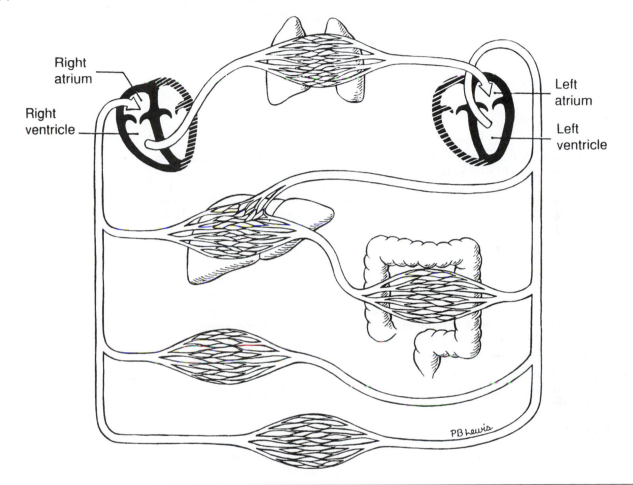

■ **Student Activities**

Color red the vessels containing blood with high levels of oxygen; color blue the vessels with blood containing high levels of carbon dioxide.

The right atrium and ventricle should be colored blue; the left atrium and ventricle should be colored red.

A. HISTOLOGY OF BLOOD VESSELS (VASCULAR STRUCTURES)

A typical blood vessel has three layers. The thickness of each will vary depending on the blood vessel type (Figure 10–4).

- **Tunica** (coat) **intima:** composed largely of a smooth, thin endothelial lining and a basement membrane. In large vessels there is also a thin layer of connective tissue.
- **Tunica media:** the relatively thick intermediate layer containing varying amounts of elastic fibers and smooth muscle fibers.
- **Tunica externa or adventitia:** an outer connective tissue layer.

B. TYPES OF BLOOD VESSELS

1. ARTERIES

These are vessels that take blood away from the heart. In the systemic circulation this blood has a high concentration of oxygen. In pulmonary and fetal circulation the arterial blood has a high concentration of carbon dioxide.

a. **Large conducting arteries.** The pulmonary trunk and the aorta and its main branches are examples of these arteries, which have a great number of elastic fibers in their tunica media. When the ventricles pump blood through these vessels they expand; when the ventricles relax, the elastic fibers recoil, sending the blood through the arterial system in an uninterrupted flow.

b. **Muscular, distributing arteries** make up the majority of the named arteries. These vessels have a thick muscular tunica media, which helps withstand the blood pressure and helps control the amount of blood being delivered to a specific body region. For instance, more blood goes to muscles during exercise.

c. **Arterioles** are the barely visible branches whose small size provides the resistance to blood flow largely responsible for blood pressure. Because of the small diameter of their **lumen** (inner cavity), the contraction of muscle cells in their media cause **constriction** (decrease in diameter of lumen) to control the amount of blood that enters the capillary beds.

2. CAPILLARIES

Capillaries are the connection between arterioles and veins, consisting of only the inner, endothelial lining layer. It is across these thin vessel walls that oxygen, nutrients, and wastes are interchanged between the blood and tissue fluid. During this process some fluid leaks into spaces between cells of the body tissues. This fluid is called *interstitial* or *intercellular* fluid and it will be discussed later with the lymphatic system.

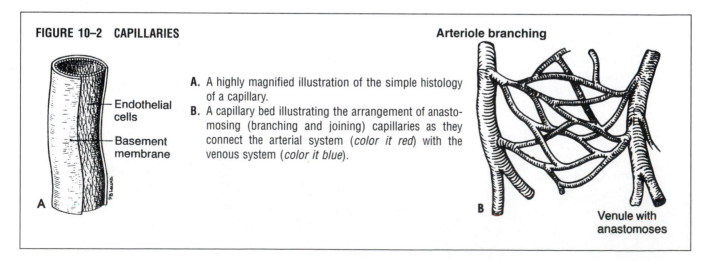

FIGURE 10–2   CAPILLARIES

Arteriole branching

— Endothelial cells

— Basement membrane

A. A highly magnified illustration of the simple histology of a capillary.

B. A capillary bed illustrating the arrangement of anastomosing (branching and joining) capillaries as they connect the arterial system (*color it red*) with the venous system (*color it blue*).

A

B

Venule with anastomoses

3. VEINS

Veins are vascular structures formed when small venules join; venules are formed when the capillaries merge. Veins return the blood to the heart. In systemic circulation the venous blood has a high concentration of carbon dioxide; in pulmonary and fetal circulation it has a high oxygen concentration.

Special characteristics of veins include the following:

a. **Thin walls.** While possessing the same three coats as arteries, the tunica media is much thinner because the veins are not exposed to the blood pressure. Therefore, the thicker walls maintain the lumen of arteries, but when empty, veins collapse.

b. **Larger diameter and more numerous** than arteries. The blood moves more slowly and so more is contained in veins. This is to compensate for rate of return so both sides of the heart have the same blood volume.

c. **Valves.** Because blood is so far from the heart there is not enough pressure to move the blood, and one-way valves help to prevent backflow (illustrated in Figure 10–3).

d. **More numerous anastomoses,** branching and joining of vessels, are found in veins than in arteries. Anastomoses are necessary in helping provide collateral circulation. *Collateral circulation* refers to more than one source of blood to a specific body part.

FIGURE 10–3
VALVES OF A VEIN

Arrows indicate that the valves are forced open by pressure from below and shut by pressure from above. This allows blood to move only toward the heart.

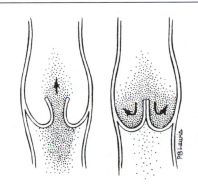

FIGURE 10–4
COMPARISON OF ARTERY AND VEIN

In this illustration of a medium-sized vein (left) and its accompanying muscular artery (right), notice the much thinner wall but larger lumen of the vein.

A small segment of the artery is shown in greater detail. The tunica externa blends with the surrounding connective tissue.

Notice the three layers: intima, media, and externa. *Color the media pink in both.*

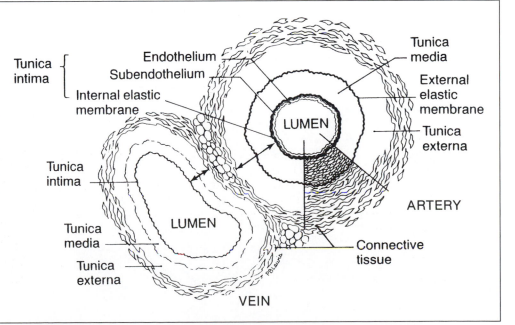

Lesson 11

Blood Vessels of the Lower Limb

Unlike nerves, blood vessels supply the structures near which they pass. For this reason, if you are familiar with the anatomy of the region, it is not necessary to learn which specific vessel supplies each muscle.

■ OBJECTIVES

1. List the vessels that take blood from the heart to each area of the lower limb and back to the heart.
2. Identify each of the major vessels of the lower limb.
3. Describe the relationships between important structures of the lower limb.

■ METHODS

1. Study the following illustrations and perform the activities indicated.
2. Observe the demonstration of each vessel and its relationship to the muscles in the area.

A. MAJOR CONDUCTING ARTERIES TO THE LOWER LIMB

As each body region is studied, we will begin at the heart and follow the blood through the arteries to the structures of that region. We will then take the blood back to the heart by way of the veins.

FIGURE 11–1
MAJOR ARTERIES

Color in red the arteries from the heart to the lower limb.

1. **Ascending aorta**—receives the highly oxygenated blood pumped by the left ventricle.

2. **Arch of the aorta**—The aorta arches and passes behind the heart.

3. **Descending aorta**—lies in the posterior thorax just left of the vertebral bodies. It descends, moves medially to lie anterior to the vertebral column, and passes behind the diaphragm. It enters the posterior abdomen, and, at the level of the fourth lumbar vertebra, it bifurcates, divides into two branches.

4. **Common iliac artery**—formed when the abdominal aorta bifurcates. Both the right and the left common iliac a. bifurcate to form external and internal iliac arteries.

5. **Internal iliac a.**—has many branches, which are highly variable. Most of these branches remain in the pelvis to supply pelvic and perineal (pelvic floor) structures, and will not be described here. Three branches that are most involved with the muscles we are studying are the **obturator a.** and the **superior** and **inferior gluteal arteries.**

6. **External iliac a.**—along the medial border of psoas major muscle. These vessels send small branches to structures along the way. They pass into the thigh at a point midway between the anterior superior iliac spine and the pubic tubercle.

7. **Femoral a.**—This is the direct continuation of the external iliac artery. The name change occurs at the inguinal ligament.

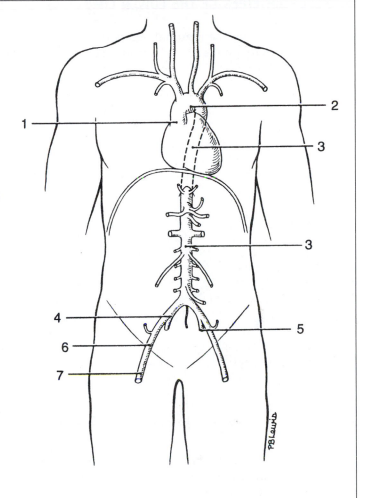

Pathway of Blood Flow: All blood that has been used by the body enters the right atrium, which pumps it to the right ventricle. The right ventricle pumps this used blood containing high levels of carbon dioxide (CO_2) through the pulmonary trunk and the right and left pulmonary arteries to the lungs. The exchange of CO_2 for a fresh supply of oxygen (O_2) occurs between the pulmonary capillaries and the alveoli of the lungs.

Pulmonary capillaries anastomose to form pulmonary venules, then veins. The pulmonary veins return freshly oxygenated blood to the left atrium, which pumps it to the left ventricle. The left ventricle pumps the blood out via the aorta to all body tissue. The O_2 passes through the thin walls of the capillaries into the body cells; CO_2 enters the capillaries and the veins then return the used blood to the right atrium.

B. MAJOR ARTERIES OF THE LOWER LIMB

After passing under the inguinal ligament, the external iliac a. changes its name to **femoral a.** The femoral a. and its branches supply the majority of the thigh and all of the leg and foot.

FIGURE 11–2
MAJOR ARTERIES OF THE LOWER LIMB

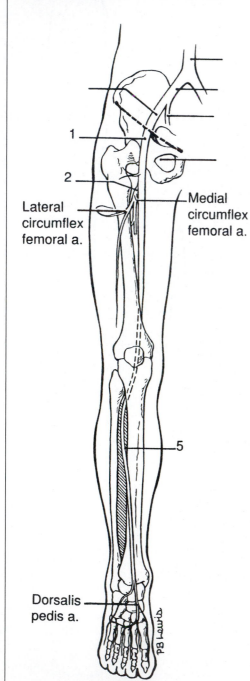

Lateral circumflex femoral a.

Medial circumflex femoral a.

Dorsalis pedis a.

A. ANTERIOR VIEW

1. **Femoral a.**—descends medially to approach the insertion of the adductor magnus muscle.

2. **Deep femoral a.**—arises dorsilaterally from the femoral a. and descends deep to it as it sends off branches to the posterior femoral muscles.

3. **Adductor hiatus**—the opening in the tendon of the adductor magnus muscle through which the femoral a. and v. pass. Vessel names change to popliteal.

4. **Popliteal a.**—continuation of femoral a. to area behind the knee.

5. **Anterior tibial a.**—branch from bifurcation of popliteal a. At the inferior border of the popliteus m. it passes through the interosseous membrane to the anterior leg. At the ankle it becomes the dorsalis pedis a.

6. **Posterior tibial a.**—passes down the leg between the posterior crural muscle groups. It terminates as medial and lateral plantar arteries.

7. **Fibular (peroneal) a.**—lateral branch of the posterior tibial a.

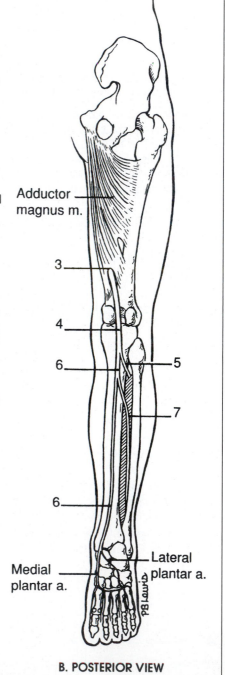

Adductor magnus m.

Medial plantar a.

Lateral plantar a.

B. POSTERIOR VIEW

C. MAJOR VEINS OF THE LOWER LIMB

The deep veins that return blood from each area of the lower limb have the same names as the arteries with which they travel. They are held together with connective tissue in a **vascular bundle.** In many places a nerve also accompanies the vessels and a **neurovascular bundle** exists. When two veins accompany one artery, the veins are referred to as **venae comitantes.** Remember, there are more veins than arteries. Venae comitantes usually exist in the leg and forearm.

To return the blood from the lower limb just reverse the order of the arterial distribution until you have formed the common iliac veins. The common iliac veins pass behind their arteries and join to form the **inferior vena cava.**

FIGURE 11–3
MAJOR VEINS

Color in blue the pathway from the lower limb to the heart.

1. Femoral vein

2. External iliac vein

3. Internal iliac vein

4. Common iliac vein

5. Inferior vena cava
   The inferior vena cava, which takes the blood back into the heart, ascends to the right of the aorta.

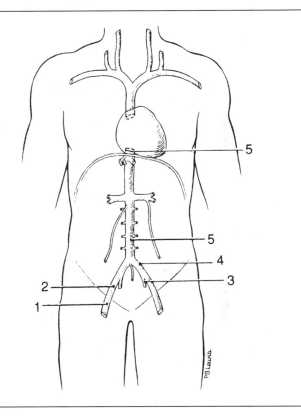

D. SUPERFICIAL VEINS OF THE LOWER LIMB

In the upper and lower limbs the veins can be divided into two groups: the deep, which were just described and which are deep to muscle, and the superficial. The superficial veins are immediately under the skin in the superficial fascia and connect to the deep veins by way of communicating veins. Valves are arranged to prevent communication of blood from deep to superficial and to prevent backflow of blood in superficial veins.

In the lower limb, most of the superficial veins are unnamed tributaries of the **greater saphenous vein** and the **lesser saphenous vein.** These veins are illustrated in Figure 11–4.

■ CLINICAL COMMENTS

Because of the lack of muscular support and the thin walls, the superficial veins often become **varicose.** A varicose vein is one in which the diameter of the lumen increases because of the pressure of the weight of the column of blood. When this occurs, the valves cannot close completely and the blood exerts even more pressure, causing the vessels to dilate.

FIGURE 11–4
SUPERFICIAL VEINS (RIGHT LOWER LIMB)

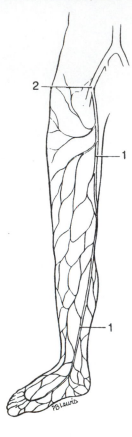

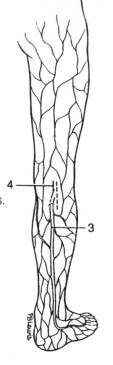

1. **Greater saphenous vein**—the longest vein in the body, originates from tributaries of the dorsum of the foot. The greater saphenous vein begins medially, crossing in front of the medial malleolus. It ascends on the medial leg, courses behind the knee, then up the medial thigh to end in the femoral vein.

2. **Femoral vein**—a deep vein, but in this position it is only deep to skin and fascia.

3. **Lesser (small) saphenous vein**—shorter, but also originating from tributaries on the dorsum of the foot; this vein is seen laterally at the ankle. It then ascends the posterior leg and dives into the popliteal fossa to enter the popliteal vein.

4. **Popliteal vein**—a deep vein, sight of drainage of lesser saphenous vein.

Note: Saphenous veins are often used in cardiac bypass surgeries.

■ **Student Activities**

In Figure 11–2, label the vessels that are unlabeled.
Without looking back at the illustrations in this chapter, use a red pencil and the illustrations on the right to draw the pattern of arteries from the heart to the toes. Label each vessel. With blue, draw and label the vessels to return the blood.

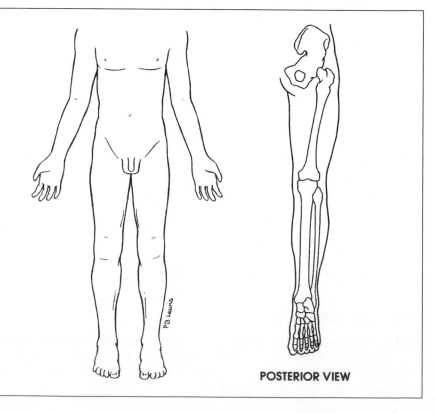

POSTERIOR VIEW

Exercise Eleven

Name _____

(Refer to Lesson 10 if needed)

1. Describe the histological characteristic that permits capillaries to perform their function: _____

2. List the *types* of vascular structures through which the blood must flow to get from the left ventricle to the right atrium.

   a. _____   d. _____

   b. _____   e. _____

   c. _____   f. _____

3. Define:

   a. artery: _____

   b. vein: _____

4. Write the name of the vessel most likely to supply each muscle listed.

   _____ a. Semitendinosus

   _____ b. Tibialis anterior

   _____ c. Popliteus

   _____ d. Vastus medialis

   _____ e. Fibularis (peroneus) longus

5. Name the nerve that would be found in a neurovascular bundle with the following:

   _____ a. Anterior tibial a.

   _____ b. Posterior tibial a.

   _____ c. Superior gluteal a.

   _____ d. Obturator a.

6. In consecutive order, name the vessels through which blood would flow to reach the indicated destination.

   a. Left ventricle   h. Capillaries of tibialis anterior m.

   b. Aorta   i. _____

   c. _____   j. _____

   d. _____   k. _____

   e. _____   l. _____

   f. _____   m. _____

   g. _____   n. Inferior vena cava to right atrium

Special Areas of the Lower Limb

In certain areas, structures have a constant, predictable relationship to each other. As you will see in this section, this can be important clinically. You have already seen how the tendons of the deep posterior crural muscles relate to the tibial nerve and the posterior tibial artery behind the medial malleolus. In this lab session you will learn the relationships of structures in other areas of the lower limb.

■ OBJECTIVES

1. Describe the areas of the lower limb where specific structures can be found in a predictable relationship.
2. Identify each structure within the special areas.
3. Name the relative position of each structure in the area.

■ METHODS

1. Using the illustrations in this unit, locate the boundaries and individual contents of the special areas in material in the lab.
2. Draw from memory each of the areas discussed. Be sure you include the correct boundaries and structures in their proper relationship.
3. Complete the student activities.

A. FEMORAL TRIANGLE

In this important area, major structures are covered by skin and fascia only. For this reason these vessels can be easily accessed, and a pulse can be felt in the femoral artery. Since the vein is positioned medial to the artery, the vein can easily be located for intravenous injections.

FIGURE 12–1
THE FEMORAL TRIANGLE (RIGHT THIGH, ANTERIOR VIEW)

Boundaries

1. **Inguinal ligament**—superior, the base of the triangle

2. **Sartorius muscle**—lateral

3. **Adductor longus muscle**—medial

4. **Iliopsoas muscle**—forms lateral part of the floor

5. **Pectineus muscle**—forms medial part of the floor

Contents
(Listed from lateral to medial.)

6. **Femoral nerve**

7. **Femoral artery**

8. **Femoral vein**

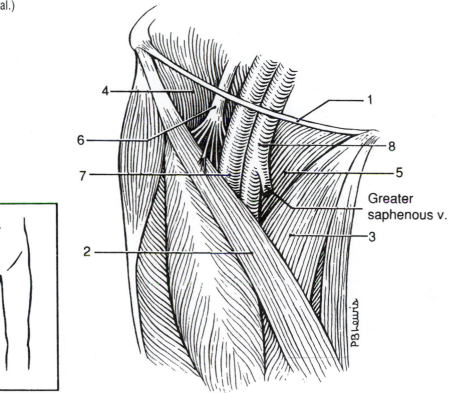
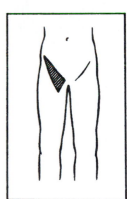

Greater saphenous v.

■ CLINICAL COMMENTS

Compressing the femoral artery during trauma of injury can prevent rapid exsanguination (loss of blood) if this large vessel is injured in the thigh.

The ease of reaching the large femoral artery and vein also make them important for **catheterizations.** For instance, a long thin catheter can be placed in the femoral artery and passed through the common iliac artery, into the aorta, and then into the vessels of the abdomen. Contrast medium can then be injected and these vessels can be studied in x-rays.

B. POPLITEAL FOSSA

The region behind the knee is referred to as the popliteal area. You have already identified many structures that have popliteus or popliteal in their names. Now you will identify the **popliteal fossa** or depression created when muscles form boundaries. In this diamond-shaped "depression," the nerves, artery, and veins are buried in fat and have a predictable relationship. It is only after dissection and removal of the fat that a fossa is apparent.

FIGURE 12--2
POPLITEAL FOSSA (RIGHT KNEE, POSTERIOR VIEW)

Boundaries

1. **Biceps femoris**—lateral and above

2. **Semitendinosus**

3. **Semimembranosus**—with semitendinosus forms upper and medial boundary

4. **Lateral head** of gastrocnemius—forms lower lateral boundary

5. **Medial head** of gastrocnemius—forms lower medial boundary

Contents

6. **Popliteal artery**—deepest in the fossa, lies against popliteal surface of femur.

7. **Popliteal vein**—intermediate

8. **Tibial nerve**—superficial and a little lateral to the vein.

9. **Common fibular (peroneal) nerve**—in same plane and lateral to the tibial n.

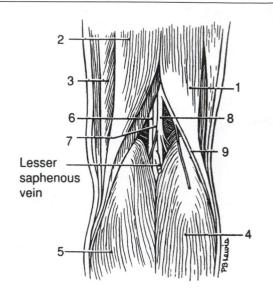

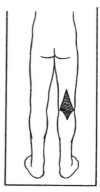

The popliteal surface of the femur and the popliteus muscle are the floor of the fossa; the roof is formed of fascia and skin.

C. ADDUCTOR CANAL

The sartorius muscle overlies this fascial compartment, which is positioned between the quadriceps femoris muscles and the medial femoral muscles in the middle one third of the thigh. Lift sartorius m. and the femoral vessels are seen in the canal. (Also seen in the canal is the saphenous n., a cutaneous branch of the femoral n. It continues onto the leg.)

FIGURE 12–3
ADDUCTOR CANAL (RIGHT THIGH, ANTERIOR VIEW)

1. Sartorius muscle (cut)

2. Femoral a. lying in the adductor canal

3. Femoral v.—posterior to the femoral artery

4. Rectus femoris m.

5. Adductor longus m.

6. Adductor magnus m.

7. Vastus medialis m.

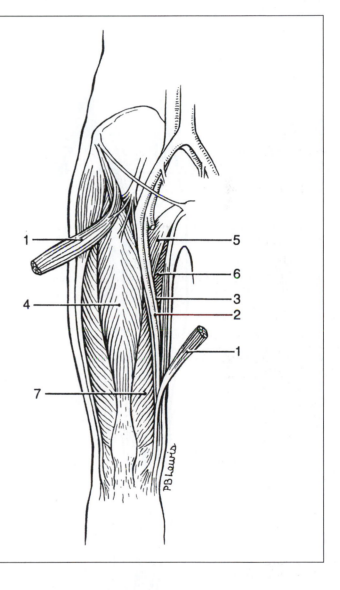

■ **Student Activities: Relationship of Arteries and Nerves of the Lower Limb**

Use this page to label each indicated structure. Photocopy it and use the copy to practice drawing the muscles that are found medial, lateral, deep, or superficial to each major structure. Color all nerves yellow.

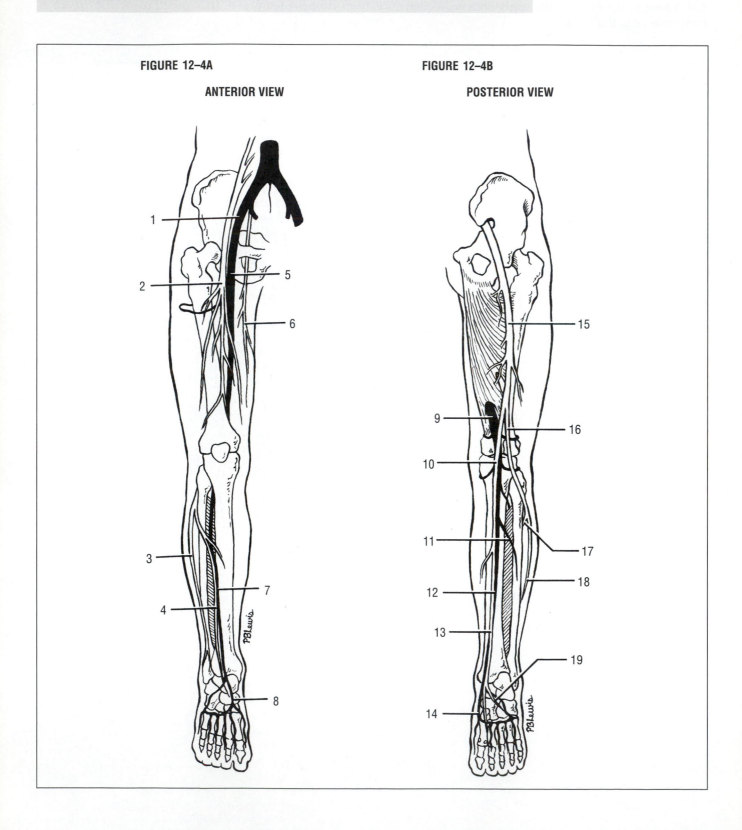

FIGURE 12–4A

ANTERIOR VIEW

FIGURE 12–4B

POSTERIOR VIEW

Name _____

1. In Figure 12–1, color the superior, lateral, and medial boundaries of the femoral triangle a pale pink. Next, color the femoral nerve yellow, the femoral artery red, and the femoral vein blue.

2. In Figure 12–2, color pale pink the medial and lateral boundaries, both upper and lower, of the popliteal fossa. Color the popliteal a. red, the popliteal v. blue, and the tibial n. and the common fibular (peroneal) n. yellow.

3. In Figure 12–3, color the quadriceps muscles yellow and the adductors green. Color the femoral a. red and the femoral v. blue.

4. Name the special areas pictured below and label their boundaries and contents.

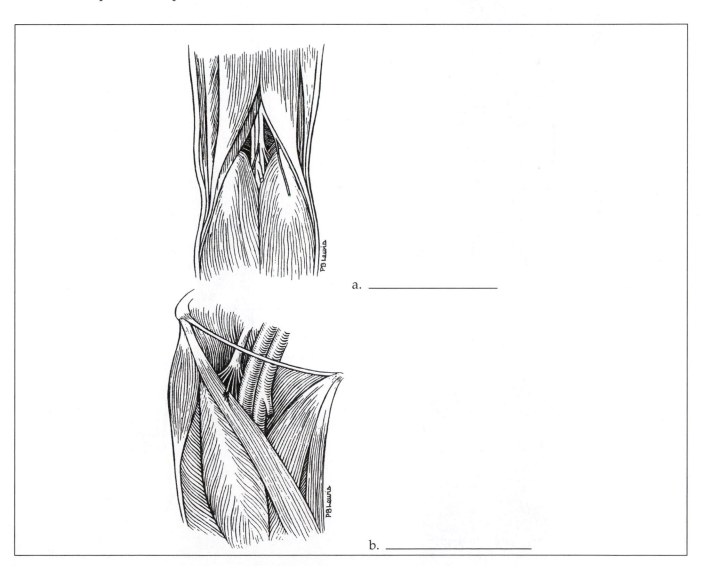

a. _____

b. _____

Exercise 13

Review of Unit I

This exercise is designed to be used after you feel fairly confident of the material you have studied. Review all student activities and lab reports; then, without using references, go through this exercise to determine your level of competence. If you have trouble, try to concentrate on the area of concern, then come back to these pages and try again.

I. Label all structures indicated.

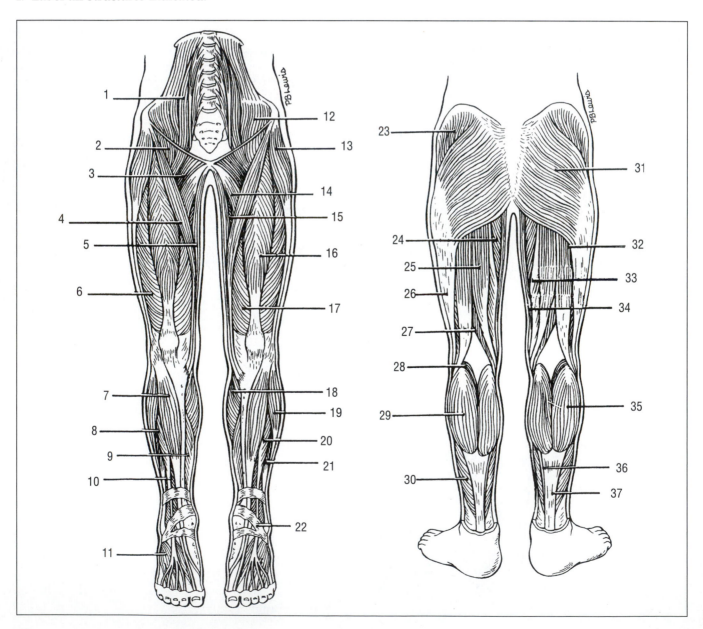

II. Organize your knowledge by filling in the muscle names that would correctly complete the chart below. If the anatomy is three-dimensional and alive for you, this exercise will help reinforce your knowledge and expand your understanding. As you add each muscle to the correct action block, try to name its origin, insertion, and innervation. This chart completed correctly can be an important reference later. To be sure it is correct, the answers have been included in the Appendix. Answers are given an asterisk if they are most important, and are in parentheses if least important.

Muscles that act on the hip to:

Flex	**Extend**	**Abduct**	**Adduct**
1.	1.	1.	1.
2.	2.	2.	2.
3.	3.	3.	3.
4.	4.	4.	4.
5.			5.

Medially rotate		**Laterally rotate**	
1.		1.	4.
2.		2.	5.
3.		3.	6.

Muscles that act on the knee to:

Flex		**Extend**
1.	5.	1.
2.	6.	2.
3.	7.	3.
4.	8.	4.

Muscles that act on the ankle and intertarsal joints to:

Dorsiflex	**Plantar flex**	**Invert**	**Evert**
1.	1.	1.	1.
2.	2.	2.	2.
3.	3.	3.	
	4.	4.	
	5.		
	6.		
	7.		
	8.		

Muscles that act on the metatarsophalangeal and interphalangeal joint to:

Flex digits	**Extend digits**	**Abduct digits**	**Adduct digits**
1.	1.	1.	1.
2.	2.	2.	2.
3.	3.	3.	
4.			

III. Answer the following questions. They may be answered orally or on paper.

1. Define the following subdivisions of anatomy: gross, histology, embryology, and neuroanatomy.
2. Name the four primary tissues of the body.
3. Define *anatomic position.*
4. Complete the following relative pairs and describe the meaning of each:

   superior — _____
   deep — _____
   medial — _____
   distal — _____

5. Name and describe the three planes through which anatomical material is cut.
6. List five functions of the skeleton.
7. Explain the difference between diaphysis and epiphysis.
8. What is the fascial covering of bone?
9. What is the name of a mature bone cell? Bone-developing cell?
10. Name the structural unit of compact bone and list its components.
11. Describe the following bone markings and give one specific example of each: process, spine, foramen, crest, fossa, condyle, and facet.
12. What pelvic bone is a part of the axial skeleton instead of the appendicular skeleton?
13. Name the three bony components of the os coxae.
14. Sketch the appropriate view of the os coxae to show the following: acetabulum, obturator foramen, anterior superior iliac spine, greater sciatic notch, ischial tuberosity, and crest of the ilium.
15. Describe the true and false pelvic cavities. What is the division between them called?
16. Draw the posterior view of the femur and include labels of at least 12 markings or structures.
17. Name the large sesamoid bone of the lower limb, and describe its position and function.
18. Name the leg bones from lateral to medial.
19. Give the anatomical term for: shin, Achilles tendon, inside ankle bone, outside ankle bone, and sole of foot.
20. Name the bones with which the femur, tibia, and fibula articulate both proximally and distally.
21. With which tarsal bone does the fifth metatarsal articulate?
22. Name the three major joint types and one example of each.
23. Name three functions of muscle tissue.
24. Name three types of muscle tissue.
25. List the connective tissue coverings that surround muscle. Start with the deepest tissue.
26. Define and perform each of the hip actions that follow: flexion, extension, abduction, adduction, rotation, and circumduction.
27. What term would you use to name a muscle that performs the action opposing the prime mover?
28. What is the major action(s) of the muscle group that attaches to:
    a. the ischial tuberosity
    b. the tibial tuberosity
    c. the calcaneus
    d. the superior part of the greater trochanter

29. Name one non-muscular structure that attaches to:
    a. the anterior superior iliac spine
    b. the ischial spine
    c. the pubic tubercle
30. What is fascia lata? The iliotibial tract?
31. When looking at the posterior thigh, what muscle would be medial to the hamstrings? lateral?
32. What muscle(s) would you have to remove to expose the deep lateral rotators of the hip?
33. What are the muscles of quadriceps femoris?
34. Name all femoral muscles that attach on the lateral leg.
35. Name two muscles of the leg whose tendons divide into four slips each.
36. Name four intrinsic foot muscles and four extrinsic foot muscles.
37. How many muscles are in the lateral crural compartment?
38. Describe the structure and function of a retinaculum.
39. Palpate your anterior tibial crest. If near the knee, what muscle would you feel just lateral to it? Just medial to it?
40. What separates the anterior from the posterior crural muscles?
41. What two muscles make up the greatest portion of the calf of the leg?
42. Name the structures (in order) behind the medial malleolus and those behind the lateral malleolus.
43. Name all intrinsic muscles on the dorsum of the foot.
44. What muscles are found "between bones" of the foot? What are the bones?
45. What is a neuron?
46. Where are the motor nerve cell bodies for the lower limb muscles found? Sensory nerve cell bodies?
47. What are the structures of the central nervous system?
48. What is a nerve? What does the term "mixed nerve" mean?
49. What is a nerve plexus? Name those involved with the lower limb.
50. What are the cord levels of origin of the plexuses you just named?
51. What are the major motor nerves of the lumbar plexus?
52. What plexus(es) are involved in muscle contractions of muscles of the leg?
53. What nerve can be palpated against the neck of the fibula? What would be the most obvious problem if that nerve were injured in that vulnerable position?
54. Name the nerve(s) that exit the true pelvis via the greater sciatic foramen.
55. What are cutaneous nerves? Where would you find the nerve cell bodies of these nerves?
56. What is the purpose of the cardiovascular system?
57. What is meant by describing the heart as a double pump?
58. Name the layers of a typical blood vessel.
59. Describe the major differences in arteries and veins.
60. The posterior tibial artery would be an example of what type artery?
61. Describe the structure and function of a capillary.
62. What is meant by the term *anastomosis? Collateral circulation?*
63. In what type blood vessel would the greatest volume of blood be found?
64. Name the vessels through which blood would flow from the heart to the extensor digitorum brevis muscle. To the abductor hallucis brevis m.?
65. Name the landmark where the external iliac a. changes its name. The femoral a.? The ant. tibial a.?
66. Name the nerve that would be found in a neurovascular bundle with each of the following: anterior tibial a., posterior tibial a., obturator a.
67. To find the femoral vein, you might palpate the femoral a. and then insert a needle _____ to it. (lateral or medial)

68. If the popliteal a. is the deepest structure in the popliteal fossa, it would lie against the _____ superiorly and against the _____ inferiorly.
69. Describe the adductor hiatus.
70. What are superficial veins superficial to?
71. Name the two largest superficial veins of the lower limb and describe the course of each. Into which vein does each drain?
72. What muscle would you have to remove to see the adductor canal?
73. If you were instructed to find the posterior tibial a. in the leg (not at the ankle), under which muscle would you look?
74. What is meant by the term *bifurcate?*
75. What are venae comitantes and where would you expect to find them?
76. This exercise should help you integrate the different components of the lower limb. Fill in the blanks in this chart. In the last column you are to find the bony marking and color it yellow; refer to figures 3–1 through 3–9, pages 18–24.

Innervation	Muscle (or group)	Bone Marking (attachment)	Artery that supplies blood	Figure # of marking used
	Quadriceps femoris	(distal)		
Obturator n.		(proximal)		
Superior gluteal n.		(distal)		
Inferior gluteal n.		(distal)		
Tibial div. of sciatic (above split)		(proximal)		
Tibial n. (below split)		(distal)		
	Ant. hip muscle	(distal)		

Unit II

The Back and the Upper Limb

With:

· Axial Skeleton
· Axial Musculature

Lesson 14

The Axial Skeleton

This lesson omits the skull, which is covered in Lesson 24.

The bones of the axial skeleton are included here because they serve as attachments for many upper limb muscles. The axial skeleton includes the skull, vertebral column, and the bones of the thorax. The lower and upper limb bones are considered appendicular skeleton.

■ OBJECTIVES

1. Identify the structures of a typical vertebra.
2. State the identifying characteristics of vertebrae from each region of the spinal column.
3. Identify the first and second cervical vertebrae; name the region for other vertebrae.
4. Identify major markings and regions of the sternum and of a typical rib.

■ METHODS

1. Compare the vertebrae in your illustrations with the bones in the lab.
2. Use skeletons and x-rays to understand where the bones articulate with each other.
3. Cover the key to the illustrations and see if you can correctly identify each marking.
4. Choose several individual vertebrae and determine their region of origin.

The **vertebral column,** the bony protection for the spinal cord (Lesson 28), consists of 33 vertebrae (Figure 14–1). At birth the column is curved with the convexity directed posteriorly. This is considered the primary direction of curvature. When the baby holds his head up, a secondary curve is developed in the cervical (neck) region, and when the baby sits up a secondary curve is formed in the lumbar (low back) area. The secondary curves are convex anteriorly. A normal vertebral column has no lateral curvature.

Normal Curves	Abnormal Curves
	(Illustrated in Exercise 14)
Primary	**Kyphosis**—exaggerated posterior
Thoracic	curve of the thoracic region
Sacrococcygeal	**Lordosis**—exaggerated anterior
	curve of the lumbar region
Secondary	**Scoliosis**—a lateral curve of
Cervical	lumbar or thoracic region
Lumbar	

FIGURE 14–1
LATERAL VIEW OF VERTEBRAL COLUMN

1. **First cervical vertebra** or atlas

2. **Second cervical vertebra** or axis

3. **Seventh cervical vertebra** (vertebra prominens) spinous process

4. **First thoracic vertebra**—body

5. **Intervertebral disc**—fibrocartilaginous disc found between bodies; compresses to absorb shock.

6. **Intervertebral foramen**—opening between vertebrae through which spinal nerves emerge.

7. **First lumbar vertebra**—body

8. **Sacrum**—a label line is on articular surface for ilium

9. **Coccyx**

10. **Cervical curve**—secondary

11. **Thoracic curve**—primary

12. **Lumbar curve**—secondary

13. **Sacrococcygeal curve**—primary curve

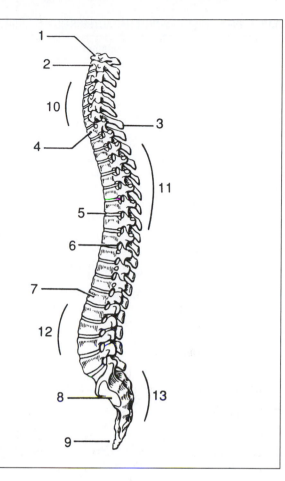

FIGURE 14–2
TYPICAL VERTEBRA (SUPERIOR VIEW)

1. Vertebral (neural) arch

2. Spinous process

3. Lamina

4. Superior articular process with articular facet

5. Transverse process

6. Pedicle

7. Vertebral foramen—when stacked, the foramina form the vertebral canal, the passageway for the spinal cord

8. Body

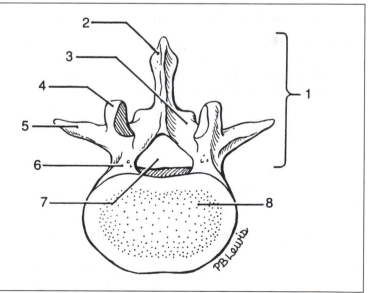

■ CLINICAL COMMENTS

Scoliosis is the most common abnormal curvature of the spine. It is most frequent in females during periods of rapid growth, and it is treated with exercise, braces, or surgery in extreme cases. The cause is unknown about 80% of the time, but early detection makes treatment most successful.

TABLE 14–1. IDENTIFYING CHARACTERISTICS OF VERTEBRAE

Region	Number	Identifying Characteristics
Cervical (typical)	7	Bifid spinous processes; foramina in transverse processes
first—atlas		No body; no spinous process
second—axis		Odontoid process (dens)
Thoracic	12	Sharp, downward pointing spinous process; articular facets for ribs
Lumbar	5	Short, blunt spinous process; large body compared to vertebral foramen

FIGURE 14–3
CERVICAL VERTEBRAE (SUPERIOR VIEWS)

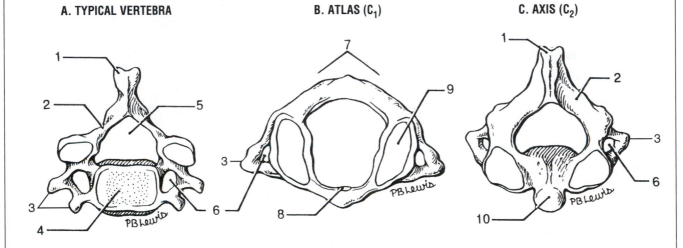

A. TYPICAL VERTEBRA   B. ATLAS (C₁)   C. AXIS (C₂)

1. **Bifid spinous process**

2. **Lamina**

3. **Transverse process**

4. **Body**

5. **Vertebral foramen**

6. **Transverse foramina**

7. Posterior arch of atlas with no spinous process.

8. Articular facet for odontoid process. Notice absence of body on atlas.

9. **Superior articular process** with facet for articulation with occipital condyle of the skull.

10. **Odontoid process or dens of axis.** The atlas rotates around this process.

FIGURE 14–4
THREE THORACIC VERTEBRAE (LATERAL VIEW)

1. **Superior articular facet.** (Note posterior orientation. This frontal plane articulation limits flexion and extension in this region.)

2. **Articular facet on transverse process. It provides articulation for tubercle of rib** of same number, i.e., vertebra T7 with rib 7.

3. _____

4. **Inferior articular facet.** (Anteriorly directed.)

5. **Articular facets for head of rib.**

6. _____

7. _____

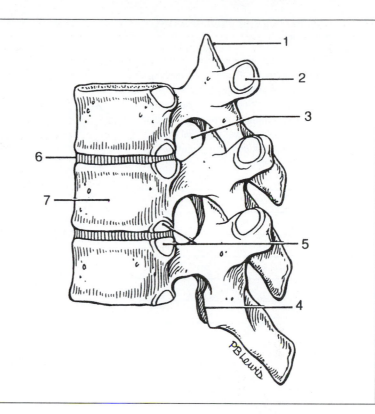

FIGURE 14–5
LUMBAR VERTEBRA (LATERAL VIEW)

(Superior view shown on Figure 14–2)

1. **Pedicle**

2. **Superior articular process** (with facet directed medially)

3. **Spinous process**

4. _____

5. **Inferior articular facet.** (Orientation of articulation is now almost in a sagittal plane and allows greater flexion and extension.)

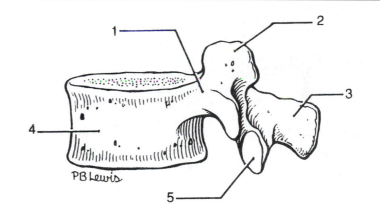

■ CLINICAL COMMENTS

In the condition called **spina bifida,** the laminae of vertebrae do not fuse and the posterior arch remains open. When this occurs, meninges and spinal cord or nerves are not protected and they bulge beneath the skin. Irreparable nerve damage often occurs.

Back pain occurs sometime in the lives of about 2/3 of all adults. Usually this pain is in the lumbosacral region (low back) and is caused by muscle strain due to overuse or injury. With rest and proper exercise, most people recover within three months. A **herniated disc** (sometimes mistakenly called a "slipped disc"), is another cause of low back pain. Each intervertebral disc is composed of a nucleus, a gel-like material, which is surrounded by a tough outer shell called the anulus. If the anulus is weakened it may develop a bulge or even break open allowing herniation of the nucleus. Most of the pain occurs when the disc presses against the nerve roots or spinal cord. Even this condition will often heal without surgery.

FIGURE 14–6
SACRUM

The sacrum, Figure 14–6, and the coccyx are the inferior bones of the axial skeleton. Of major significance is the fact that the sacrum provides the attachment for the appendicular skeleton bones of the lower limb. Fill in the KEY for these illustrations. (See Figure 3–2, page 19, if you need help).

1. _____
2. _____
3. _____
4. _____
5. _____
6. _____
7. _____
8. _____

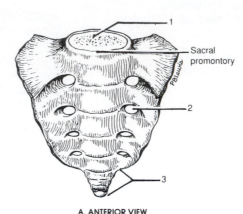

Sacral promontory

A. ANTERIOR VIEW

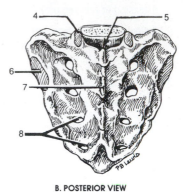

B. POSTERIOR VIEW

THE THORAX

The bones of the thorax (chest) help protect the heart and the lungs. The 12 thoracic vertebrae provide attachment for 12 pairs of ribs, which form the posterior, lateral, and part of the anterior thorax. The sternum (breastbone), composed of a manubrium, body, and xiphoid process, completes the anterior thorax. Ribs attach to the sternum by way of costal cartilages.

FIGURE 14–7
THORAX (ANTERIOR VIEW)

1. **Body of the sternum**

2. **Intercostal space**

3. **Costal cartilage.** Rib pairs 1–7 attach directly to the sternum via their own costal cartilage and are called true ribs. Pairs 8–12 are called false ribs; 8–10 attach via cartilage of other ribs; pairs 11 and 12 have no sternal attachment and are, therefore, called floating ribs.
   Beginning at the top of Figure 14–6, number the left ribs from 1–12. Notice that rib 5 is numbered for you.

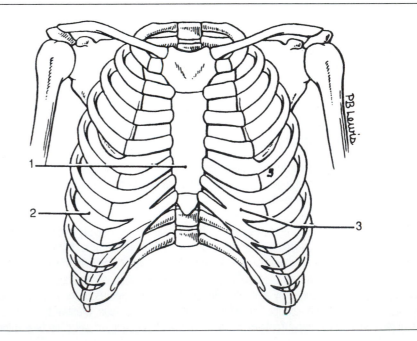

FIGURE 14–8
STERNUM

1. **Jugular notch**

2. **Clavicular notch**—provides the only bony articulation between the axial skeleton and the upper extremity.

3. **Manubrium** of the sternum.

4. **Sternal angle**—where the manubrium meets the body. The second rib articulates here.

5. **Body**

6. **Xiphoid process**—landmark for locating attachment of diaphragm, superior surface of the liver, and right margin of the heart.

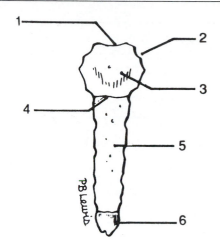

FIGURE 14–9
RIBS

1. **Head** with facets for articulation with vertebral bodies.

2. **Tubercle** with facet for articulation with transverse process.

3. **Body.** The region of greatest curve is called the angle.

4. **Costal groove.** Located on the inferior surface of the ribs, the grooves are formed by the intercostal nerves, arteries, and veins.

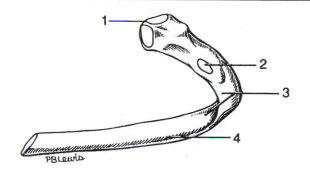

A. Inferior view of rib

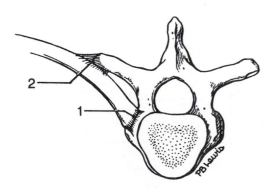

B. Articulation between rib and thoracic vertebra

Exercise Fourteen

Name _____

1. Complete the keys for Figures 14–4 and 14–5.

2. In Figure 14–6, color the true ribs blue and the floating ribs red.

3. In Figure 14–8B, color in red the two articulations between rib and vertebra.

4. Label the illustrations using the appropriate term for the abnormal curve shown.

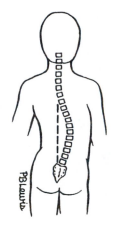 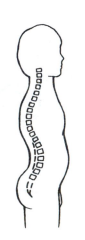 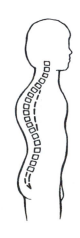

a. _____ b. _____ c. _____

5. Use the identifying characteristics to identify the following vertebrae:

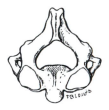 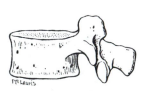 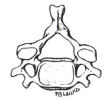 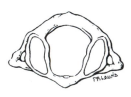

a. _____ b. _____ c. _____ d. _____

6. Match the following:

_____	1. floating	a. paris 1–7
_____	2. axis	b. large body
_____	3. thoracic	c. dens
_____	4. true	d. facets for ribs
_____	5. atlas	e. pairs 11–12
_____	6. cervical	f. pairs 8–12
_____	7. lumbar	g. no body
_____	8. false	h. transverse foramina

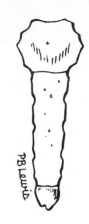

7. Draw the second rib in the appropriate position on the sternum at the right. Color the manubrium red and the xiphoid process blue.

Lesson 15

Muscles of the Axial Skeleton

The muscles of the deep back (post-vertebral), those covered by superficial muscles of the upper limb (which will be discussed in Lesson 18), consist of many converging and diverging fibers that are given individual names. Although very important, since these muscles do not act independently as do the muscles of the limbs, they will not be dealt with individually here. The more superficial muscles, which have longer fibers and less complicated origins and insertions, will be discussed.

The true back muscles are primarily extensors and rotators of the vertebral column and head, and when the body is erect, their major function is to resist gravity. When you bend forward, all the deep back muscles come into play to resist gravity so that you do not fall forward. Most of the lateral flexion is produced by posterior and anterolateral abdominal muscles, which will be included in Unit IV.

■ OBJECTIVES

1. Be aware of the complexity of the deep back muscles.
2. Identify the three columns of the erector spinae group of deep back muscles.
3. State the function and innervation of the deep back muscles.

■ METHODS

1. Find the three columns of the erector spinae muscles in the mid-thoracic regions.
2. Complete the activities in this lesson.

A. ERECTOR SPINAE MUSCLES

This largest muscle mass of the deep back muscles can be seen originating from the sacrum, iliac crest, and spinous processes of lumbar vertebrae. The fibers are directed upward and laterally, and by the mid-thoracic region three columns can be distinguished. From lateral to medial they are: iliocostalis, longissimus, and spinalis.

INNERVATION OF DEEP BACK MUSCLES

Dorsal rami of spinal nerves. There are no plexuses formed by dorsal rami.

A.

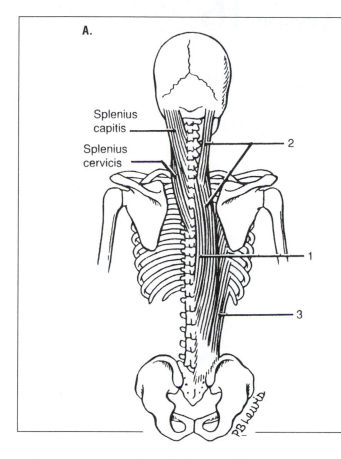

Splenius capitis

Splenius cervicis

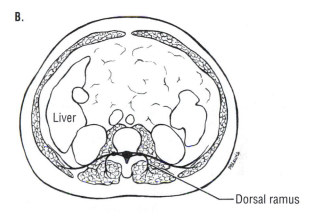

FIGURE 15–1A, B
DEEP BACK MUSCLES

The erector spinae muscles are numbered. Most of the small complex muscles are not pictured. For more information, see a reference book.

1. **Spinalis** (located only in the thoracic region)

2. **Longissimus**

3. **Iliocostalis**

B.

Liver

Dorsal ramus

B. **Transverse Section. Inferior view.** Dorsal rami of spinal nerves enter deep back muscles; ventral rami enter intercostal and abdominal muscles.

B. SPLENIUS CAPITIS AND CERVICIS

The most superior and superficial of the deep back muscles, the splenius capitis originates on the lower half of the ligamentum nuchae and spinous processes of the seventh cervical and upper three or four thoracic vertebrae and inserts on the skull. The splenius cervicis originates on the spinous processes of about the third to the sixth thoracic vertebrae and inserts on the upper two to four cervical transverse processes. These muscles help in extension and lateral flexion of the head and neck.

C. TRANSVERSOSPINALIS, INTERSPINALES, AND INTERTRANSVERSALES

These short muscle fibers are found between vertebrae and contract with the other deep back muscles to perform antigravity, extension, and rotatory functions.

■ **Student Activities**
1. Color each of the three columns of erector spinae with a different color.
2. Fill in the blanks.
   a. Deep back muscles have both their origins and insertions on bones of the _____ skeleton.
   b. The erector spinae muscles can be subdivided into _____ columns.
   c. Innervation of all deep back muscles is: _____ _____ of _____ _____.
   d. The major actions of the deep back muscles are: _____ and _____ of _____.

Bones of the Pectoral Girdle
and Upper Limb

The bones of the upper limb are not as large or heavy as those of the lower limb, the weight-bearing bones. The markings are still important for muscle attachments. Review Lesson 2 and the bone-marking information on pages 12–15. If the bone markings in this unit have an asterisk, feel these markings on your own body.

■ OBJECTIVES

1. Recognize both articular and non-articular bone markings.
2. Identify specific markings of the upper limb bones as indicated in the lesson.
3. Determine whether the following bones are from the right or left side of the body: scapula, humerus, radius, ulna, hand.

■ METHODS

1. Compare the markings in your illustrations with the upper limb bones provided.
2. Use skeletons and x-rays to see how the individual bones articulate with each other.
3. Cover the key to each illustration and see if you can identify each marking.
4. Feel on your own body the bone markings indicated by an asterisk.

A. PECTORAL GIRDLE

The pectoral girdle (shoulder girdle) provides attachment of the upper limb to the axial skeleton. Made up of the (1) **clavicle** and (2) **scapula,** it has only one bony articulation with the axial skeleton, the **sternoclavicular joint.** This allows great range of movement, but not the great strength of the pelvic girdle. The clavicle, a long thin bone, is frequently broken because (1) it is in a superficial position and (2) the weight of the body is borne by it when the arms are used to break a fall.

FIGURE 16–1
SHOULDER REGION (ANTERIOR VIEW)

1. **Clavicle.*** The medial end articulates with the sternum and the lateral end with the acromion process of the scapula. A ligament connects the clavicle to the coracoid process.

2. **Sternoclavicular joint.*** The only bony attachment of the upper limb with the axial skeleton.

3. **Scapula.** Lies posterior to the ribs, but has no bony attachment to the axial skeleton.

4. **Acromion.*** "Corner" of the shoulder.

5. **Acromioclavicular joint.** Attachment of clavicle with scapula.

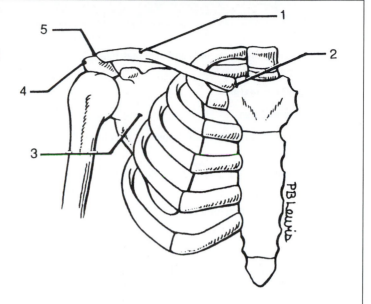

FIGURE 16–2
THE RIGHT SCAPULA

1. **Lateral angle**—most lateral projection of scapula.

2. **Coracoid process**

3. **Lateral (axillary) border.** The area under the arm is named the axilla.

4. **Inferior angle***

5. **Subscapular fossa**—the anterior surface of the bone.

6. **Medial (vertebral) border**

7. **Suprascapular notch**

8. **Superior angle**

9. **Acromion process***

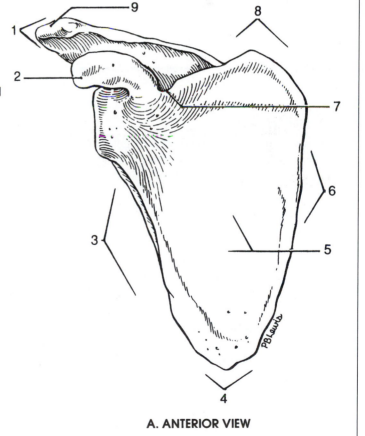

A. ANTERIOR VIEW

**FIGURE 16–2
CONTINUED**

10. **Spine***—attached posteriorly and becomes free to form the acromion process.

11. **Supraspinous fossa**

12. **Infraspinous fossa**

13. **Supraglenoid tubercle** for attachment of long head of biceps brachii.

14. **Glenoid fossa.** Articulates with the head of the humerus.

15. **Infraglenoid tubercle** for attachment of the long head of triceps brachii.

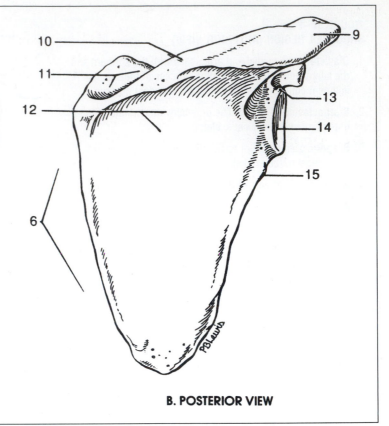

B. POSTERIOR VIEW

■ **Student Activities**

With your books closed, quickly sketch both anterior and posterior view of the scapula (a triangle will get you started) and humerus. Include the markings that are found in each view.

B. UPPER LIMB

The upper limb consists of 30 bones arranged as follows:

The arm or brachium	1	humerus
The forearm or antebrachium	2	radius and ulna
The wrist	8	carpals
The hand	5	metacarpals
The digits	14	phalanges

HUMERUS

The proximal end of the humerus articulates with the glenoid fossa of the scapula at the glenohumeral or shoulder joint. Distally, the humerus articulates with the radius and ulna at the humero-radial and humero-ulnar or elbow joint.

FIGURE 16–3
RIGHT HUMERUS

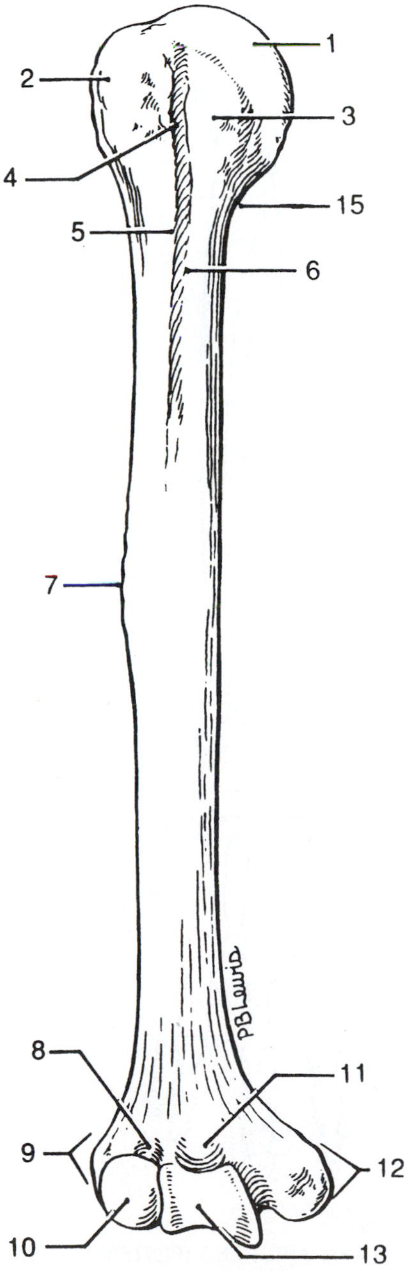

1. **Head.** Articulates with the glenoid fossa.

2. **Greater tubercle**

3. **Lesser tubercle**

4. **Intertubercular sulcus** (bicipital groove). Contains: tendon of long head of the biceps brachii muscle between tubercles; attachment for latissimus dorsi muscle between crests of tubercles.

5. **Crest of greater tubercle**

6. **Crest of lesser tubercle**

7. **Deltoid tuberosity**

8. **Radial fossa.** Receives the head of radius when elbow is fully flexed.

9. **Lateral epicondyle***

10. **Capitulum.** Round articular process for head of the radius.

11. **Coronoid fossa.** Receives the coronoid process of the ulna in elbow flexion.

12. **Medial epicondyle***

13. **Trochlea.** Spool-shaped articular process around which the trochlear notch of the ulna articulates.

14. **Anatomical neck**

15. **Surgical neck**

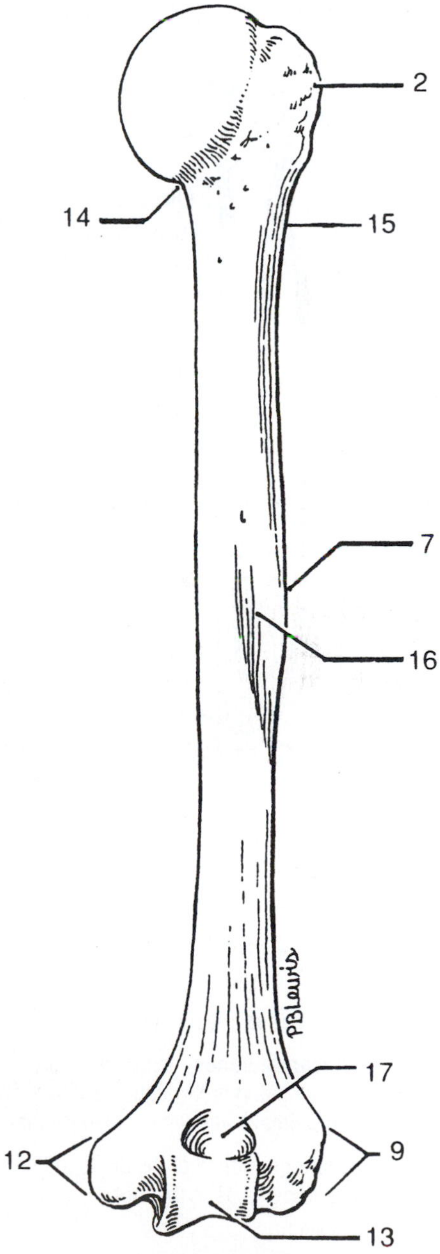

A. ANTERIOR VIEW

B. POSTERIOR VIEW

16. **Radial groove** (spiral groove), gentle depression on the posterior surface of the humerus indicates the position where the radial n. and the deep brachial a. pass against the bone.

17. **Olecranon fossa.** Receives the olecranon process in elbow extension.

THE FOREARM AND HAND

The **radius** is the lateral bone of the forearm; the ulna is medial. They articulate with each other both proximally and distally. The radius articulates with the wrist distally.

FIGURE 16–4
RIGHT RADIUS AND ULNA (ANTERIOR VIEW)

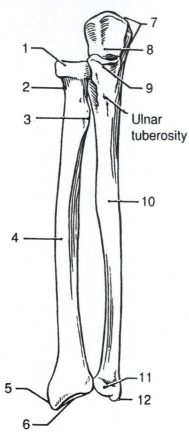

1. **Head of radius.** Cup-like end receives the capitulum; perimeter fits into the radial notch of the ulna.

2. **Neck of** radius

3. **Radial tuberosity**

4. **Shaft of radius.** Note the smooth anterior surface of the distal end of the bone and the ulnar notch medially.

5. **Styloid process of radius**

6. **Articular surface** for carpal bones

7. **Olecranon process*** of ulna (in olecranon fossa in Fig. 16-5)

8. **Trochlear notch**

9. **Coronoid process**

10. **Shaft of ulna**

11. **Head of ulna**

12. **Styloid process of ulna**

13. **Head of radius** articulating with both the capitulum of the humerus and the radial notch of the ulna.

14. Posterior radius with grooves caused by extensor tendons. (Helps identify posterior.)

15. The **carpal bones.** There are eight carpal bones in the wrist.

16. The **metacarpal bones,** hand bones, are numbered from lateral to medial, one through five. They articulate with carpals proximally and with phalanges distally.

17. The **phalanges,** bones of the digits, named proximal, middle, and distal as in the foot.

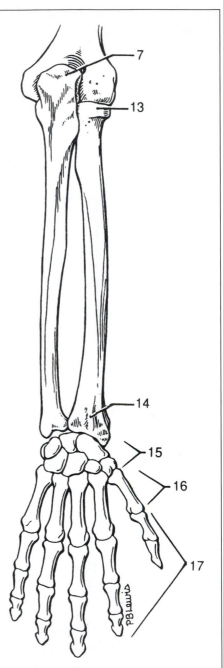

FIGURE 16–5
RIGHT FOREARM AND HAND (POSTERIOR VIEW)

BONES OF THE HAND

The only articulation between the antebrachium (forearm) and the hand is that of distal radius with scaphoid and lunate, two of the carpal bones.

a. The **carpal bones.** There are eight small bones in the wrist. The four bones in the proximal row, from lateral to medial, are: **scaphoid, lunate, triangular (triquetrum),** and **pisiform.** The distal row (from lateral to medial) are: **trapezium, trapezoid, capitate,** and **hamate.**

b. The **metacarpal bones.** These five hand bones are numbered from lateral to medial, one through five. They articulate with carpals proximally and with phalanges distally.

c. The **phalanges** (one is a **phalanx**) are the bones of the digits. There are five digits numbered from lateral to medial, one through five. In that order they are named: **pollex** (thumb), **index, medius, annularis, minimus.**

Digits two through five each have three phalanges: a proximal (articulates with a metacarpal at the metacarpo-phalangeal or M-P joint), a middle, and a distal phalanx.

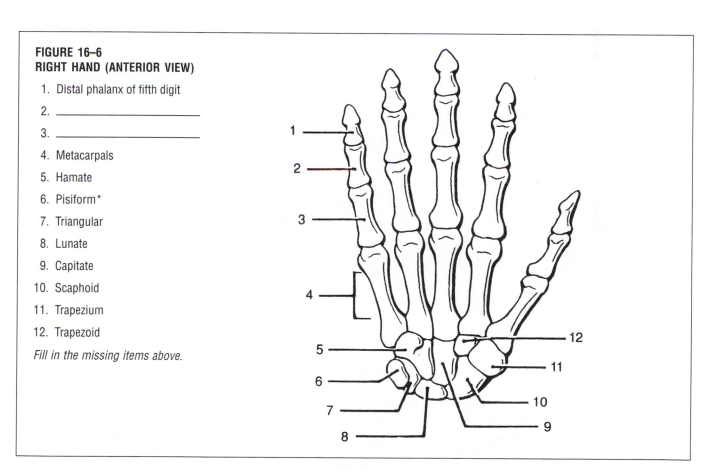

FIGURE 16–6
RIGHT HAND (ANTERIOR VIEW)

1. Distal phalanx of fifth digit

2. _____

3. _____

4. Metacarpals

5. Hamate

6. Pisiform*

7. Triangular

8. Lunate

9. Capitate

10. Scaphoid

11. Trapezium

12. Trapezoid

Fill in the missing items above.

■ **Student Activities**

1. In Fig. 16–4, use a yellow pencil to color both the proximal and distal radio-ulnar joints.

2. List all bones that articulate with the radius.

Name _____

1. Fill in the blanks with the name of the appropriate upper limb bone.

   a. The pectoral girdle bone that has no bony connection with the axial skeleton is the _____.
   b. At the elbow, the bone that has the most stable articulation with the humerus is the _____.
   c. At the wrist, the ulna articulates directly with the _____; the radius articulates directly with the _____ and the _____.
   d. Name all the bones of the brachium: _____.
   e. The lateral forearm bone is the _____.

2. On the drawings at the right:

   a. Label the acromioclavicular joint with an "a".
   b. Label the glenohumeral joint with a "b".
   c. Label manubrium, body, and xiphoid process of sternum.
   d. On (B), the lateral view of the scapula, label the following:
      1. glenoid fossa
      2. axillary border
      3. coracoid process
      4. acromion process
      5. supraspinous fossa

A   **B**

3. In the space provided, write the name of the bone on which you would find the marking. In the first column use the appropriate letter to indicate whether the marking is anterior (A), posterior (P), lateral (L), or medial (M) when the bone is in the anatomical position.

A,P,L,M	Name of Bone	Marking
_____	_____	1. deltoid tuberosity
_____	_____	2. olecranon fossa
_____	_____	3. lesser tubercle
_____	_____	4. coronoid process
_____	_____	5. subscapular fossa
_____	_____	6. medial epicondyle
_____	_____	7. radial groove
_____	_____	8. styloid process

Arthrology of the Upper Limb

Refer to Lesson 4 for general information on arthrology.

The major joints of the upper limb are synovial joints (diarthroses). Detailed anatomy of the joints is not included in this book.

■ OBJECTIVES

1. Name the joints of the upper limb.
2. Identify the bones involved at each joint.
3. Classify the major joints of the upper limb.

■ METHODS

1. Observe the joint models on display.
2. Find each upper limb joint on both the skeleton and x-ray.

TABLE 17–1. JOINTS OF THE UPPER LIMB

Joint	Type (subtype)	Movement
Sternoclavicular	Diarthrosis (gliding)	Gliding
Acromioclavicular	Diarthrosis (gliding)	Gliding and rotation of scapula on clavicle
Glenohumeral (shoulder)	Diarthrosis (ball and socket)	Flexion, extension, abduction, adduction, circumduction, medial and lateral rotation
Humero-ulnar and Humeroradial (both = elbow)	Diarthrosis (hinge)	Flexion and extension
Radio-ulnar (proximal and distal)	Diarthrosis (pivot)	Pivot in long axis to pronate and supinate
Radiocarpal (wrist) radius with scaphoid and lunate	Diarthrosis (condyloid)	Flexion, extension, abduction, adduction, and circumduction
Intercarpals	Diarthrosis (gliding)	Gliding
Carpometacarpal	Diarthrosis (gliding)	Gliding
Metacarpophalangeal (MP joint)	Diarthrosis (condyloid)	Flexion, extension, abduction, adduction, and circumduction
Interphalangeal (IP joint)	Diarthrosis (hinge)	Flexion and extension

■ Student Activities

In Figure 2–3, label all joints of the upper limb: (Anterior view) . . . the joint name. (Posterior view) . . . the subtype. All the labeled joints are _____ (type).

Lesson **18**

Muscles of the Shoulder and Arm

Muscles of the shoulder and arm act on the pectoral girdle, shoulder, and elbow. The general information concerning muscle action can be reviewed in Lesson 5. It is helpful to learn the muscles by grouping them according to action or position.

■ OBJECTIVES

1. Describe the actions of the joints of the upper limb.
2. Recognize all shoulder and arm muscles. (These are seen together on page 116.)
3. Describe the attachments of each muscle as indicated.
4. Define the major actions of each muscle.

■ METHODS

1. Observe demonstrations of the muscles.
2. Identify each of the shoulder and arm muscles until you can name each muscle.
3. Looking at bones and the skeletons, imagine each muscle on the appropriate bone markings.
4. Cover the keys in the illustrations and correctly identify each labeled structure.

A. ACTIONS OF THE PECTORAL GIRDLE, SHOULDER, AND ELBOW

PECTORAL GIRDLE

Because the scapula is attached to the axial skeleton by muscle only, it can move in many directions. When the vertebral border is pulled closer to the vertebral column it is retracted; protraction occurs when the vertebral border is pulled closer to the anterior body. When the shoulders are "shrugged" the scapula is elevated; the opposite is depression. Rotation of the scapula occurs when the arm is lifted above the head.

FIGURE 18–1
SHOULDER JOINT

The shoulder joint is a ball and socket joint and has the following wide range of motions:

    (a) Flexion
    (b) Extension
    (c) Abduction
    (d) Adduction
    (e) Medial rotation
    (f) Lateral rotation
    (g) Circumduction (not shown)

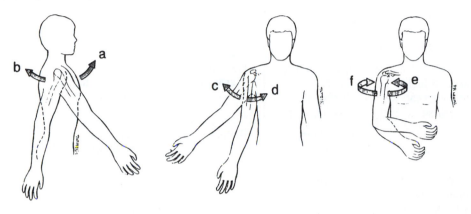

FIGURE 18–2
ELBOW

The elbow undergoes
    (a) Flexion
    (b) Extension
When the head of the radius turns in the radial notch of the ulna,
the distal radius moves into a position medial to the distal ulna
causing pronation (c).
    The reverse of pronation is supination (d).

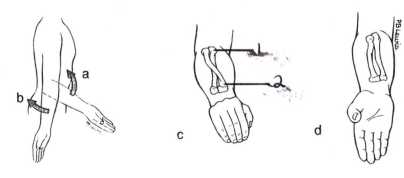

In addition to the specific actions listed in Table 18–1, these muscles are important in the fixation and rotation of the scapula.

TABLE 18–1. MUSCLES FROM THE AXIAL SKELETON TO THE SHOULDER GIRDLE

Name	Origin	Insertion	Action	Innervation
Trapezius	Superior nuchal line, external occipital protuberance, lig. nuchae, spinous proc. C7 & T1–T12	Lateral 1/3 of clavicle; acromion and spine of the scapula	Elevates, retracts scapula	Accessory n. (CN XI)
Levator scapulae	Transverse proc. of first 3 or 4 cervical vertebrae	Superior part, medial border of scapula	Elevates scapula	Dorsal scapular n.
Rhomboid minor and major	Minor: ligamentum nuchae, spinous processes C7, T1. Major: spinous processes T2–T5	Medial border of scapula from spine to inferior angle	Retracts scapula	Dorsal scapular n.
Serratus anterior	Outer surface of lateral part of first 8 ribs	Anterior surface of medial border of scapula	Protracts & holds scapula to body	Long thoracic n.
Subclavius	Junction of first rib and its costal cartilage	Inferior surface of clavicle	Fixes clavicle. Cushions vessels	N. to subclavius
Pectoralis minor	Ribs 3–5	Medial portion of coracoid process	Protracts scapula	Med. & lat. pectoral n.

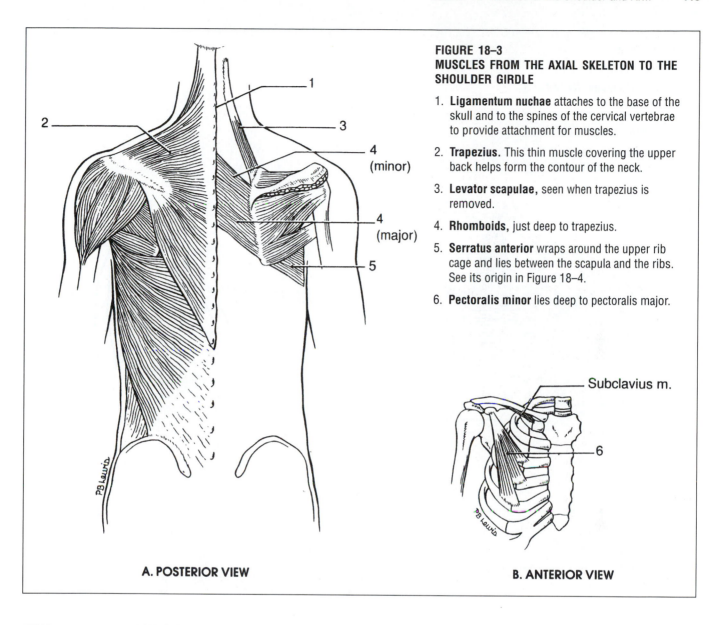

FIGURE 18–3
MUSCLES FROM THE AXIAL SKELETON TO THE SHOULDER GIRDLE

1. **Ligamentum nuchae** attaches to the base of the skull and to the spines of the cervical vertebrae to provide attachment for muscles.

2. **Trapezius.** This thin muscle covering the upper back helps form the contour of the neck.

3. **Levator scapulae,** seen when trapezius is removed.

4. **Rhomboids,** just deep to trapezius.

5. **Serratus anterior** wraps around the upper rib cage and lies between the scapula and the ribs. See its origin in Figure 18–4.

6. **Pectoralis minor** lies deep to pectoralis major.

A. POSTERIOR VIEW

B. ANTERIOR VIEW

TABLE 18–2. MUSCLES FROM THE AXIAL SKELETON TO THE HUMERUS

Name	Origin	Insertion	Action	Innervation
Pectoralis major	Medial one half clavicle, sternum, and costal cartilage of ribs 2–6	Crest of the greater tubercle	Adducts, medially rotates humerus (arm)	Medial and lateral pectoral n.
Latissimus dorsi	Spinous process of lower six thoracic vertebrae; thoracolumbar fascia; crest of ilium	Floor of the intertubercular sulcus	Adducts, extends, and medially rotates humerus	Thoracodorsal n.

FIGURE 18–4
PECTORALIS MAJOR AND LATISSIMUS DORSI

1. **Pectoralis major.** *Color it pink.*

2. _____

3. **Latissimus dorsi.** *Color it pink.*

4. **Thoracolumbar fascia.** A fascial sheet attaching to the lumbar and sacral spines.

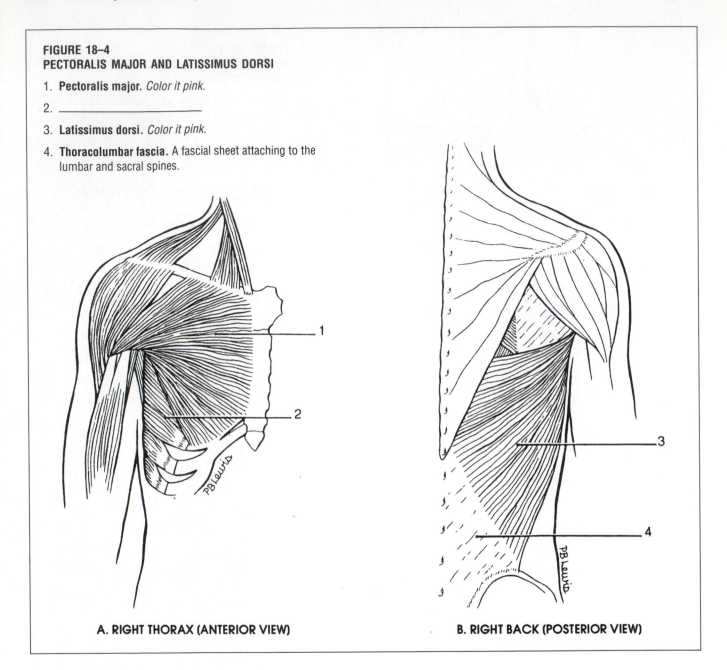

A. RIGHT THORAX (ANTERIOR VIEW)   **B. RIGHT BACK (POSTERIOR VIEW)**

■ CLINICAL COMMENTS

The **rotator cuff,** composed of the tendons of subscapularis, supraspinatus, infraspinatus, and teres minor, is frequently injured in repetitive motions of the shoulder joint such as those used when pitching a baseball. Even with the help of these four muscles, this remains the most commonly dislocated joint in the body because of the shallow glenoid fossa and lack of strong ligaments, specifically along the inferior region of the cuff.

FIGURE 18–5
ROTATOR CUFF MUSCLES

A. RIGHT SHOULDER (ANTERIOR VIEW)

B. RIGHT SHOULDER (POSTERIOR VIEW)

First four muscles listed in Table 18–3 surround the proximal end of the humerus and help prevent dislocation of the shoulder joint. For this reason they are collectively called *"rotator cuff muscles."*

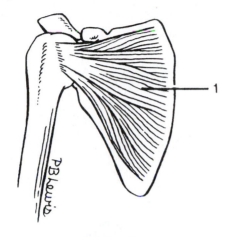

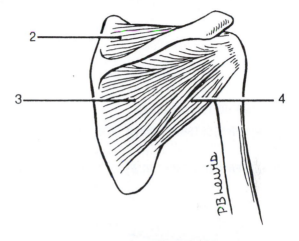

A. ANTERIOR VIEW

B. POSTERIOR VIEW

1. **Subscapularis m.** The serratus anterior muscle lies between subscapularis and the ribs.

2. **Supraspinatus m.** initiates abduction at the shoulder.

3. **Infraspinatus m.** fills infraspinous fossa.

4. **Teres minor m.** fibers blend with the lower fibers of infraspinatus.

TABLE 18–3. MUSCLES FROM THE PECTORAL GIRDLE TO THE HUMERUS

Name	Origin	Insertion	Action	Innervation
Subscapularis	Subscapular fossa	Lesser tubercle of humerus	Medial rotation of humerus (arm)	Upper and lower subscapular n.
Supraspinatus	Supraspinous fossa	Greater tubercle of humerus (superior facet)	Abducts humerus (arm)	Suprascapular n.
Infraspinatus	Infraspinous fossa	Greater tubercle of humerus (middle facet)	Lateral rotation of humerus (arm)	Suprascapular n.
Teres minor	Lateral part, dorsal surface of scapula	Greater tubercle of humerus (inferior facet)	Lateral rotation of humerus	Axillary n.

TABLE 18–3. (CONT.)

Name	Origin	Insertion	Action	Innervation
Teres major	Dorsal surface of inferior angle of scapula	Crest of lesser tubercle of humerus	Adducts, extends, and medially rotates arm	Lower subscapular n.
Deltoid	Lateral 1/3 clavicle; acromion and spine of scapula	Deltoid tuberosity of humerus	Anterior—flexes, medially rotates arm Middle—abducts arm Posterior—extends and laterally rotates arm	Axillary n.

FIGURE 18–6
TERES MAJOR AND DELTOID MUSCLES

A. RIGHT SHOULDER (POSTERIOR VIEW) WITH DELTOID REMOVED

B. RIGHT SHOULDER (POSTERIOR VIEW) WITH ONLY DELTOID

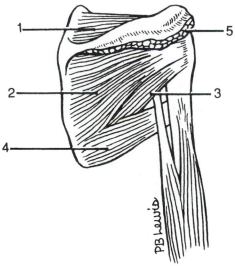

1. _____

2. _____

3. _____

4. **Teres major.** A thicker, heavier muscle than teres minor.

5. **Deltoid muscle.** The middle fibers are the major abductors of the shoulder but need the supraspinatus to initiate the action because of the angle of pull.

■ **Student Activities:**
Color teres major and deltoid pink; color all the rotator cuff muscles blue (Figures 18–5 and 18–6).

TABLE 18–4. MUSCLES OF THE ARM

Name	Origin	Insertion	Action	Innervation
Coracobrachialis	Tip of coracoid process	Medial surface of the middle of the humerus	Flexion and adduction of arm	Musculocutaneous n.
Biceps brachii a. short head b. long head	Tip of coracoid process Supraglenoid tubercle of scapula	Radial tuberosity	Supinates forearm; flexes forearm. (Slight arm flexion)	Musculocutaneous n.
Brachialis	Lower half of anterior humerus	Tuberosity of ulna	Flexes elbow (forearm)	Musculocutaneous n.
Triceps brachii a. long head b. lateral head c. medial head	Infraglenoid tubercle of scapula Posterior shaft of humerus Posterior shaft of humerus	Olecranon process of the ulna	Extension of elbow (forearm)	Radial n.

These are the muscles whose bellies lie around the humerus. Three are anterior muscles; only one is posterior.

FIGURE 18–7
ANTERIOR ARM MUSCLES

1. **Coracobrachialis**

2. **Biceps brachii**—the short head originates with the coracobrachialis m. on the tip of the coracoid process. Pectoralis minor insertion is medial to it.
   The tendon of the long head originates on the supraglenoid tubercle and creates the intertubercular sulcus. Latissimus dorsi inserts in the sulcus distal to the tubercles.

3. **Brachialis.** A major flexor of the elbow.

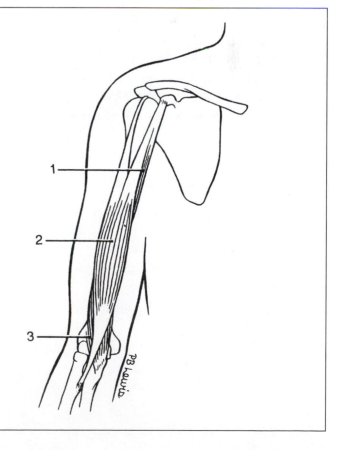

FIGURE 18–8
ANTERIOR ARM

1. Short head of biceps brachii

2. Long head of biceps brachii

3. Coracobrachialis

4. Brachialis

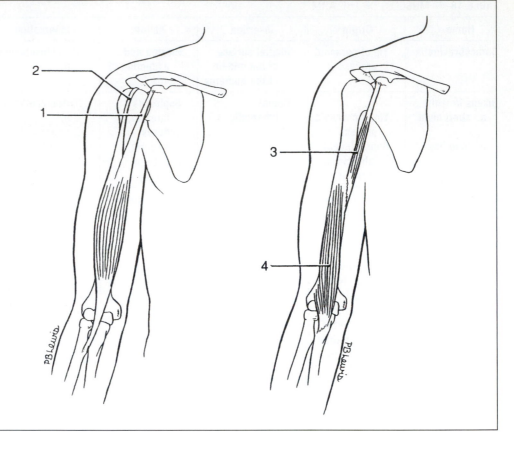

FIGURE 18–9
POSTERIOR ARM: TRICEPS BRACHII

1. **Long head of triceps brachii,** passes between teres minor and major as it leaves the infraglenoid tubercle.

2. **Lateral head of triceps brachii.** The origin is above the radial groove. The space between the medial and lateral heads provides passage for the radial n. and deep brachial a. This is the position of the radial groove.

3. **Medial head of triceps brachii.** The origin on the humerus is inferior to the radial groove, and the belly is covered by the other heads; therefore the lateral head is cut to show the medial head.

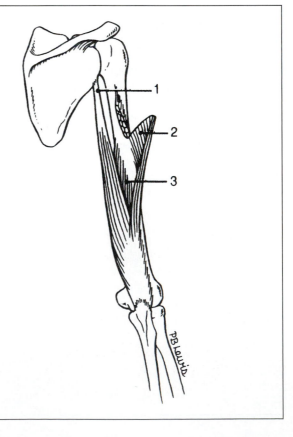

FIGURE 18–10
SHOULDER AND ARM (POSTERIOR VIEW WITH TRAPEZIUS REMOVED)

1. _____
2. _____
3. _____
4. _____
5. _____
6. **Triceps brachii**—long head
7. **Triceps brachii**—lateral head

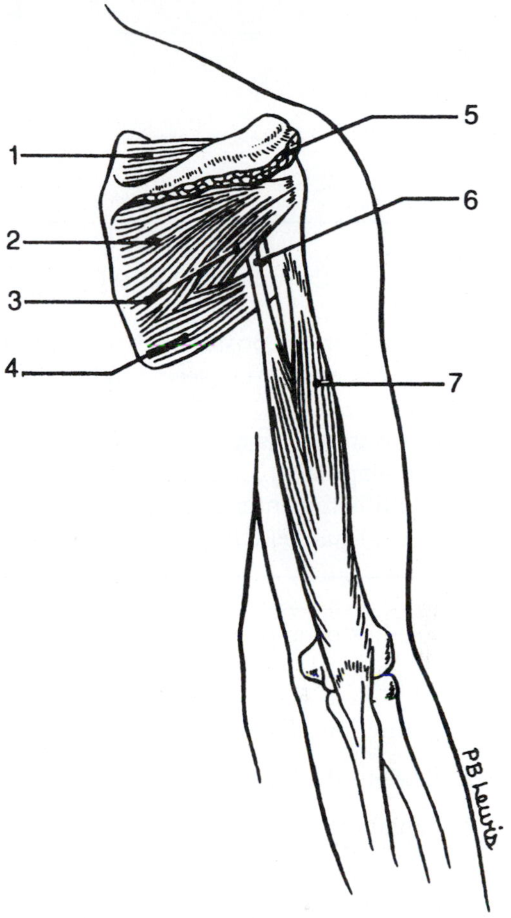

■ CLINICAL COMMENTS

Bursitis is an inflammation of a *bursa,* a small, flat, fluid-filled sac that cushions a joint to prevent friction at the point of contact between the bones, tendons and ligaments. There are more than 150 bursae in the body, but the joints that are most commonly affected are the shoulder, elbow, wrist, hip, knee and ankle. Aging, overuse, repeated movements or trauma can cause this painful condition. It will usually heal by itself. Bursitis is usually treated with rest, ice packs, and pain relievers. Stiffness can be prevented with stretching and gentle exercises.

■ Student Activities

1. Perform each action illustrated in Figures 18–1 and 18–2; complete all blank keys for illustration labels.
2. Using Figure 18–3, color the six muscles that go from the axial skeleton to the shoulder girdle.
3. The portion of the triceps brachii not visible in Figure 18–10 is the _____ head.
4. In Figure 18–7, label the greater tubercle and the lesser tubercle; color the three anterior arm muscles pink.

Exercise Eighteen

Name _____

1. Write the answers to the following questions.

   a. When looking at a posterior view of the back, what are the two muscles which would be seen superficially? _____ and _____.

   b. If the trapezius muscle is removed, what muscles would be seen deep to it and medial to the scapula? _____ and _____.

   c. What muscle fills the anterior scapula? _____

   d. What three muscles have attachments on the coracoid process? _____, _____ and _____.

   e. What muscle lies deep to the biceps brachii belly? _____

2. Matching. Use the letters of the muscles as often as needed.

   _____ 1. abduction of shoulder
   _____ 2. flexion of elbow
   _____ 3. elevation of scapula
   _____ 4. extension of humerus
   _____ 5. medial rotation of arm
   _____ 6. extension of elbow
   _____ 7. flexion of arm
   _____ 8. lateral rotation of arm

   a. teres major
   b. supraspinatus
   c. biceps brachii
   d. teres minor
   e. trapezius

   f. deltoid
   g. triceps brachii
   h. latissimus dorsi
   i. brachialis
   j. subscapularis

3. Name the labeled muscles.

   a. _____
   b. _____
   c. _____
   d. _____
   e. _____
   f. _____
   g. _____
   h. _____
   i. _____
   j. _____

122

Muscles of the Forearm and Hand

Most students will find it unnecessary to know the origins and insertions of all the forearm and hand muscles. You should remember that the superficial posterior muscles originate on the lateral side of the arm and the superficial anterior muscles originate on the medial side. In order to understand actions, you must also remember whether the muscle inserts on the forearm, carpals, or phalanges. The name of the muscle may give much of the needed information. Very few of these muscles have major action at the elbow. They act primarily on the wrist, hand, and digits.

■ OBJECTIVES

1. Describe the actions of the joints of the wrist, hand, and digits.
2. Recognize all the forearm and hand muscles as indicated.
3. Describe the general attachments of each muscle group.
4. Define the major actions of each muscle indicated.

■ METHODS

1. Watch the demonstration of the muscles.
2. Look at the bones to understand attachments of muscles.
3. Cover the keys in the illustrations until you can correctly identify labeled structures.

A. ACTIONS OF THE WRIST, HAND, AND DIGITS

In flexion of the hand (wrist), the palm of the hand moves toward the anterior forearm; extension returns it and pulls the dorsum of the hand toward the posterior forearm. Because of the many joints of the wrist, the hand can also move toward the body, adduction, and away from the body, abduction. (Those actions are not shown.)

FIGURE 19–1
ACTIONS OF THE DIGITS

The digits
    (a) Flex
    (b) Extend
    (c) Abduct
    (d) Adduct
Notice the position of the thumb in abduction and adduction. In opposition (e), the thumb and little finger oppose each other; this action gives the human a great advantage over other animals.

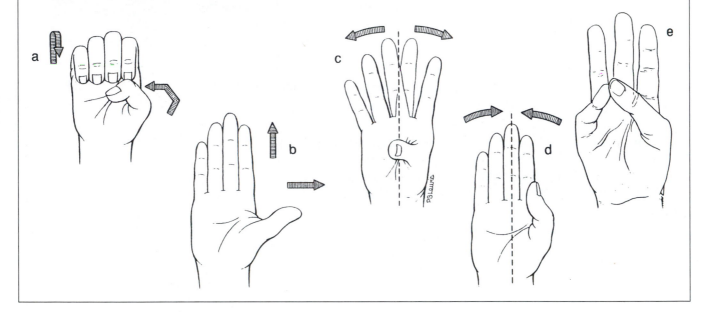

B. MUSCLES OF THE ANTERIOR FOREARM

The anterior forearm has a superficial group of five muscles and a deep group of three. The superficial group originates in the region of the medial epicondyle; the deep group originates on the anterior surfaces of the radius, ulna, and interosseous membrane. Considered as a group, the muscles of the anterior forearm are the major flexors of the wrist and digits. See Figure 19–2.

■ CLINICAL COMMENTS

"Tennis elbow" is an inflammation of the connective tissue surrounding the tendons of the muscles that attach on the lateral epicondyle of the humerus. It is one example of **tendinitis.**

FIGURE 19–2
ANTERIOR FOREARM: SUPERFICIAL MUSCLES

To locate these muscles, find the tendon of insertion of the biceps brachii muscle. Medial to the tendon you will find the origin of these superficial muscles.

1. **Pronator teres.** The only muscle of this group that has its primary action on the elbow.

2. **Flexor carpi radialis.**

3. **Palmaris longus.** This muscle is small, not very strong, and is often absent.

4. **Flexor carpi ulnaris.** As its name implies, it is a flexor of the wrist, and it is also an important adductor.

5. **Flexor digitorum superficialis.**

6. **Flexor retinaculum.** The thickened band of fascia that holds flexor tendons to the wrist.

7. **Palmar aponeurosis.** Tough connective tissue that serves as muscle attachment.

   Brachioradialis* (8) appears to be an anterior muscle, but its origin and innervation are with the posterior muscles.

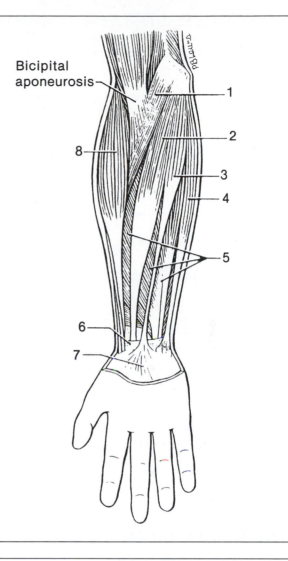

FIGURE 19–3
DEEP MUSCLES OF THE ANTERIOR FOREARM

1. **Flexor digitorum profundus.** The tendons of flexor digitorum superficialis split to allow the deep tendons to reach the distal phalanges.

2. **Flexor pollicis longus**

3. **Pronator quadratus**

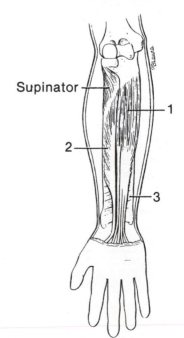

The following tables need not be committed to memory; however, they should be used as reference in understanding a specific muscle. Necessary information is provided about actions and innervations.

TABLE 19–1. ANTERIOR FOREARM MUSCLES: SUPERFICIAL GROUP

Name	Origin	Insertion	Action	Innervation
Pronator teres	Medial epicondyle of humerus; coronoid process of ulna	Middle of lateral surface of radius	Pronates forearm and flexes elbow	Median n.
Flexor carpi radialis	Medial epicondyle of humerus	Base of second metacarpal	Flexes wrist and abducts hand	Median n.
Palmaris longus	Medial epicondyle of humerus	Palmar aponeurosis	Flexes wrist	Median n.
Flexor carpi ulnaris	Medial epicondyle of humerus; olecranon and post. border ulna	Pisiform bone, hook of hamate, 5th metacarpal	Flexes wrist and adducts hand	Ulnar n.
Flexor digitorum superficialis	Medial epicondyle, humerus; coronoid process of ulna; upper ant. radius	Bodies of middle phalanges of digits 2–5	Flexes digits 2–5 and flexes wrist	Median n.

TABLE 19–2. ANTERIOR FOREARM MUSCLES: DEEP GROUP

Name	Origin	Insertion	Action	Innervation
Flexor digitorum profundus	Anterior surface, prox. 3/4 ulna; interosseous membrane	Base of distal phalanges 2–5	Flexes digits 2–5 and flexes wrist	Ulnar half by ulnar n.; rest by median n.
Flexor pollicis longus	Anterior surface radius; interosseous membrane	Base of distal phalanx of first digit (pollex)	Flexes first digit and flexes wrist	Median n.
Pronator quadratus	Distal 1/4 anterior surface of ulna	Distal 1/4 of anterior surface of radius	Pronates forearm	Median n.

C. MUSCLES OF THE POSTERIOR FOREARM

The posterior forearm can be divided into a superficial group of seven muscles and a deep group of five muscles. The superficial group originates in the region of the lateral epicondyle and the deep group from the posterior surface of the radius, ulna, and interosseous membrane. Considered as a group, these muscles are the major extensors of the wrist and digits.

To identify the superficial muscles, locate the tendon of the biceps brachii muscle; lateral to it you will find the muscles in the order in which they are listed in Figure 19–4.

FIGURE 19–4
RIGHT POSTERIOR FOREARM

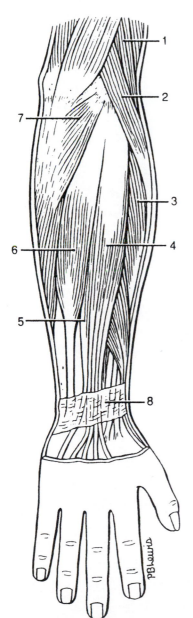

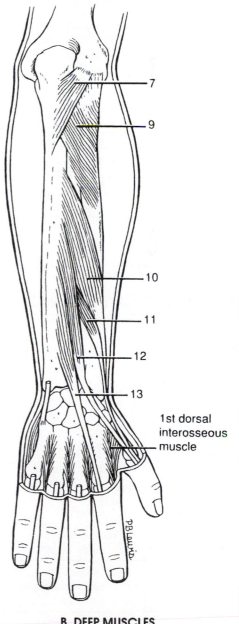

1. **Brachioradialis.** More of this muscle can be seen in Figure 19–2 because its belly actually lies on the anterior forearm. Because of its position, it is one of the three **major flexors** of the forearm even though we consider it with the extensors.

2. **Extensor carpi radialis longus**

3. **Extensor carpi radialis brevis**

4. **Extensor digitorum** (communis)

5. **Extensor digiti minimi.** This is actually a slip from the extensor digitorum.

6. **Extensor carpi ulnaris**

7. **Anconeus** is actually a part of triceps brachii and acts in extension of the elbow.

8. **Extensor retinaculum**

9. **Supinator** wraps around the upper 1/3 of the radius.

10. **Abductor pollicis longus**

11. **Extensor pollicis brevis**

12. **Extensor pollicis longus.** With the tendon of extensor pollicis brevis, this muscle forms one boundary of "the anatomical snuff box" when the thumb is fully extended.

13. **Extensor indicis**

1st dorsal interosseous muscle

A. SUPERFICIAL MUSCLES

B. DEEP MUSCLES

Because *all the muscles of the posterior forearm are innervated by the radial nerve,* the muscles of the posterior forearm are listed in Table 19–3 without the innervation. Once again, it will not be necessary to commit these origins and insertions to memory.

TABLE 19–3. POSTERIOR FOREARM MUSCLES: SUPERFICIAL GROUP

Name	Origin	Insertion	Action
Brachioradialis	Proximal 2/3 of supracondylar ridge of humerus	Lateral surface of distal end of radius	Flexes forearm (elbow)
Extensor carpi radialis longus	Lateral supracondylar ridge of humerus	Base of second metacarpal bone	Extends and abducts hand
Extensor carpi radialis brevis	Lateral epicondyle of humerus	Base of 3rd metacarpal bone	Extends and abducts hand
Extensor digitorum	Lateral epicondyle of humerus	Bases of middle phalanges via extensor expansion	Extends fingers; extends wrist
Extensor digiti minimi	Lateral epicondyle of humerus	Extensor expansion of 5th digit	Extends digiti minimi and wrist
Extensor carpi ulnaris	Lateral epicondyle of humerus; proximal part, border of ulna	Base of 5th metacarpal bone	Extends and adducts hand
Anconeus	Lateral epicondyle of humerus	Lateral surface of olecranon; proximal part, posterior ulna	Assists in extension of forearm

TABLE 19–4. POSTERIOR FOREARM MUSCLES: DEEP GROUP

Name	Origin	Insertion	Action
Supinator	Lateral epicondyle of humerus; crest of ulna	All surfaces of proximal 1/3 of radius	Supinates forearm
Abductor pollicis longus	Posterior surfaces of ulna and radius and interosseous membrane	Base of first metacarpal	Abducts and extends thumb
Extensor pollicis brevis	Posterior surface of radius and interosseous membrane	Base of proximal phalanx of thumb	Extends thumb
Extensor pollicis longus	Posterior surface of middle 1/3 ulna	Base of distal phalanx of thumb	Extends thumb
Extensor indicis	Posterior surface of ulna; interosseous membrane	Extensor expansion of index finger	Helps extend index finger

D. MUSCLES OF THE HAND

There are 19 (20) intrinsic hand muscles. They are easy to learn because groups of muscles have the same or similar names. The origins and insertions of these muscles are included in this book, for your reference.

The fleshy mound at the base of the little finger is called the **hypothenar eminence.** It contains three important muscles: an abductor, a flexor, and an opponens muscle. These *may* be covered by a thin muscle called *palmaris brevis,* a very thin muscle that will not be illustrated.

The fleshy mound at the base of the thumb is called the **thenar eminence.** It also contains three important muscles: an abductor, a flexor, and an opponens. *Deep* to this eminence is the adductor pollicis.

The remaining muscles include four *lumbricals* and the interosseous muscles. There are four dorsal interossei and three or four palmar interossei. (A portion of adductor pollicis is sometimes described as the fourth palmar interosseous.)

FIGURE 19–5
MUSCLES OF THE HAND (PALMAR VIEW)

Tendons of flexor digitorum profundus (a) and flexor digitorum superficialis (b) are labeled. *Carefully color those of flexor digitorum profundus yellow; be sure to color to the flexor retinaculum. Color the superficial tendons green.*

1. **Abductor pollicis brevis,** most lateral superficial muscle.

2. **Opponens pollicis.** Deepest of the thenar muscles, it abducts, flexes, and rotates the first metacarpal for opposition of the thumb.

3. **Flexor pollicis brevis.** More medially positioned to flex the thumb.

4. **Adductor pollicis.** Deep to the eminence, the only thenar muscle innervated by the ulnar nerve. It has both an oblique head and a transverse head.

5. **Abductor digiti minimi**

6. **Flexor digiti minimi brevis**

7. **Opponens digiti minimi.** Abducts, flexes, rotates 5th metacarpal.

8. **First lumbrical m.** These four "wormlike" muscles arise from the radial side of each of the four tendons of flexor digitorum profundus; they insert into the expanded tendon of extensor digitorum. Action: flex metacarpophalangeal joints and extend interphalangeal joints.

9. **Flexor retinaculum**

Note: There are no intrinsic muscles on the dorsum of the hand. However, the tendons of insertion of the extensor digitorum muscle spread to form *extensor expansions* over the posterior surface of each of the four medial digits. Tendons of the interosseous muscles and lumbrical muscles insert into these extensor expansions.

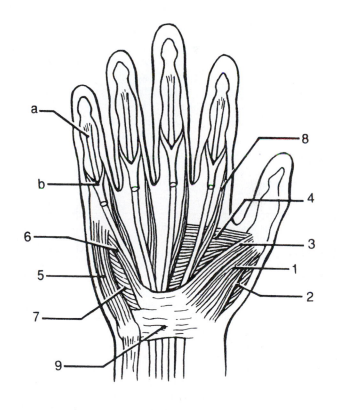

The **interossei** bellies are found between the metacarpal bones. The palmar interossei adduct the digits and the dorsal interossei abduct the digits. The **palmar interossei** can be seen when the other muscles and tendons of the palm are removed. The **dorsal interossei,** numbered in the same order as the digits, are seen in Figure 19–4B.

TABLE 19–5. MUSCLES OF THE PALMAR ASPECT OF THE HAND (THE DETAILS OF THESE MUSCLES ARE FOR REFERENCE)

Name	Origin	Insertion	Action	Innervation
Abductor pollicis brevis	Scaphoid and trapezium; flexor retinaculum	Base of proximal phalanx of thumb	Abducts thumb	Median n.
Opponens pollicis	Flexor retinaculum; trapezium	Whole length, 1st metacarpal bone	Abducts, flexes, rotates first metacarpal	
Flexor pollicis brevis	Flexor retinaculum; trapezium	Base of proximal phalanx of 1st digit (thumb)	Flexes thumb	
Adductor pollicis	Oblique head: Base of 2nd and 3rd metacarpals; capitate bone. Transverse head: Lower 2/3 of 3rd metacarpal bone	Base of proximal phalanx of the thumb	Adducts the thumb	Ulnar n.
Palmaris brevis	Palmar fascia	Skin of palm	Wrinkles skin (May help protect ulnar n. and a.)	
Abductor digiti minimi	Pisiform bone	Base of proximal phalanx of 5th digit	Abducts 5th digit (little finger)	Ulnar n.
Flexor digiti minimi brevis	Hook of hamate and flexor retinaculum	Base, proximal phalanx of 5th digit	Flexes 5th digit	
Opponens digiti minimi	Hook of hamate and flexor retinaculum	Whole length ulnar side 5th metacarpal	Abducts, flexes, rotates 5th metacarpal	
Lumbricals (4)	Tendons of flexor digitorum profundus	Tendons of extensor digitorum	Flex MP joints 2–5; extend IP 2–5	Median n. = 1&2 Ulnar n. = 3&4
Dorsal interossei (4)	Bases metacarpals 1–5	Proximal phalanx of same digit	Abduct fingers	Ulnar n.
Palmar interossei (3 or 4)	(1st), 2nd, 4th, and 5th metacarpals	Bases of proximal phalanges of digits 1, 2, 4, 5	Adduct fingers	

Exercise Nineteen

Name _____

1. Flex, extend, abduct, and adduct all five digits.

2. Color the pronator teres muscle in Figure 19–2. Use a different color for the other superficial muscles. They all originate on the _____.

3. Using a different pencil for each, color the superficial posterior forearm m. in Figure 19–4A and underline the name of each muscle with that color; underline the names of all *deep posterior forearm m.* with a pink pencil, and color the deep muscles in Figure 19–4B with pink.

4. In Figure 19–5, color all the lumbricales pink, the flexors blue, the abductors red. The muscles you did not color are the: _____, _____, and _____.

5. Label the structures indicated in the illustration at the right without looking back in the text. Under the name of each muscle, write its action and its innervation. Check your work and complete those you could not remember.

6. Name the illustrated action:

a. _____   b. _____   c. _____   d. _____

Lesson 20

Nerves of the Upper Limb

Review Lesson 8 for general nervous system information.

The nerves that stimulate contraction of the muscles of the upper limb are **brachial plexus** nerves. The only exception: trapezius muscle is innervated by cranial nerve XI, the accessory nerve.

■ OBJECTIVES

1. Draw the brachial plexus; include the major branches.
2. Identify the three cords of the brachial plexus with their terminal branches.
3. State the cord levels of origin of the five terminal branches of the brachial plexus.
4. Name the nerves of major upper-limb muscles.
5. State the relationship between each nerve and the muscle action made possible because of it.
6. State which cutaneous nerves innervate general regions of the upper limb.

■ METHODS

1. Perform the indicated activities as you study the exercise.
2. Observe the demonstration of the major nerves of the upper limb.
3. After the demonstration, identify the indicated nerves on your own.
4. Working with another student, point out a specific nerve and have your partner state which actions would not be possible if that nerve were injured at the point indicated.

A. THE BRACHIAL PLEXUS

This is formed from ventral rami of spinal nerves, *cord levels of origin,* C5, C6, C7, C8, and T1. The roots of C5 and C6 join, C7 continues alone, and C8 and T1 join to begin formation of the plexus in the neck. These trunks then divide under the clavicle. Nerves with an intermingling of different cord levels are then formed in the axillary region (see Figure 20–1).

Notice that there are eight cervical nerves but only seven cervical vertebrae. The first cervical nerve emerges between the skull and cervical vertebra number one; therefore, C8 spinal nerve emerges between vertebrae C7 and T1; each remaining spinal nerve emerges below the vertebra of its number.

Figure 20–1 includes the *five important terminal branches* of the brachial plexus. You can see the position of the structures and understand how the major nerves of the arm and forearm are formed. Additional nerves of the plexus are included in the schematic drawing in Exercise 20.

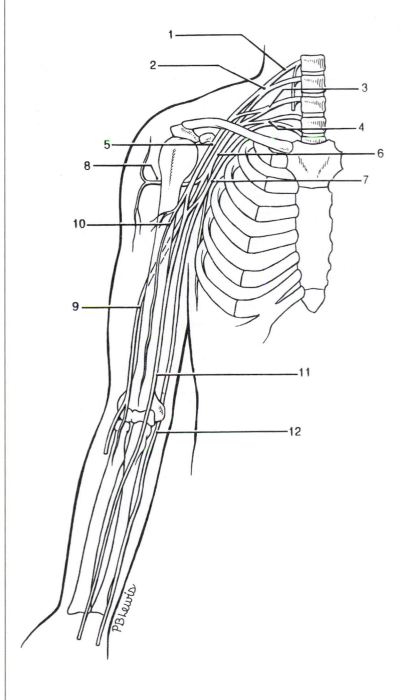

FIGURE 20–1
RIGHT BRACHIAL PLEXUS (ANTERIOR VIEW)

1. **Ventral ramus** of spinal nerve C5; emerges from the intervertebral foramen between vertebrae C4 and C5. (Label other rami.)

2. **Upper trunk,** ventral rami of C5 and C6 join.

3. **Middle trunk,** continuation of C7.

4. **Lower trunk,** ventral rami of C8 and T1 join.

5. **Lateral cord,** anterior divisions of the upper and middle trunk join.

6. **Posterior cord,** posterior divisions of all three trunks join. (Color this green to its origin and distally to the nerves.)

7. **Medial cord,** continuation of the anterior division of the lower trunk.

8. **Axillary n.,** a terminal branch of posterior cord; it circles behind the axillary region to innervate deltoid and teres minor muscles.

9. **Radial n.,** direct continuation of the posterior cord. It passes posterior to the humerus and lies between the lateral and medial heads of triceps brachii in the radial groove. It then passes anterior to the lateral epicondyle and splits. It innervates all the posterior arm and forearm muscles.

10. **Musculocutaneous n.,** continuation of the lateral cord, passes through coracobrachialis, enters biceps brachii, and brachialis muscles. Innervates all anterior arm m.

11. **Median n.** Formed from a branch of both lateral and medial cords, it enters the forearm by passing through the cubital fossa. It is the major nerve of the forearm, and innervates the three thenar eminence muscles (but *not* adductor pollicis) and lumbricales 1 and 2.

12. **Ulnar n.** The direct continuation of the medial cord, it is the only nerve that passes behind the elbow. It can be palpated between the medial epicondyle of the humerus and the olecranon process. It innervates the flexor carpi ulnaris and the ulnar half of the flexor digitorum profundus before entering the hand by passing just lateral to the pisiform bone. The major nerve of the hand, it innervates all intrinsic hand muscles except those listed for median n.

As you study Figure 20–3, notice that, with the exception of the axillary nerve (C5, 6), each terminal branch can be followed back to its correct cord levels of origin.

TERMINAL BRANCHES OF BRACHIAL PLEXUS

1. Radial n . . . . cord levels _____.
2. Axillary n . . . . cord levels _____.
3. Musculocutaneous n . . . . _____.
4. Median n. . . . . _____.
5. Ulnar n . . . . _____.

■ Student Activities

Learn to draw the plexus; include the five terminal branches, the long thoracic n., and the thoracodorsal n. (Figure 20–3). Fill in blanks (above) with correct cord levels.

B. NERVES FROM VENTRAL RAMI, TRUNKS, AND CORDS

These nerves of the brachial plexus supply the innervation for the other upper-limb muscles and for the cutaneous innervation not supplied by the terminal branches. Notice that the five terminal branches are not included in Table 20–1.

TABLE 20–1. NERVES FROM VENTRAL RAMI, TRUNKS, AND CORDS

Nerve	Muscles Innervated	Origin
Dorsal scapular	Rhomboids and levator scapulae	Ventral ramus of C5
Long thoracic	Serratus anterior	Ventral rami C5, 6, 7
Suprascapular	Supraspinatus and infraspinatus	Upper trunk
N. to subclavius	Subclavius	Upper trunk
Lateral pectoral	Pectoralis major	Lateral cord
Medial pectoral	Pectoralis major and minor	Medial cord
Medial brachial and medial antebrachial cutaneous	No muscles; these are sensory	Medial cord
Upper subscapular	Subscapularis	Posterior cord
Thoracodorsal	Latissimus dorsi	Posterior cord
Lower subscapular	Teres major and subscapularis	Posterior cord

■ CLINICAL COMMENTS

Carpal tunnel syndrome results when the median nerve is compressed within the carpal tunnel, the space between the carpal bones and the flexor retinaculum. Usually due to thickening of synovial sheaths of the flexor tendons, this syndrome results in pain in the lateral three and one half digits, numbness in the palm, and weakness in the muscles of the thenar eminence. Repetitive motions such as using a computer keyboard or a hammer often result in carpal tunnel syndrome.

C. CUTANEOUS INNERVATION OF THE UPPER EXTREMITY

See Figure 20–2.

Many of the nerves that contain motor fibers send cutaneous fibers to the skin overlying the muscles involved. Others, such as musculocutaneous (also called lateral antebrachial cutaneous in the forearm), have sensory distribution to a different region. The medial brachial cutaneous and medial antebrachial cutaneous nerves come off the plexus without motor fibers.

It is not necessary to be concerned with specific boundaries of regions innervated by a specific nerve, but you should have a general idea of the distribution.

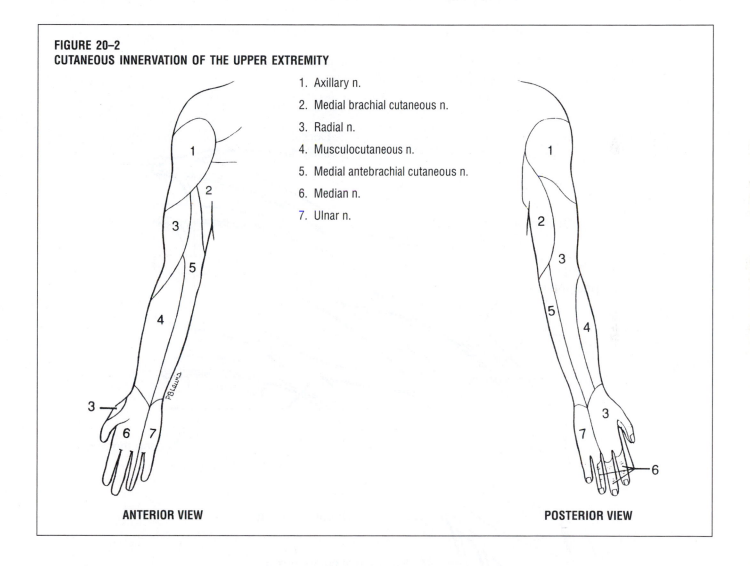

FIGURE 20–2
CUTANEOUS INNERVATION OF THE UPPER EXTREMITY

1. Axillary n.
2. Medial brachial cutaneous n.
3. Radial n.
4. Musculocutaneous n.
5. Medial antebrachial cutaneous n.
6. Median n.
7. Ulnar n.

ANTERIOR VIEW   POSTERIOR VIEW

Name _____

1. a. Label the illustration below.
   b. Color the median n. yellow and continue to color proximally (toward its origin!) all the way to the rami.
   c. Put an "A" on all three anterior divisions; a "P" on all three posterior divisions.
   d. Color the posterior cord green; color all the nerves of the posterior cord green; use the same color to color proximally to the rami.

FIGURE 20–3

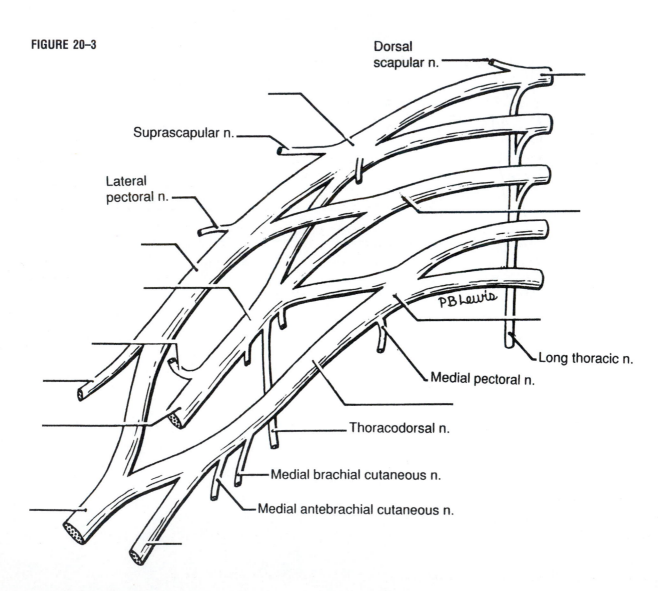

Dorsal scapular n.

Suprascapular n.

Lateral pectoral n.

PB Lewis

Long thoracic n.

Medial pectoral n.

Thoracodorsal n.

Medial brachial cutaneous n.

Medial antebrachial cutaneous n.

2. Label the illustration at the right with the name of the nerve that would innervate the muscle indicated.

a. _____

b. _____

c. _____

d. _____

e. _____

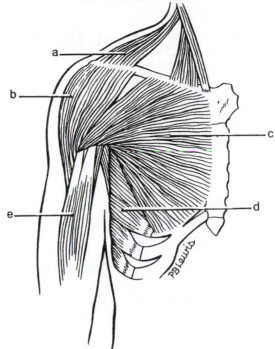

3. Complete the chart below.

Name	Muscle Innervated	Origin
_____ n.	1. Deltoid	_____ cord
Radial n.	1. _____ 2. (group) _____ _____	_____ cord
Musculocutaneous n.	1. _____ 2. _____ 3. _____	_____ cord
Median	1. (group) _____ 2. (group) _____	_____ and _____ cord
Ulnar	1. (group) _____	_____ cord

4. Complete the following:
   a. The nerve that could be considered the extensor nerve is the

   _____.

   b. The nerves involved in flexion of the forearm (elbow) are:

   _____ and _____.

   c. If you cannot flex your thumb, you may have lost the _____ n.

   d. The tingling in the little finger when the elbow is hit is caused by injury to the

   _____ n.

   e. When you shrug your shoulders the nerve most involved would be the

   _____.

5. Use a piece of notebook paper to draw a simple brachial plexus. Include rami, trunks, divisions, cords, and the five terminal nerves. Practice until you can do it.

Blood Vessels of the Upper Limb

Review Lesson 10 before studying this lesson.

The vessels of the upper limb provide the transportation of nutrients and oxygen to the cells and the removal of waste of cellular metabolism. These vessels will carry the blood from the left ventricle of the heart and return it to the right atrium. As you learn the vessels it is important to relate them to the muscles and nerves. There are several areas of the upper limb where the relationship of various structures have important clinical significance.

Remember that vessels supply all structures that lie around them.

■ OBJECTIVES

1. List, in sequence, the vessels that take blood from the heart to the upper limb and back to the heart.
2. Identify each of the major arteries of the upper limb.
3. Describe the relationship between the vessels and the upper limb structures you have already learned.

■ METHODS

1. Study the following illustrations performing the tasks indicated.
2. Observe the demonstration of the major vessels on the lab material.
3. Find each vessel yourself.
4. Cover the keys in the lab guide illustrations and name each structure.

A. MAJOR CONDUCTING ARTERIES TO THE UPPER LIMB

After being pumped by the left ventricle, the blood leaves the heart by way of the ascending aorta. The aorta arches to the left, and the major vessels to the upper limb branch from the arch.

FIGURE 21–1
BRANCHES FROM THE AORTIC ARCH

1. **Left ventricle**

2. **Ascending aorta**

3. **Brachiocephalic trunk.** Found only on the right side, this vessel is needed to shunt the blood to the right side while the aorta passes to the left.

4. **Right subclavian a.** A branch of the brachiocephalic trunk.

5. **Left subclavian a.** A branch from the aortic arch.

Notice that the pattern of the vessels from the heart to the subclavian artery is different on the left and on the right.

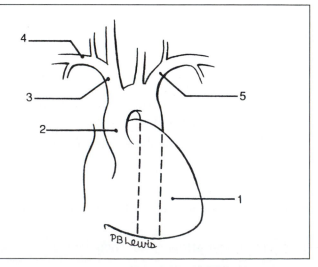

B. MAJOR ARTERIES OF THE UPPER LIMB

The subclavian artery exists on each side under the sternoclavicular joint. It arches just superior to the clavicle (deep to it) and when it reaches the lateral border of the first rib it changes its name to the *axillary artery.* The branches of the axillary a. supply blood to the upper limb.

FIGURE 21–2
ARTERIES OF THE RIGHT UPPER LIMB

1. **Subclavian a.**

2. **Axillary a.**

3. **Thoracoacromial a.** for shoulder and thorax.

   (See lateral thoracic a. also coming off under pectoralis minor m.)

4. **Subscapular a.**, a short trunk that continues as thoracodorsal a. and circumflex scapular a. that circles the scapula and emerges posteriorly through the triangular space.

5. **Thoracodorsal a.**, lies with the thoracodorsal n.

6. **Posterior circumflex humeral a.**

7. **Anterior circumflex humeral a.**

8. **Deep brachial a.** Branches from the posterolateral aspect of the brachial a.; travels in the radial groove with the radial n.

9. **Brachial a.** A direct continuation of the axillary a.; name changes at the tendon of insertion of teres major muscle. A blood pressure cuff stops blood flow in this artery by pressing it against the medial shaft of the humerus.

10. **Ulnar a.** The medial branch of the brachial a., this vessel is found with the ulnar n. in the distal 2/3 of the forearm.

11. **Common interosseous a.**, a branch of the ulnar a., it branches to supply the muscles that arise from the anterior and posterior surfaces of the interosseous membrane.

12. **Superficial palmar arterial arch**, direct continuation of the ulnar a. onto the superficial hand, anastomoses with the deep arch.

13. **Radial a.** This lateral branch of the brachial a. is normally used in taking the pulse rate. Feel it on the anterior surface of the wrist lateral to the flexor tendons. It circles the first metacarpal bone and enters the deep palm as the deep palmar arterial arch.

14. **Deep palmar arterial arch.** This has a branch that passes through the thenar eminence to anastomose with the superficial arterial arch.

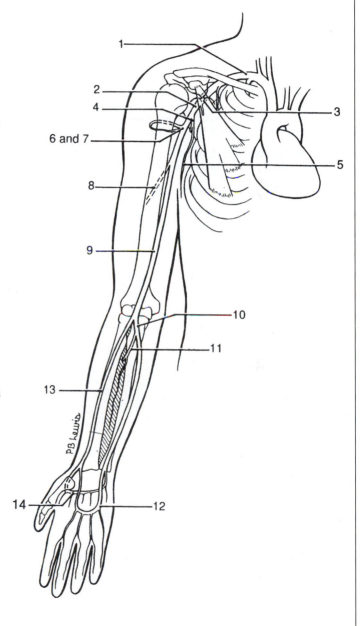

■ CLINICAL COMMENTS

In severe trauma where the axillary a. or brachial a. is severely damaged, blood flow can be stopped with strong pressure by compressing the subclavian artery against the first rib.

C. MAJOR VEINS OF THE UPPER LIMB

Each artery of the upper limb has a vein of the same name. The capillaries become venules, which then anastomose to form veins. These veins travel with the arteries and so are found deep to muscles. In the forearm there are usually two veins per artery and they are called *venae comitantes*.

In addition to the deep veins there are veins that lie superficial to the muscles. All the superficial veins originate from anastomoses on the dorsum of the hand. They form a major vein on the lateral side of the forearm, the **cephalic vein,** and one on the medial side, the **basilic vein.**

FIGURE 21–3
SUPERFICIAL VEINS OF THE UPPER LIMB

1. **Cephalic v.** Shown in both the forearm and the arm, it can be followed to where it empties into the axillary vein.

2. **Basilic v.** Seen in the forearm and arm, it dives to join the brachial venae comitantes to form the axillary vein.

3. **Median cubital v.** A superficial vein, it lies over the cubital fossa and serves as an anastomosis between the cephalic and basilic vs.

4. **Brachial v.** Deep vein(s).

5. **Axillary v.** A deep vein.

6. **Subclavian v.** A deep vein.

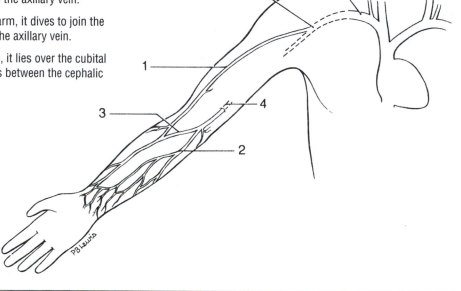

FIGURE 21–4
FORMATION OF SUPERIOR VENA CAVA

1. **Internal jugular v.** Brings blood from the head.

2. **Subclavian v.** Brings blood from the upper limb.

3. **Brachiocephalic v.** Forms on both the right and left.

4. **Superior vena cava.** Formed when the right and the left brachiocephalic veins join. Takes the blood into the right atrium.

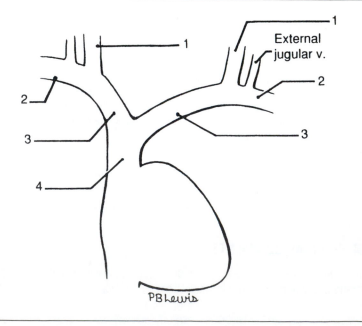

Name _____

1. In Figure 21–1, use a red pencil to color the brachiocephalic trunk and the right subclavian a. With the same pencil, color the left subclavian a.

2. Feel your pulse in the brachial a. against the medial humerus; in the radial artery lateral to the flexor tendons on the anterior forearm.

3. In Figures 21–2 and 21–3, color arteries red and veins blue. Be careful to see the unlabeled circumflex scapular artery in Figure 21–2.

4. Now that you know the nerves and vessels, go back to Figure 18–9 and use red and yellow to draw the radial n. and the deep brachial a. in the radial groove. Label each. What do they now lie between?

5. a. Carefully study the pattern of vessels in the illustration below. If the vessels are arteries (high oxygen content) use red to color the subclavian on both sides. If the vessels are veins (high carbon dioxide content) color the subclavians blue.

   b. The labeled vessels are:

   1. _____

   2. _____

   3. _____

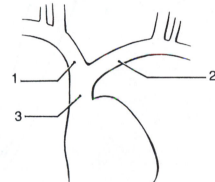

6. Blood vessels that are used clinically include:

   a. _____ to count the pulse rate.

   b. _____ in determination of the blood pressure.

7. On the illustration below:

Use side (A) to draw in red the pattern of blood flow from the heart to the fingers by way of the deep palmer arterial arch. Label all the vessels needed.

Use side (B) to draw in blue the pattern of blood returning from the fingers by way of the superficial palmar venous arch. Label all the vessels needed.

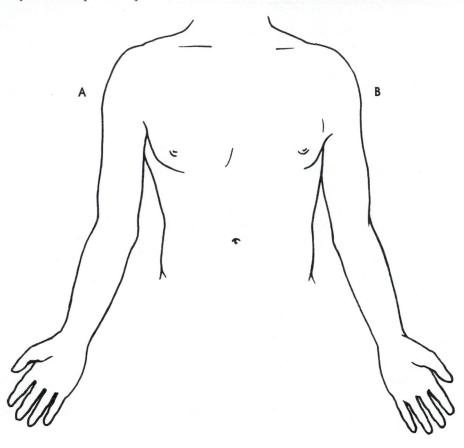

Special Areas of the Upper Limb

There are several areas of the upper limb where the relationship of various structures has important clinical significance.

■ OBJECTIVES

1. Describe the boundaries of clinically important regions within the upper limb.
2. Identify each structure within a special area and the relative position of each.
3. State the significance of each special area.

■ METHODS

1. Cover the keys in the illustrations and name the area and identify each structure labeled.
2. Quickly sketch each described special area and its contents.
3. Complete the activities.

A. TRIANGLE OF AUSCULTATION

To auscultate, or listen to, the sounds of various organs is often important in diagnoses. When the scapula is protracted, a triangle is formed with the trapezius above, the latissimus dorsi below, and the medial border of the scapula laterally. The rhomboids are the floor. This allows sounds of the heart and lungs to be heard between the sixth and seventh ribs.

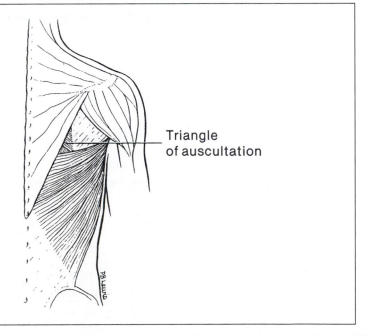

FIGURE 22–1
TRIANGLE OF AUSCULTATION

1. **Superior border** = trapezius m.

2. **Lateral boundary** = medial border of scapula

3. **Inferior border** = latissimus dorsi m.

Triangle of auscultation

B. TRIANGULAR AND QUADRANGULAR SPACES

Several major vessels and nerves pass from anterior sources to the posterior shoulder region by passing through the axilla. They emerge posteriorly through spaces between muscles.

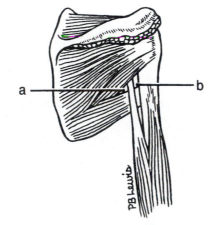

FIGURE 22–2
TRIANGULAR AND QUADRANGULAR SPACES (RIGHT SHOULDER POSTERIOR VIEW)

a. Triangular Space Boundaries:

1. Teres minor

2. Teres major

3. Long head, triceps brachii

Contents:

• Circumflex scapular vessels

b. Quadrangular Space Boundaries

1. Teres minor

2. Teres major

3. Long head, triceps brachii

4. Shaft of humerus

Contents:

• Axillary n., posterior circumflex humeral a. & v.

C. CUBITAL FOSSA (ANTECUBITAL FOSSA)

This area anterior to the elbow is important for several reasons. It contains the brachial artery, used in determining blood pressure. The superficial veins most frequently used for removal of blood or for intravenous injections of medicines and other fluid lie above this area.

The depression (fossa) is created by the bellies of muscles of the forearm.

Boundaries

Lateral = brachioradialis m.
Medial = pronator teres m.
Superior = line between
epicondyles of humerus

Contents (from lateral to medial)

Tendon of biceps brachii m.
Brachial artery
Median nerve

Superficial to the contents
is the median cubital vein

FIGURE 22–3
RIGHT CUBITAL FOSSA (ANTERIOR VIEW)

1. **Brachialis.** With supinator, floor of cubital fossa.

2. **Tendon of biceps brachii.** Most lateral of contents.

3. **Brachioradialis**—lateral boundary.

4. **Pronator teres**—medial boundary.

5. **Brachial artery.** Used here to listen for sounds of pulse when determining the blood pressure. The flow of blood is stopped in this vessel by placing the cuff around the arm and pressing the brachial artery against the humerus.

6. **Median nerve.** Most medial of cubital fossa contents.

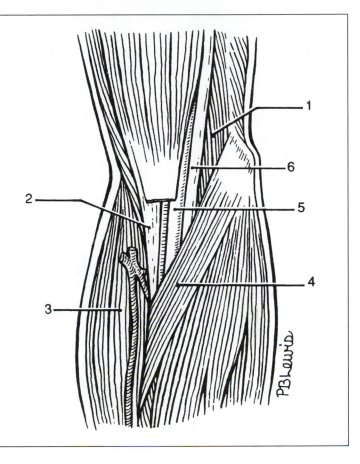

■ **Student Activities**

1. In Figure 22–1, color the triangle of auscultation.

2. In Figure 22–2, color the quadrangular space yellow; color the triangular space red.

   The _____ a. emerges here.

   The _____ a. and the _____ n. emerge from the quadrangular space.

3. In Figure 22–3, color the brachial artery red, the brachial vein blue, and the median nerve yellow.

4. Use this page to label each indicated structure. Photocopy it and use the copy to practice drawing the muscles that are found medial, lateral, deep, or superficial to each major structure. Color the nerves yellow.

RELATIONSHIP OF ARTERIES AND NERVES OF THE UPPER LIMB

FIGURE 22–4A
ANTERIOR VIEW

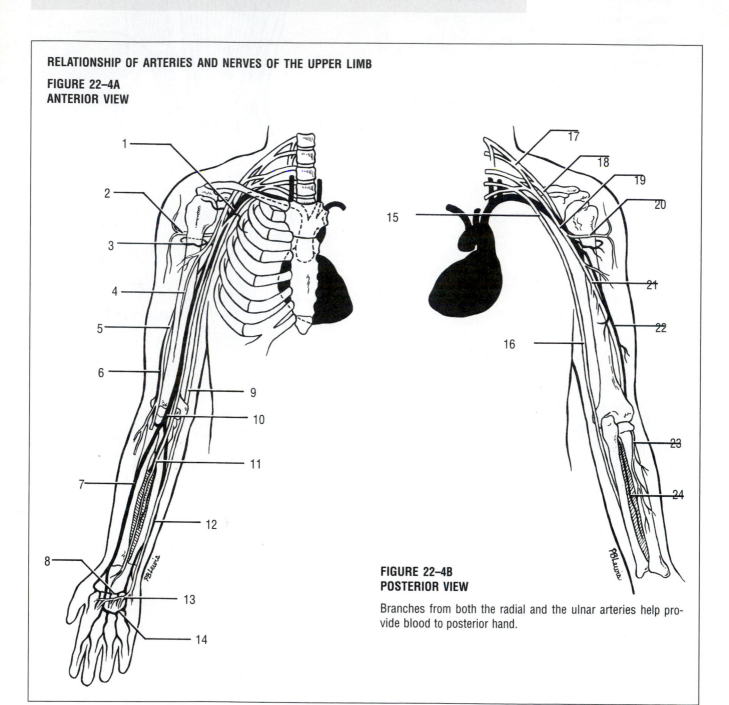

FIGURE 22–4B
POSTERIOR VIEW

Branches from both the radial and the ulnar arteries help provide blood to posterior hand.

Review of Unit II

This exercise is designed to be used after you feel fairly confident of the material you have studied. Review all student activities and lab reports, then, without using references, go through this exercise to determine your level of competence. If you have trouble, try to concentrate on the area of concern, then come back to these pages and try again.

1. Label all structures indicated in both illustrations.

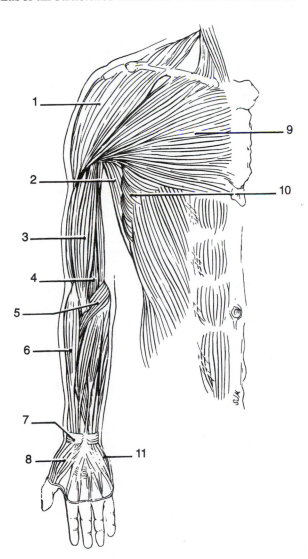

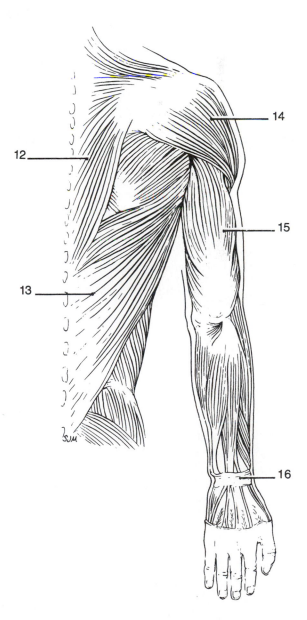

II. Organize your knowledge by filling in the muscle names that would correctly complete the chart below. This exercise should help reinforce your knowledge and expand your understanding. As you add each muscle to the correct action block, try to name its origin, insertion, and, if applicable, other actions. Completed correctly, this chart can be an important reference later. To be sure it is correct, the answers have been included in the Appendix. The most important muscles for the action are given with an asterisk; those in parentheses are least important.

Muscles that act on the shoulder (glenohumeral) joint to:

Flex the arm	Extend the arm	Abduct the arm	Adduct the arm
1.	1.	1.	1.
2.	2.	2.	2.
3.	3.		3.
4.	4.		4.

Medially rotate arm (humerus)	Laterally rotate arm
1.	1.
2.	2.
3.	
4.	
5.	

Muscles that act on the elbow to:

Flex forearm	Extend forearm
1.	1.
2.	
3.	

Supinate	Pronate
1.	1.
2.	2.

Muscles that act on the wrist to:

Flex	Extend	Abduct	Adduct
1.	1.	1.	1.
2.	2.	2.	2.
3.	3.	3.	
4.	4.	4.	
5.	5.		
6.	6.		

Muscles that act on the metacarpophalangeal and interphalangeal joints to:

Flex digits	Extend digits	Abduct digits	Adduct digits
1.	1.	1.	1.
2.	2.	2.	2.
3.	3.	3.	
4.	4.	4.	
5.	5.		
6.	6.		

III. Complete the chart below by filling in the names of the terminal branches of the brachial plexus; name all muscles innervated by each.

Name of Nerve

1. Musculocutaneous	**2.**	**3.**	**4.**	**5.**
a.	a.	a.	a.	a.
b.	b.	b.	b.	b.
c.	c.	c.	c.	
	d.	d.	d.	

IV. Answer the following questions. They may be answered orally or on paper.

1. List three regions of the vertebral column made up of individual vertebrae. State the number of vertebrae in each region and give two distinguishing characteristics of each region.
2. Name two primary and two secondary curves of the adult spinal column.
3. What is the name of the pathological lateral curve of the spine?
4. Why are rib pairs 11 and 12 called "floating" ribs?
5. Where are the erector spinae muscles located? What is their action and their innervation?
6. Name all (three) bony attachments involving pectoral girdle bones.
7. Quickly sketch an anterior and a posterior view of the scapula. Label on the appropriate view the angles, borders, spine, acromion, and coracoid process. Did you draw a right or a left bone?
8. Excluding the pectoral girdle, how many bones are in one upper limb?
9. Sketch an anterior and a posterior humerus. Include 17 markings with labels.
10. Name the medial and the lateral forearm bone and both the proximal and distal articulations of each.
11. What bone has the greatest range of movement at the elbow?
12. Name the bony connection between the upper limb and the axial skeleton.
13. Name the pair of muscles that work together in abduction of the arm; in extension of the elbow.
14. Which of the actions in question 13 could be totally eliminated with the loss of one nerve? Which nerve?
15. What action is being described when the distal end of the radius moves medial to the head of the ulna?
16. Name two muscles that can elevate the scapula.
17. What clinical symptom would indicate injury to the long thoracic n.?
18. Name the muscles you would encounter from superficial to deep if you stuck a pin in the posterior shoulder region just below the spine of the scapula. Do not stop until you reach the ribs. (**Hint:** There are four.)
19. Name three muscles that retract the scapula.
20. Name the four rotator cuff muscles and give their significance.
21. A groove developed in the proximal humerus to accommodate the tendon of what muscle?
22. Total loss of flexion of the digits would indicate injury to which nerves(s)?
23. Total loss of extension of the digits would indicate injury to which nerve(s)?
24. The fleshy mound at the base of the thumb is called _____ ; of the little finger? _____ .
25. Name the three major flexors of the forearm (elbow). How many nerves are involved in their innervation?

26. Where would you find the radial n. and the deep brachial a. together? What do they lie between?
27. Where would you find the ulnar n. and ulnar a. together?
28. What is the typical vessel used to determine pulse rate?
29. What vessel(s) is(are) needed to determine blood pressure? The one compressed with the cuff? The one used to hear the beat?
30. What flexor of the forearm is considered a posterior forearm muscle because of origin and nerve?
31. What action(s) would be lost if the radial n. were cut at the elbow?
32. What action would be lost if the median n. were cut in the cubital fossa?
33. The loss of what nerve(s) would prevent flexion of the wrist? Of the thumb?
34. What nerve(s) would have to be lost to lose abduction of the thumb?
35. What two muscle groups are separated by the interosseous membrane only?
36. What muscles have the distinction of being able to both flex and extend joints of the digits?
37. What is the difference in the blood supply to the right and the left upper limb?
38. In return of blood to the heart from the upper limb, what vessel actually enters the heart?
39. Name the lateral superficial vein found in the forearm.
40. Name the vessel that terminates as the deep palmar arterial arch.
41. Draw the pattern of arteries from the heart to the hand. Where applicable, draw a yellow line parallel to the vessel where a large nerve would lie with the vessel.
42. List all the muscles that would move the thumb.
43. Where would you find each of the following in its most superficial position?
    a. ulnar n. ——————————— b. brachial a. ———————————
    c. median n. ——————————— d. ligamentum nuchae ——————————
44. Why would latissimus dorsi be referred to as the "swimming" muscle?
45. What muscle of the upper limb is innervated by a cranial n.?
46. Draw and label the brachial plexus. Be sure to include the long thoracic n. and the thoracodorsal n.

Unit III

The Head and Neck

With:

· Nervous System

Lesson 24

The Skull

This laboratory section is written as a self-study of the skull. The skull is the bony protection for the brain. Because the cranial nerves and spinal cord serve as the communication between the brain and all other body structures, it is important to understand how each nervous structure either enters or leaves the skull. Each bone or marking should be found and understood as you study the text. Use of colored pencils is important to make each bone stand out.

■ OBJECTIVES

1. Describe the eight cranial cavity bones.
2. Identify the 14 facial bones and the important markings on each.
3. Identify the four major sutures of the cranial cavity.
4. Locate the paranasal sinuses.
5. Identify the foramina through which all cranial nerves and major vessels are transmitted.

■ METHODS

1. Study the text, performing activities as described.
2. Use skulls provided as you follow the text. Please remember to use *only* pipe cleaners on the skulls. Pencils, pens, and probes damage the expensive, delicate skulls.
3. With pipe cleaners, identify a foramen for passage of each cranial nerve.
4. Locate bones, major markings, and sinuses on x-rays.

A. BONES OF THE CRANIAL CAVITY

These eight bones form a box to protect the brain. The immovable joints between the bones are called **sutures.** *As you locate the bones in either the frontal view, Figure 24–1, or the lateral view, Figure 24–2, color them lightly with a pencil of the color indicated.*

Frontal—in both views (green)
Parietal (2)—lateral view (red)
Occipital—lateral view (yellow)
Temporal (2)—lateral view (blue)
Sphenoid—lateral view (brown). This irregular bone extends across the skull behind the orbits. It helps form the floor of the brain case; many of the foramina are found there.
Ethmoid—frontal view (orange). Another irregular bone; very little of it can be seen without removing nasal and maxillary bones. Most of this bone is not seen in this view.

Sutures, the lines of fusion, can all be named, but we will only learn the major ones:

1. **Coronal**—where frontal bone meets parietal bones
2. **Squamosal (squamous)**—between parietal and temporal bones
3. **Sagittal**—between parietal bones
4. **Lambdoidal (lambdoid)**—between parietal and occipital bones

B. BONES OF THE FACE

The 14 facial bones are immovable except for the mandible. *Locate them in either Figure 24–1 or Figure 24–2 and color them as indicated.*

Nasal (2)—both views (red)
Maxillae (2)—both views (blue)
Zygomatic (2)—both views (yellow)
Mandible—both views (green)

Lacrimal (2)—frontal view (yellow)
Palatine (2)—in Figure 24–3 only (red)
Inferior nasal conchae (2)—frontal view (brown)
Vomer—frontal view (yellow)

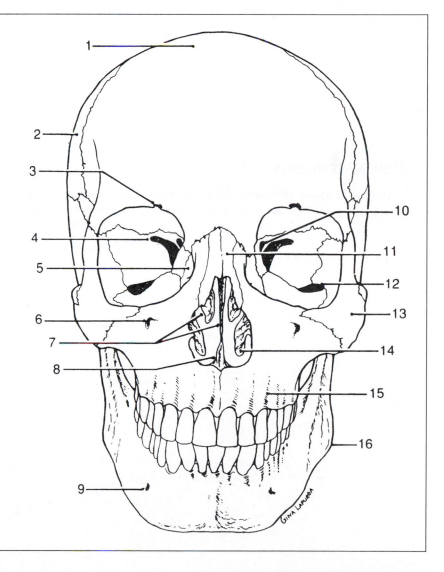

FIGURE 24–1
SKULL (FRONTAL VIEW)

1. **Frontal bone**

2. **Parietal bone**

3. **Supraorbital foramen,** or **notch,** on superciliary arch

4. **Superior orbital fissure** in sphenoid bone

5. **Lacrimal bone**

6. **Infraorbital foramen** in maxillary bone

7. **Middle nasal concha** and **perpendicular plate,** both ethmoid bone

8. **Vomer bone,** the inferior portion of nasal septum

9. **Mental foramen** in body of mandible

10. **Optic foramen**

11. **Nasal bone**

12. **Inferior orbital fissure**

13. **Zygomatic bone**

14. **Inferior nasal concha**

15. **Alveolar processes** of maxillary bone

16. **Angle of mandible**

FIGURE 24–2
SKULL (LATERAL VIEW)

1. **Coronal suture**

2. **Sphenoid bone**—greater wing

3. **Temporal bone**

4. **Zygomatic arch**

5. **Condyloid process** in the mandibular fossa

6. **Sagittal suture**

7. **Parietal bone**

8. **Squamosal suture**

9. **Lambdoidal suture**

10. **External occipital protuberance** of occipital bone

11. **External acoustic meatus**

12. **Mastoid process** of the temporal bone

13. **Styloid process** of the temporal bone

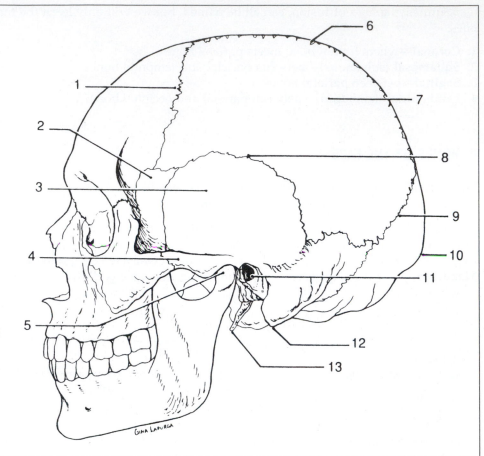

■ **CLINICAL COMMENTS**

Fontanels are the areas of fibrous connective tissue between the developing skull bones. During birth the fontanels allow the bones to move closer together to ease the passage of the head through the birth canal. Until the brain is fully developed these fontanels remain. If brain development stops too soon (due to a genetic or developmental problem), growth of the skull is arrested, and the sutures form. As a result, the baby has **microcephaly,** a small head.

C. MARKINGS OF THE SKULL

Now that you can identify and locate the 22 bones of the skull, proceed by identifying the bony markings in each view of the skull. You should be able to identify all structures in bold print.

1. FRONTAL VIEW OF SKULL (FIGURE 24–1)

a. Frontal bone forms the eyebrow ridges or **superciliary arches.** On or near these ridges can be seen the **supraorbital foramina** or notches. The frontal bone extends into the orbit (eye socket) to form its roof.

b. The orbit is bounded laterally by the zygomatic bone and inferiorly and medially by the maxillary bone. Looking into the orbit you can see three openings in the sphenoid bone: the **optic foramen,** or passageway of the optic nerve from the eye to the brain, and the **superior** and **inferior orbital fissures.** The most medial bone of the orbit, the **lacrimal bone,** has a groove that communicates below with the nasal cavity through the **nasolacrimal canal.** Between the lacrimal bone and the optic foramen, a portion of the ethmoid bone can be seen.

c. The **zygomatic bone** forms the prominent part of your cheek and articulates medially with the maxillary bone. In the **maxillary bone** the **infraorbital foramen** is inferior to the orbit, and the **alveolar processes** house the upper teeth.

d. The **nasal cavity** is formed by the maxillary bones laterally and the nasal bones superiorly. The nasal cavity is divided by the **nasal septum,** which consists of the **vomer bone** and the **perpendicular plate** of the ethmoid bone. From the lateral walls of the nasal cavity extend three pairs of nasal conchae. The **inferior nasal conchae** are separate bones. Superior to these are the **middle nasal conchae** and superior nasal conchae, all part of the ethmoid bone. The superior conchae are hard to find and need not be seen.

e. The **mandible** is the last bone to be seen from this view. Its **alveolar processes** house the lower teeth. The **mental foramina** lie on either side of the midline in the body of the mandible.

2. LATERAL VIEW OF SKULL (FIGURE 24–2)

In this view the frontal bone is still visible, but now you can see the parietal bone and the occipital bone. The irregularly shaped bone inferior to the parietal is the temporal bone. It has a free process, the **zygomatic process,** which joins the **temporal process** of the **zygomatic bone** to form the **zygomatic arch.** Just posterior to this arch is the **external acoustic meatus.** The **mastoid process** is below the meatus and the **styloid process** projects from a region just anterior and medial to the mastoid process. The **mandibular fossa** of the temporal bone provides an articulation for the mandible, the only movable joint of the skull. The irregular sphenoid bone can be seen between the temporal and frontal bones.

The area superior and deep to the zygomatic arch is referred to as the **temporal fossa;** the area inferior and deep to the zygomatic arch is called the **infratemporal fossa.**

3. INFERIOR VIEW OF BASE OF THE SKULL (FIGURE 24–3)

Hold the skull as indicated in the illustration and look for each labeled structure.
Look for the large, jugular foramen between the carotid canal and the occipital condyle.

FIGURE 24–3
BASE OF THE SKULL (INFERIOR VIEW)

1. **Palatine process** of the maxillary bone. The upper teeth are lateral. Moving down (posteriorly) you can see the suture line with the palatine bones.

2. **Palatine bones** complete the hard palate. The **palatine foramina** can be seen in these bones.

3. **Medial pterygoid plate,** on which you can see a hook or **hamulus.**

4. **Pterygoid fossa,** a part of the sphenoid bone, is seen where the tooth sockets end posteriorly. The fossa, in a plane perpendicular to the teeth, is bounded by medial and lateral plates of bone.

5. **Lateral pterygoid plate** can be followed superiorly to the greater wing of the sphenoid bone between the temporal and frontal bones.

6. **Mandibular fossa,** for articulation with the condyle of the mandible.

7. **Styloid process** of the temporal bone is very thin and breaks off easily.

8. **Stylomastoid foramen** between the **mastoid and styloid processes.**

9. **Mastoid process** of the temporal bone. Contains air cells or sinuses.

10. **Foramen magnum,** through which the spinal cord, vertebral a., and anterior and posterior spinal arteries enter the skull. It is between the occipital condyles.

11. **External occipital protuberance** has superior nuchal lines extending laterally.

12. **Foramen lacerum.** This inferior aspect is plugged with cartilage in the living skull.

13. **Carotid canal,** anterior and lateral to the occipital condyle. Internal carotid a. enters here, passes through the canal, and enters the cranial vault from foramen lacerum.

14. **Occipital condyle,** bilateral structures articulate with the atlas (1st cervical vertebra).

15. **Inferior nuchal lines** are closer to foramen magnum.

■ CLINICAL COMMENTS

A **cleft palate** results when the palatine processes of the maxillary bones fail to fuse. This usually occurs between weeks 10 and 12 of embryonic development.

FIGURE 24–3
BASE OF THE SKULL (INFERIOR VIEW) (CONTINUED)

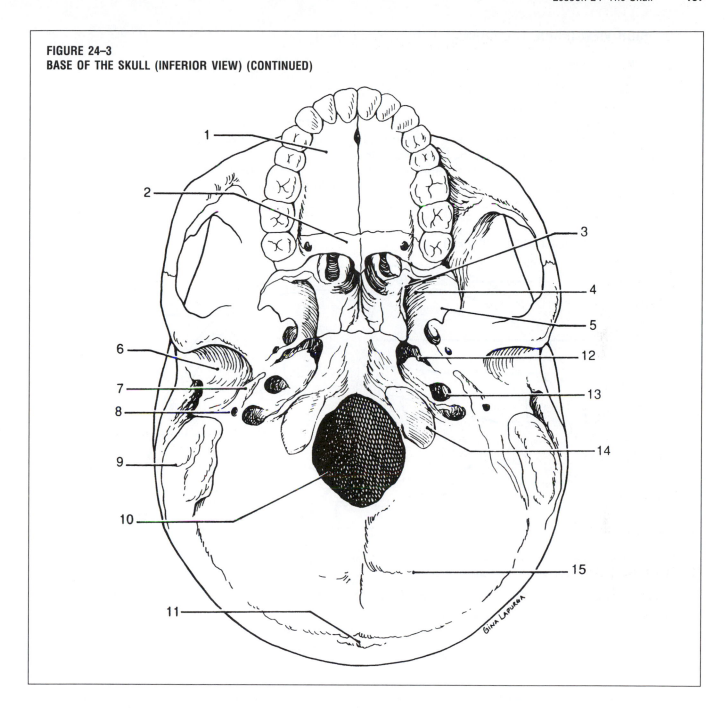

4. SUPERIOR VIEW INSIDE THE CRANIAL VAULT (FIGURE 24–4)

With the **calvaria**, skull-cap, removed, look into the cranium and see three levels or fossae. The **anterior cranial fossa** is formed largely from frontal bone (some **ethmoid bone** in the midline) and the **lesser wing of the sphenoid bone.** The frontal lobe of the brain lies in this plane.

Moving posteriorly you will notice a step down into the **middle cranial fossa.** It is composed of the **body** and the **greater wing of sphenoid bone,** and part of the **temporal bone.** The temporal lobe of the brain lies in this plane.

The deepest fossa is the **posterior cranial fossa.** It is formed of **temporal** and **occipital bones.** The cerebellum and part of the brain stem lie in this fossa.

FIGURE 24–4
INSIDE THE CRANIAL VAULT (SUPERIOR VIEW)

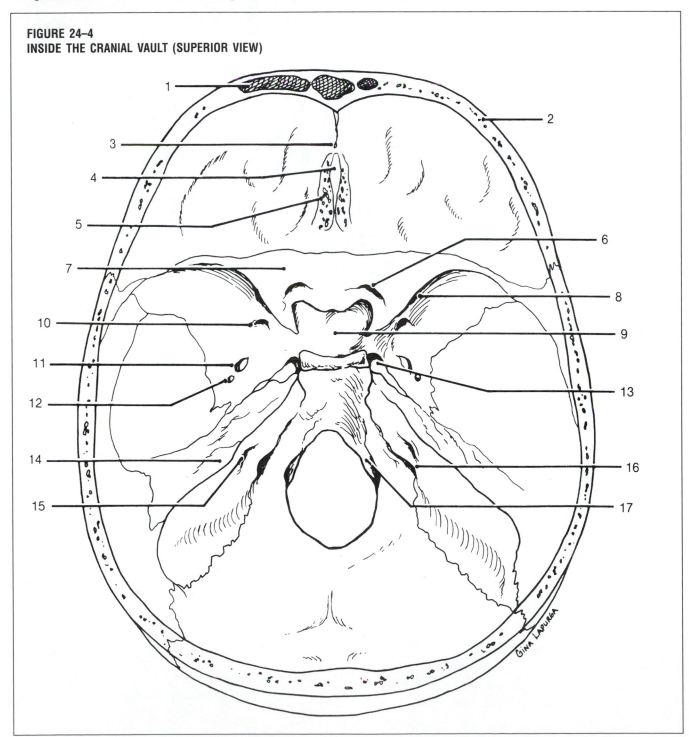

FIGURE 24–4
INSIDE THE CRANIAL VAULT (SUPERIOR VIEW)
(CONTINUED)

1. **Frontal sinus.**

2. **Diploe,** cancellous bone between two layers of flat, compact bone.

3. **Foramen cecum,** provides an opening for a nasal vein to drain into the superior sagittal sinus.

4. **Crista galli**—a process of ethmoid bone to which the falx cerebri attaches.

5. **Cribriform plate** of the ethmoid bone has tiny foramina for passage of olfactory nerve processes.

6. **Optic foramen,** transmits CN II and the ophthalmic artery.

7. **Lesser wing of sphenoid bone**

8. **Superior orbital fissure,** between the lesser and greater wings of sphenoid bone; transmits CNs III, IV, VI, and ophthalmic branch of CN V.

9. **Hypophyseal fossa (sella turcica)**—depression in body of sphenoid bone; houses the pituitary gland.

10. **Foramen rotundum**—directed toward the maxillary bone; transmits maxillary division of CN V.

11. **Foramen ovale**—transmits mandibular branch of CN V.

12. **Foramen spinosum**—for passage of the middle meningeal artery.

13. **Foramen lacerum,** internal carotid a. enters cranial vault. (The foramina numbered 10–13 are in the **greater wing of the sphenoid bone.**)

14. **Petrous ridge of temporal bone** divides the middle and posterior fossae and is thick because it houses the middle and inner ear structures.

15. **Internal acoustic (auditory) meatus,** transmits CNs VII and VIII.

16. **Jugular foramen,** at the base of the petrous ridge. Named for the internal jugular vein that forms here; transmits CNs IX, X, and XI.

17. **Hypoglossal canal,** obliquely directed; at the edge of foramen magnum. Transmits CN XII.

5. THE MANDIBLE

This is the only movable bone of the skull and it must move during speech as well as for ingestion and chewing of food.

FIGURE 24–5
THE MANDIBLE (POSTEROLATERAL VIEW)

1. **Condyloid process**—posterior, articulates with the mandibular fossa of the temporal bone to form the temporomandibular (TM) joint.

2. **Coronoid process**—anterior process of the superior end of the ramus.

3. **Mandibular foramen**—inside surface of the ramus. Transmits alveolar n. for the lower teeth.

4. **Angle**—where the body joins the ramus. It is roughened for muscle attachments.

5. **Genoid tubercle**—process for muscle attachments.

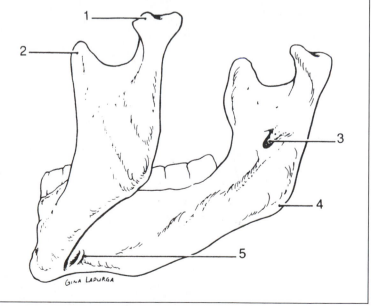

GINA LAPURGA

6. PARANASAL SINUSES

These are spaces within the bones of the skull. These cavities help make the bones lighter and are important in resonance of the voice. These sinuses are lined by a mucous membrane, which is continuous with that of the nasal cavity. They all open into the nasal cavity.

FIGURE 24–6
PARANASAL SINUSES

The **hyoid bone,** not a skull bone, does not articulate with any other bone. It does serve as a site of attachment for several muscles.

    It is found between the mandible and the thyroid cartilage.

1. **Frontal sinus**—in the frontal bone, superior to the eyes.

2. **Ethmoid air cells**—several compartments separated by thin walls of bone. These are located in the ethmoid bone deep to the nasal bones.

3. **Sphenoid sinus**—within the body of the sphenoid bone, inferior to sella turcica. This is a midline structure posterior to the ethmoid air cells.

4. **Maxillary sinus**—inferior to the eyes; in the maxillary bones, these are the largest sinuses.

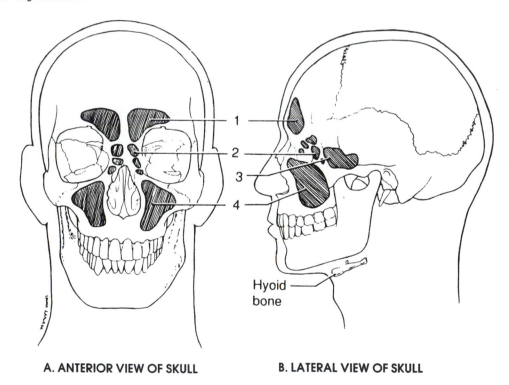

A. ANTERIOR VIEW OF SKULL   **B. LATERAL VIEW OF SKULL**

D. STRUCTURES TRANSMITTED THROUGH FORAMINA

The purpose of the cranial vault is protection of the brain. The brain has to communicate with the rest of the body and it must receive nutrients and eliminate wastes. The many foramina allow the passage of nerves and vessels to serve this purpose. To help you understand the foramina you must learn the names and numbers of the 12 pairs of cranial nerves because each one must find its way into or out of the skull. They will be discussed in detail in Exercise 29, but they are listed here. Notice that Roman numerals are used when using numbers instead of names. You should know both.

CN I	olfactory n.	CN VI	abducens n.
CN II	optic n.	CN VII	facial n.
CN III	oculomotor n.	CN VIII	vestibulocochlear n.
CN IV	trochlear n.	CN IX	glossopharyngeal n.
CN V	trigeminal n.	CN X	vagus n.
Division I	ophthalmic n. (CN V_1)	CN XI	accessory n.
Division II	maxillary n. (CN V_2)	CN XII	hypoglossal n.
Division III	mandibular n. (CN V_3)		

■ Student Activities

In Figure 24–4, lightly color each bone the same color used on that bone in Figures 24–1 and 24–2.

The foramina you should learn are those with important structures passing through. Complete the table below by naming the correct foramen for each of the listed structures. This will be important information, so use the preceding text to complete it carefully.

Foramen	Transmitted Structure(s)
1.	Olfactory nerve fibers
2.	Optic n., ophthalmic a.
3.	CN III, IV, VI, and ophthalmic n. (CN V_1)
4.	Maxillary n. (CN V_2)
5.	Mandibular n. (CN V_3)
6.	Middle meningeal a.
7.	Internal carotid a. enters cranial vault here
8.	Internal jugular v., CN IX, X, and XI
9.	CN VII and VIII
10.	CN VII
11.	CN XII
12.	Vertebral arteries; spinal cord
13.	Internal carotid a. enters skull here

Name _____

1. In the cranial vault below draw all foramina needed for the 12 pairs of cranial
   nerves. In the space on the left, label the foramen with its name; on the right,
   label the foramen with structure(s) transmitted. See example.

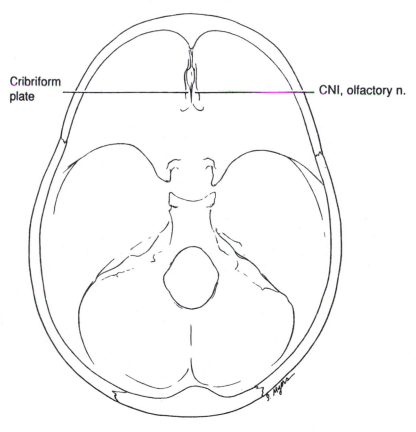

Cribriform
plate

CNI, olfactory n.

2. Matching exercise: Use each letter only once.

_____ 1. temporal bone   a. a sinus under the eye

_____ 2. sella turcica   b. unpaired bone of vault

_____ 3. calvaria   c. houses ear structures

_____ 4. occipital bone   d. contains foramen magnum

_____ 5. maxillary   e. only movable bone

_____ 6. crista galli   f. joint between parietal bones

_____ 7. sphenoid   g. defines an area

_____ 8. sagittal   h. part of ethmoid bone

_____ 9. infratemporal   i. top of skull

_____ 10. mandible   j. houses pituitary gland

The Brain

Before you begin this unit you should review Lesson 8.

The central nervous system begins its development about $2\frac{1}{2}$ weeks after the ovum is fertilized. Rapidly proliferating cells of the dorsal embryo fold over to form a neural tube. The caudal end of the neural tube becomes the spinal cord; the cranial end develops three enlargements, which will be the future brain.

■ OBJECTIVES

1. Describe the gross development of the brain.
2. Identify the adult structures of each embryological enlargement of the cranial neural tube.
3. Identify the major lobes, gyri, and sulci of the brain.
4. Locate each structure of the brainstem.

■ METHODS

1. Perform the suggested activities as you preview the exercise.
2. Observe a demonstration of the human brain if available.
3. Use the brains and/or models to identify the structures listed in the lab guide.
4. Sketch medial and lateral views of the brain.

FUNCTIONS OF THE BRAIN

The brain is more complicated than the most powerful computer and has billions of neurons, each of which may connect to thousands of other neurons. It is our major communications and integration control center. The job of the beginning student is to understand the brain in the simplest of terms while remembering that everything we do or think depends on this fascinating organ. This book tries to keep this in mind by simplifying the material as much as possible while conveying a basic understanding of the brain and nervous system.

- **Stimulates movement**—requires coordination of sensory and motor information.
- **Maintains homeostasis**—integrates internal and external environment.
- **Origin of conceptual thought**—(intelligence) creativity, imagination, memory, learning, calculation, prediction, abstract reasoning, altruism, free will, and personality.

NEURAL TUBE DEVELOPMENT

This involves a folding of embryonic ectoderm that leaves a central hollow core, the central canal. In Figure 25–1, the spinal cord portion is not complete.

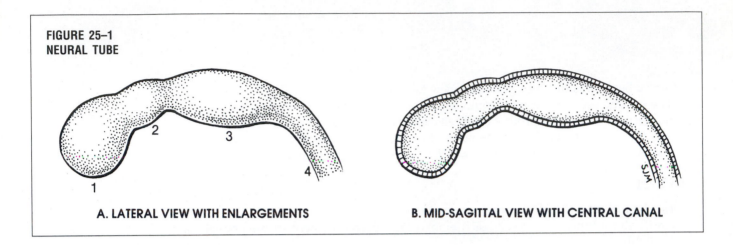

FIGURE 25–1
NEURAL TUBE

A. LATERAL VIEW WITH ENLARGEMENTS   B. MID-SAGITTAL VIEW WITH CENTRAL CANAL

TABLE 25–1. NEURAL TUBE DEVELOPMENT

Original Enlargement	Derivatives		Central Canal Development
1. Forebrain (prosencephalon)	(telencephalon)	Cerebral hemispheres	Right and left lateral ventricle
	(diencephalon)	Thalamus Hypothalamus	Third ventricle
2. Midbrain (mesencephalon)	(mesencephalon)	Midbrain	Cerebral aqueduct
3. Hindbrain (rhombencephalon)	(metencephalon)	Cerebellum Pons	Fourth ventricle
	(myelencephalon)	Medulla oblongata	
4. Spinal cord			Central canal

NOTE: The ***brainstem*** consists of the midbrain, pons, and medulla oblongata.

■ CLINICAL COMMENTS

Hydrocephalus is a condition in which cerebrospinal fluid builds up within the ventricles. When this occurs in a developing fetus, the brain and bones expand and the baby's head is enlarged. While the fetus is still in the uterus, a shunt can be used to drain the excess fluid and prevent mental retardation. If it occurs in an adult, the intracranial pressure causes headaches and can lead to brain damage unless a shunt is used to drain the excess fluid.

LATERAL VIEW OF THE BRAIN: LEFT HEMISPHERE

As you begin this study you must first orient yourself to the specific specimen to determine which is the anterior (rostral) and which is the posterior (caudal) extremity of the cerebral hemisphere. Also, decide whether you are looking at the ventral or the dorsal brainstem. Until you can do this, do not proceed. Remember which structures are found in each location.

FIGURE 25–2
BRAIN (LATERAL VIEW)

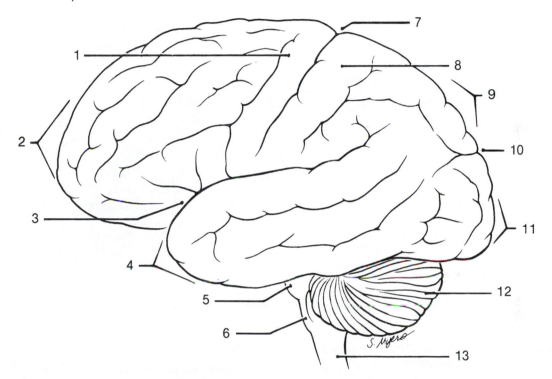

1. **Precentral gyrus**—the elevated portion of a brain fold is called a **gyrus.** This one is "before" or rostral to the central sulcus. It is part of the frontal lobe, and fine motor control is its function.

2. **Frontal lobe**—natural divisions created by brain folds divide the brain into sections called **lobes.** This "front" one lies in the anterior cranial fossa on the frontal bone.

3. **Lateral fissure**—separation of temporal lobe from frontal. Fissures are deeper than sulci.

4. **Temporal lobe**—lies in the middle cranial fossa and is important in hearing, olfaction, memory and learning.

5. **Pons**—superior enlargement of ventral hindbrain.

6. **Medulla oblongata**—inferior enlargement of ventral hindbrain.

7. **Central sulcus**—a sulcus is the depression created by the folding of the brain. This one is in a central position on the lateral brain.

8. **Postcentral gyrus**—caudal to the central sulcus. It is part of the parietal lobe and is the primary sensory reception area.

9. **Parietal lobe**—extends from central sulcus to occipital lobe.

10. **Parieto-occipital sulcus**—between parietal and occipital lobes; easily seen in a medial view.

11. **Occipital lobe**—most caudal lobe. Important receptor of visual information.

12. **Cerebellum**—connected to pons, medulla oblongata, and midbrain; it is essential for coordination of motor activity. It lies in the posterior cranial fossa.

13. **Spinal cord**

MEDIAL VIEW OF THE BRAIN—RIGHT HEMISPHERE

The longitudinal fissure (Figure 25–5) separates the two hemispheres of the brain. If a knife passes through this fissure to separate the hemispheres, the first brain tissue that will be cut is the **corpus callosum.**

FIGURE 25–3
BRAIN (MEDIAL VIEW)

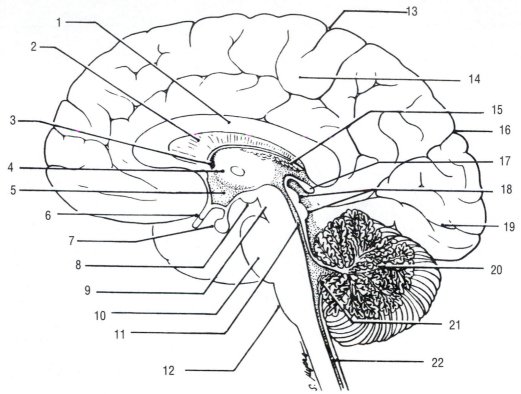

1. **Corpus callosum**—commissural fibers; structural and functional connection of hemispheres.

2. **Septum pellucidum**—thin tissue separating the lateral ventricles.

3. **Interventricular foramen**—opening between lateral and third ventricles.

4. **Thalamus**—oval-shaped enlargement formed of nuclei: groups of nerve cell bodies. The two sides may touch at the massa intermedia. One of its many functions is to serve as a relay for most sensory information.

5. **Hypothalamus**—delineated from thalamus by hypothalamic sulcus; involved in functions of autonomic nervous system, limbic system and endocrine system.

6. **Optic chiasma**—the crossing of some of the optic fibers.

7. **Hypophysis** or **pituitary gland**—extends from the infundibulum (stalk); secretes hormones important in maintaining homeostasis. Rests in the hypophyseal fossa of the sphenoid bone.

8. **Mammillary body**—a nucleus related to emotional function (limbic system).

9. **Cerebral peduncle of midbrain**—motor processes are located here.

10. **Pons**

11. **Cerebral aqueduct**—passageway between the third and fourth ventricles.

12. **Medulla oblongata**—inferior part of the brain stem, for autonomic reflex control of heart beat and respiration.

13. **Central sulcus**—separates frontal lobe from parietal lobe.

14. **Paracentral lobule**—U-shaped continuation of pre- and postcentral gyri.

15. **Choroid plexus** within third ventricle—produces cerebrospinal fluid (CSF).

16. **Parieto-occipital sulcus**

17. **Pineal gland**—involved in sleep/wake cycles

18. **Superior and inferior colliculi**—midbrain structures relay visual and auditory information.

19. **Calcarine fissure**—primary visual cortex surrounds this sulcus.

20. **Arbor vitae of cerebellum**—tree-like arrangement of white matter.

21. **Choroid plexus** in fourth ventricle—produces CSF.

22. **Central canal** of spinal cord.

BASE OF THE BRAIN: VENTRAL BRAINSTEM

The structures of the brainstem and the cranial nerves can be more easily studied by using this ventral view of a whole brain. The nerves will be identified here, but discussed in Exercise 29.

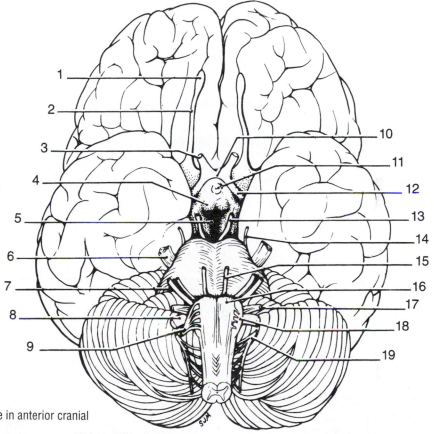

FIGURE 25–4
BASE OF BRAIN (VENTRAL BRAINSTEM)

1. **Olfactory bulb**—rests on cribriform plate in anterior cranial fossa.

2. **Olfactory tract,** fibers from cell bodies in the bulb.

3. **CN II, optic n.** enters through optic foramen.

4. **Mammillary body**—part of the limbic system.

5. **Interpeduncular fossa,** depression between the two cerebral peduncles.

6. **Trigeminal n.,** emerges from the side of pons.

7. **CN VIII, vestibulocochlear n.; CN VII, facial n.** just medial; corner of pontomedullary junction.

8. **CN X, vagus n.**

9. **CN XII, hypoglossal n.**—fibers can be seen in the sulcus just lateral to the pyramids.

10. **Optic chiasma**—crossing of fibers carrying peripheral vision.

11. **Infundibulum,** stalk of the hypophysis, torn off when brain is removed from skull.

12. **Optic tract**—continuation of optic fibers from the chiasm to brain.

13. **CN III, oculomotor n.**—emerges from interpeduncular fossa.

14. **CN IV, trochlear n.**—very small; originates dorsally but wraps around the midbrain.

15. **CN VI, abducens n.**—emerges from junction of pons with medulla.

16. **Pyramid of medulla**—made of motor processes or "pyramidal" tracts.

17. **CN IX, glossopharyngeal n.**—hard to identify; easily confused with vagus n. on brain.

18. **Olive**—oval nucleus just lateral to medullary pyramids.

19. **CN XI, accessory n.**—fibers easily confused with those of vagus n.

DORSAL VIEW OF BRAIN AND BRAINSTEM

Because of the growth of the cerebral hemispheres and cerebellum, little is seen of brainstem structures in this view. If the cerebral hemispheres and cerebellum were separated, you would be able to see the colliculi of the dorsal midbrain. There are some very important structures on the dorsal medulla you should understand.

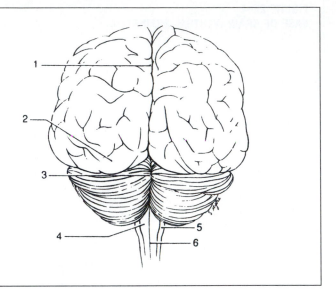

FIGURE 25–5
BRAIN AND BRAINSTEM (DORSAL VIEW)

1. **Longitudinal fissure**—separates cerebral hemispheres.

2. **Occipital lobe**—most caudal lobe.

3. **Vermis of cerebellum**—the tissue between the two cerebellar hemispheres.

4. **Gracile tubercle**—a nucleus that relays sensory information from the lower body

5. **Cuneate tubercle**—a nucleus that relays sensory information from the upper body

6. **Dorsal median sulcus of medulla**

CORONAL SECTION THROUGH THE BRAIN

The position of many brain structures can be understood only in a coronal section. Identify familiar structures and relate them to each other.

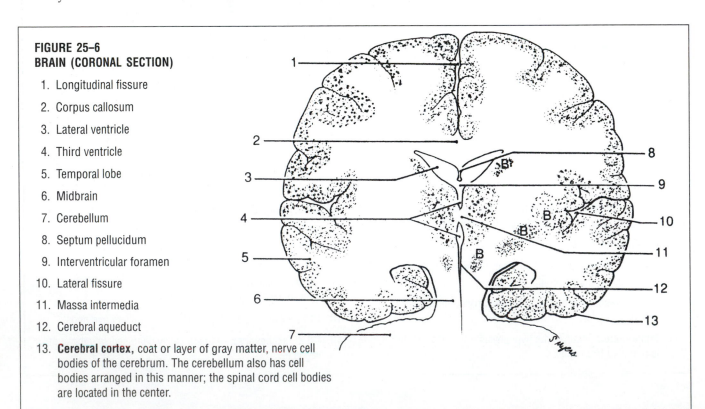

FIGURE 25–6
BRAIN (CORONAL SECTION)

1. Longitudinal fissure

2. Corpus callosum

3. Lateral ventricle

4. Third ventricle

5. Temporal lobe

6. Midbrain

7. Cerebellum

8. Septum pellucidum

9. Interventricular foramen

10. Lateral fissure

11. Massa intermedia

12. Cerebral aqueduct

13. **Cerebral cortex,** coat or layer of gray matter, nerve cell bodies of the cerebrum. The cerebellum also has cell bodies arranged in this manner; the spinal cord cell bodies are located in the center.

Basal nuclei, marked with a (B) on the right side of Figure 25–6, are groups of nerve cell bodies deep to the cortex. These are not to be identified in the lab, but recognize their names and be aware of general function. They inhibit skeletal muscle contraction and help maintain motor control. If not functioning properly, involuntary motor activity results. The muscle rigidity and tremors of Parkinson's disease are examples. Names of the basal nuclei are: caudate nucleus, putamen, globus pallidus, and amygdaloid nucleus.

VENTRICLES OF THE BRAIN

All the ventricles contain choroid plexus (Figure 25–3), capillary-like structures that continually produce cerebrospinal fluid (CSF). The CSF fills all the ventricles and subarachnoid space (described in Lesson 26). The CSF functions to:

1. Serve as a shock absorber
2. Help transport nutrients to cells and to remove waste products
3. Help maintain the ion balance within the nerve tissue

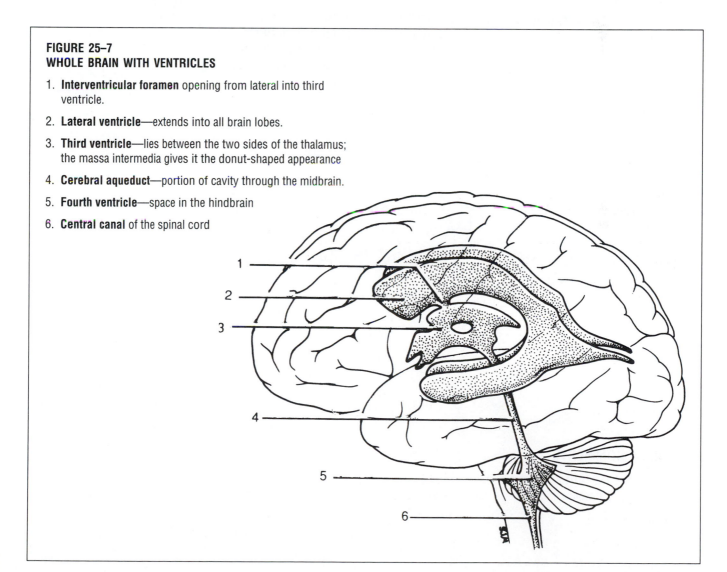

FIGURE 25–7
WHOLE BRAIN WITH VENTRICLES

1. **Interventricular foramen** opening from lateral into third ventricle.

2. **Lateral ventricle**—extends into all brain lobes.

3. **Third ventricle**—lies between the two sides of the thalamus; the massa intermedia gives it the donut-shaped appearance

4. **Cerebral aqueduct**—portion of cavity through the midbrain.

5. **Fourth ventricle**—space in the hindbrain

6. **Central canal** of the spinal cord

The Limbic System is made up of nuclei and tracts that are found around the diencephalon (thalamus, hypothalamus) and basal nuclei. The word limbic means border. The limbic system structures include the cingulate gyrus, located just above the corpus callosum, the mammillary bodies, and the parahippocampal gyrus and the uncus, on the medial surface of the temporal lobe; most other structures of this system (e.g., amygdala, and hippocampus) are deep. This system is closely related to olfactory function.

The limbic system is important in regulation of emotions such as pleasure, and, by way of communication with the hypothalamus, helps control the behavioral changes in the body (such as rapid heartbeat) related to emotion. The limbic system also communicates with the prefrontal cortex and therefore links intellectual and emotional functions such as feelings and perceptions. One part of the limbic system, the **hippocampus** (located deep in the medial part of the temporal lobe) is very important in the storage and retrieval of memory.

■ Student Activity

Because the **coronal section** is used in understanding many structures and functions of the brain, this activity is included to be sure you are learning to recognize all structures in this view. In the highly schematic illustration below, label each listed structure with the letter of its name. The first label is done for you. If you need help, refer to Figure 25–6 on page 168.

a. longitudinal fissure
b. lateral fissure
c. corpus callosum
d. 3rd ventricle
e. midbrain
f. cerebellum
g. 4th ventricle
h. cerebral aqueduct
i. septum pellucidum
j. thalamus
k spinal cord

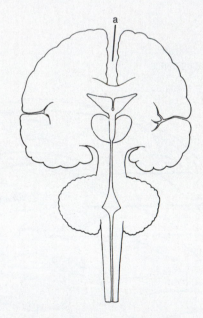

■ CLINICAL COMMENTS

Alzheimer's disease (AD) first develops in the hippocampus. Some researchers are beginning to use MRI (magnetic resonance imaging) to determine the amount of activity in the hippocampus as a way to diagnose AD.

Exercise Twenty-Five

Name _____

1. In the space below, sketch a lateral view of the brain and include the following: frontal, parietal, occipital, and temporal lobes; precentral and postcentral gyri; lateral fissure; cerebellum; pons; and medulla oblongata.

2. Label the following illustration.

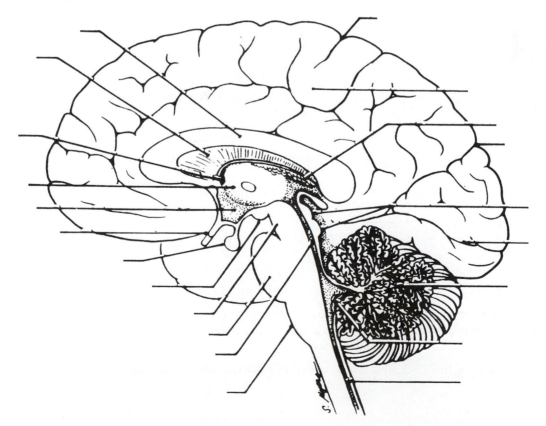

3. Matching exercise: Use each letter only once.

_____ 1. midbrain   a. commissural fibers

_____ 2. occipital lobe   b. crossing fibers

_____ 3. corpus callosum   c. hindbrain

_____ 4. nucleus   d. dorsal midbrain

_____ 5. optic chiasma   e. vagus n.

_____ 6. colliculi   f. trigeminal n.

_____ 7. medulla oblongata   g. cerebral aqueduct

_____ 8. CN V   h. groups of nerve cell bodies

_____ 9. arbor vita   i. cerebellum

_____10. CN X   j. caudal

4. In what view of the brain, lateral (L), medial (M), ventral (V), or dorsal (D), would you best see the following:

_____ 1. interpeduncular fossa   _____ 6. parieto-occipital sulcus

_____ 2. septum pellucidum   _____ 7. vermis

_____ 3. calcarine fissure   _____ 8. temporal lobe

_____ 4. paracentral lobule   _____ 9. lateral fissure

_____ 5. CN III   _____10. pyramid of medulla

5. Nerve cell bodies in the cerebrum are found either:
   a. in _____, or

   b. in the _____ _____

6. Name the *ventricle* that is described:

_____ a. It is found between halves of the thalamus.

_____ b. It develops from the central canal within the original
                            hindbrain enlargement.

_____ c. Bilateral structures within the cerebrum.

7. Using structures of the cerebrum, complete the following without looking in the text.

   Lobes   **Gyri**   **Fissures and Sulci**

   1. _____   1. _____   1. _____

   2. _____   2. _____   2. _____

   3. _____   3. _____

   4. _____   4. _____

8. In Figure 25–2, color the precentral gyrus pink and the postcentral gyrus blue.
   The precentral gyrus is part of the _____ lobe; the postcentral
   gyrus is part of the _____ lobe.

9. From information in Figure 25–3, find the definition of a nucleus and write it here:

Lesson 26

Meninges and Circulation of the Brain

The meninges are three layers of membranes covering the brain and spinal cord. Each has a special functional significance.

■ OBJECTIVES

1. Describe and identify the three layers of meninges.
2. State the relationship of the meningeal layers and the significance of each.
3. Identify the dural venous sinuses.
4. Describe the pattern and distribution of arteries supplying the brain.
5. Identify the major arteries on the brain.

■ METHODS

1. Complete the activities described as you study this lesson.
2. Observe demonstrations of meninges and arteries on human brains and/or models.
3. Find each meningeal layer, specified arteries, and dural venous sinuses on the brains and models available in the lab.
4. Use the human skulls to identify indentations caused by dural venous sinuses.

A. MENINGES OF THE BRAIN WILL BE DESCRIBED FROM DEEP TO SUPERFICIAL

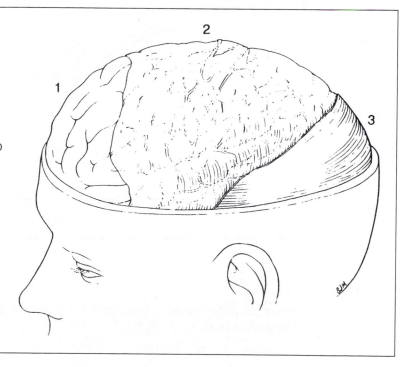

FIGURE 26–1
BRAIN WITH MENINGES

1. **Pia mater,** the innermost layer. This covering dips into all sulci and fissures of the brain and spinal cord. Grossly, it cannot be distinguished from nervous tissue.

2. **Arachnoid,** the middle layer. Named for its spider web-like, transparent appearance. It inserts only into the longitudinal and transverse fissures. (The transverse fissure separates cerebrum and cerebellum.)

3. **Dura mater,** the opaque outer covering, is a single layer around the spinal cord but is a double layer inside the skull.
   The outermost layer, the one against the skull, is called the **periosteal dura;** the innermost layer, the **meningeal dura,** lies just superficial to the arachnoid membrane.

FIGURE 26–2
SPECIALIZATIONS OF THE MENINGES

The enlarged illustration is of the coronal section of the skull and brain from the boxed area shown below.

1. **Pia mater**

2. **Subarachnoid space** with connective tissue strands from pia to arachnoid. CSF and blood vessels are found here.

3. **Arachnoid mater**—transparent cobweb-like membrane.

4. **Meningeal dura mater**—the layer of dura that is against the other meninges.

5. Subdural space, potential space (dark line).

6. **Periosteal dura mater**—adheres to the skull as the inner lining of the bone. This is the layer that will not exist around the spinal cord.

7. **Dura mater**—periosteal and meningeal layers are fused at this location.

8. **Superior sagittal sinus**—space between layers of meninges.

9. **Arachnoid granulations**—special villous extensions of arachnoid membrane that insert through dura mater into superior sagittal sinus. The CSF passes through these structures and returns to venous blood.

10. **Falx cerebri**—a double fold of meningeal dura inserted into the longitudinal fissure. It attaches to crista galli.

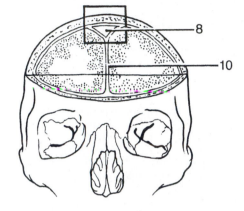

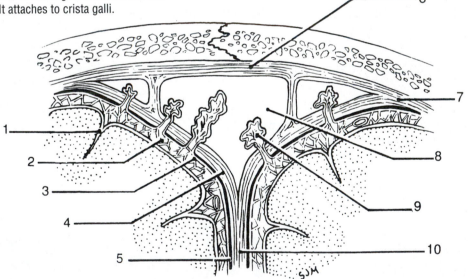

■ **Student Activities**

In Figure 26–2, color pia mater, green; subarachnoid space, yellow; arachnoid membrane, red; superior sagittal sinus, blue.

B. DURAL VENOUS SINUSES

These are spaces between two layers of dura mater into which the small veins of the brain return the used blood. These spaces occur where the meningeal layer separates from the periosteal layer as well as between two layers of meningeal dura.

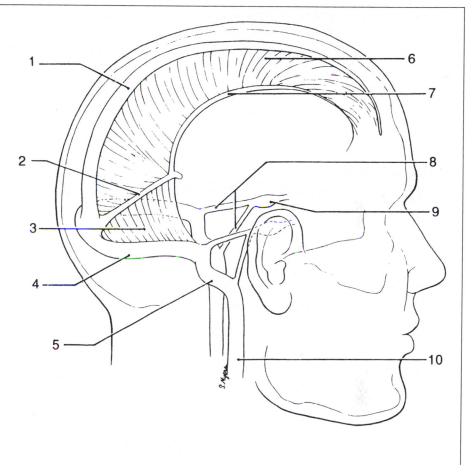

FIGURE 26–3
DURAL SPECIALIZATIONS
(POSTEROLATERAL VIEW)

1. **Superior sagittal sinus**

2. **Straight sinus** (rectus)—where falx cerebri and tentorium cerebelli meet.

3. **Tentorium cerebelli**—separates cerebrum from cerebellum.

4. **Transverse sinus**—in lateral boundary of tentorium cerebelli.

5. **Sigmoid sinus**—S-shaped

6. **Falx cerebri**—a double fold of meningeal dura that attaches to the crista galli and is inserted into the longitudinal fissure.

7. **Inferior sagittal sinus**—found in the free edge of falx cerebri.

8. **Superior and inferior petrosal sinuses**

9. **Cavernous sinus**—on margins of hypophyseal fossa.

10. **Internal jugular v.**—a direct continuation of sigmoid sinus; receives all blood from inside the skull.

■ Student Activities

In Figure 26–3, color the venous sinuses and the internal jugular vein blue. Color the other specializations of dura mater yellow.
    The direction of blood flow in the dural sinuses is toward the internal jugular vein. Draw small arrows to indicate the direction of flow from each of the sinuses.

■ CLINICAL COMMENTS

Subdural (between the dura and arachnoid) **hemorrhaging** can occur after a blow to the head that displaces the brain and ruptures a blood vessel. If not repaired, the buildup of blood, **hematoma,** can press against brain tissue and cause brain damage. Less frequently, bleeding will occur between the skull and dura and an epidural hematoma results.

Meningitis, an infection of the meninges of brain and spinal cord that can be caused by a variety of bacteria, viruses, or fungi, damages or kills nervous tissue in the infected areas. Initially, it causes headaches and stiff neck, but it can progress to high fevers and disorientation, and even result in death if untreated.

C. ARTERIES OF THE BRAIN

Two major pairs of arteries supply blood to the brain:

Vertebral arteries are branches of the subclavian arteries. They ascend through the transverse foramina of cervical vertebrae (Figure 31–6) and enter the skull via foramen magnum.

Internal carotid arteries are the posterior branches from the common carotid arteries (Figure 31–6). They enter the base of the skull through the carotid canal and, after passing through the canal, enter the cranial vault through foramen lacerum.

Circle of Willis is the name given to the pattern formed when the vertebral and internal carotid sources of blood join at the base of the brain, Figure 26–5. The arteries in this list are those arteries you should be able to identify on the base of the brain; the arteries marked with an asterisk are a part of the circle.

■ **Student Activities**

Using Figure 26–4, label and color the starred vessels red.

FIGURE 26–4
CIRCLE OF WILLIS

1. Anterior cerebral a.*

2. Anterior communicating a.*

3. Internal carotid a.*

4. Middle cerebral a.

5. Posterior communicating a.*

6. Posterior cerebral a.*

7. Superior cerebellar a.

8. Basilar a.

9. Vertebral a.

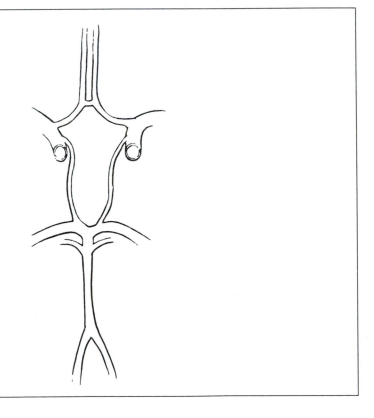

This anastomosis is very important to provide collateral blood supply to the brain. If specific cerebral arteries are occluded, however, blood still does not reach important areas and a stroke occurs. For clinical purposes it is important to know what areas are supplied by each vessel.

FIGURE 26–5
ARTERIES OF THE BRAIN

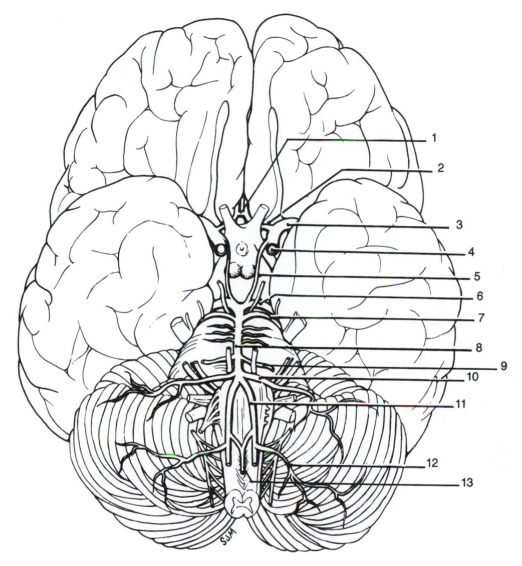

1. **Anterior communicating a.**—connects the right and left anterior cerebral arteries.

2. **Anterior cerebral a.**—a terminal branch of internal carotid a.; enters longitudinal fissure.

3. **Middle cerebral a.**—a terminal branch of the internal carotid a.; passes between the temporal and frontal lobes to reach the lateral brain.

4. **Internal carotid a.**—Lumen of the cut vessel.

5. **Posterior communicating a.**—between the internal carotid and the posterior cerebral a.

6. **Posterior cerebral a.**—bifurcation of basilar a.; end of vertebral contribution of blood.

7. **Superior cerebellar a.**—named for its position on the cerebellum.

8. **Basilar a.**—lies on the pons. Pontine branches supply pons.

9. **Labyrinthine a.** (internal auditory)—enters internal auditory meatus.

10. **Anterior inferior cerebellar a.**

11. **Vertebral a.**—enters skull by way of foramen magnum and lies on medulla oblongata.

12. **Posterior inferior cerebellar a.**

13. **Anterior spinal a.**

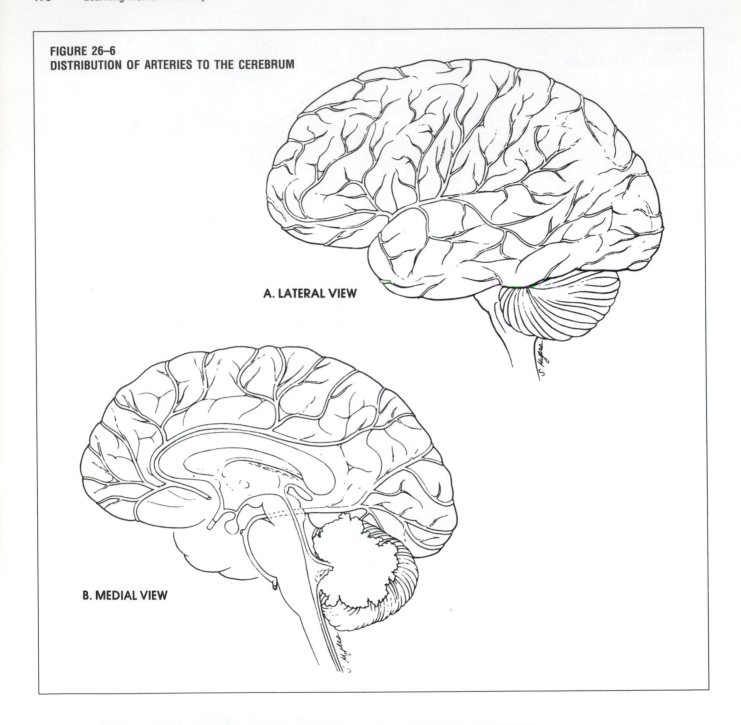

FIGURE 26–6
DISTRIBUTION OF ARTERIES TO THE CEREBRUM

A. LATERAL VIEW

B. MEDIAL VIEW

■ **Student Activities**

1. Label each of the three cerebral arteries.
   a. **Middle cerebral a.** emerges from between the frontal and temporal lobes. It distributes blood to most of the lateral brain. Color it red.
   b. **Anterior cerebral a.** is found in the longitudinal fissure. Its branches supply most of the medial view of the brain and end just over the top of each hemisphere. Color it pink.
   c. **Posterior cerebral a.** is a terminal branch of the basilar a. It is distributed to the occipital lobe. Color it red.
2. Label the basilar a. It is easy to find because it always lies on the _____.

Exercise Twenty-Six

Name _____

1. On a separate paper, draw the major blood vessels of the brain until you can do so without looking at any illustration. Label all vessels.

2. Answer the following:

    a. The blood supply to the temporal lobe is largely from the _____ artery.

    b. Blood to the occipital lobe is mainly from the _____ artery.

    c. The paracentral lobule is largely supplied by the _____ artery.

3. Arteries that supply the cerebrum are from two sources. List the four arteries from the internal carotid source on the left, and the one from the vertebral source on the right.

Internal Carotid Source   **Vertebral Source**

a. _____   c. _____   e. _____

b. _____   d. _____

4. On the base of the brain illustrated below, draw the major arteries. Be sure you have them in the correct position. Label the arteries.

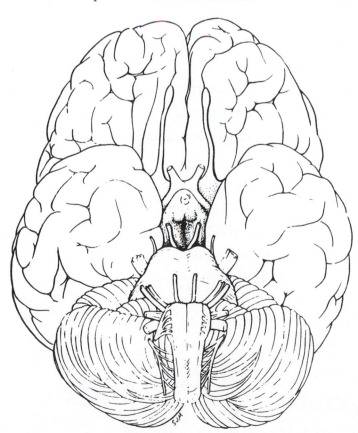

5. On the coronal section of the brain, brain stem and spinal cord illustrated below, draw the meninges using the following color code: pia mater = green; arachnoid = red; dura = blue; with yellow, color all space where CSF is found. (Refer to Figure 26–1 if you need help. Remember that the arachnoid membrane has space deep to it.)

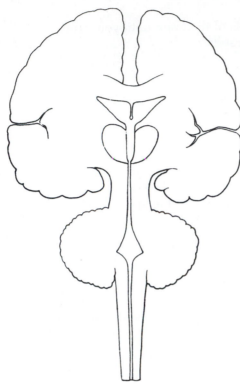

6. Matching exercises: Use each letter only once.

_____ 1. choroid plexus	a. CSF resorption
_____ 2. dura mater	b. venous blood
_____ 3. tentorium cerebelli	c. location of choroid plexus
_____ 4. arachnoid granulations	d. falx cerebri
_____ 5. subarachnoid space	e. arterial blood
_____ 6. superior sagittal sinus	f. CSF production
_____ 7. lateral ventricle	g. CSF circulation
_____ 8. circle of Willis	h. straight sinus

Functions of the Cerebrum

This lesson includes no new gross structures. It is included to reinforce an understanding of each structure by including some function.

■ OBJECTIVES

1. Identify lobes and gyri according to Brodmann numbers.
2. Describe the functions of specific brain areas.
3. Define the term *homunculus;* identify general regions for specific body parts on the brain.
4. Associate brain function and the homunculus with the blood supply.

■ METHODS

1. Complete the suggested activities as you study this exercise.
2. Identify the specified Brodmann areas on a brain in the lab.

A. CONTRALATERAL BRAIN FUNCTION

The left hemisphere controls most of the motor function of the right side of the body and receives most of the sensory information from the right side of the body. The right side of the brain controls the left side of the body and receives left-side information.

The **dominant** hemisphere, the left in right-handed people, is more involved in complex communication and calculation. The right hemisphere is more important in spatial orientation. Because of the complexity of the brain, it is important that areas within hemispheres communicate and that the hemispheres communicate with each other.

1. **Commissural fibers**—nerve cell processes by which hemispheres communicate.
   Example: corpus callosum
2. **Association fibers**—communicate within a hemisphere.
3. **Projection fibers**—communicate from cortex to other parts of the CNS.
   Example: tracts, discussed in Lesson 28.

B. BRODMANN NUMBERS

These were assigned to many functional areas of the brain early in the 20th century.
A few of the major areas are included here.

FIGURE 27–1
BRODMANN'S CYTOARCHITECTURAL MAP OF THE HUMAN CORTEX

Illustrations are simplified.

    Key to the map: begin at the central sulcus and progress clockwise.

3,1,2, postcentral gyrus and its continuation onto the paracentral lobule. This is the primary sensory area and receives general sensory information from all over the body. General sensory information includes: pressure, vibration, spacial orientation of body parts, touch, appreciation of texture, two-point discrimination, localization of pain and temperature.

17, area immediately surrounding the calcarine sulcus. It is the primary visual reception area where visual stimuli are received.

18, secondary visual area, surrounds 17 and helps associate visual impulses with prior experience.

41, posterior and inferior to the lateral fissure. It is the primary auditory cortex where auditory stimulation is received.

42, surrounds 41 and is the secondary auditory cortex.

44, 45 motor speech area, dominant hemisphere only.

9,10,11, the prefrontal cortex. It is the center for personality and character traits.

4, the precentral gyrus. It is the primary motor area and is responsible for fine motor control.

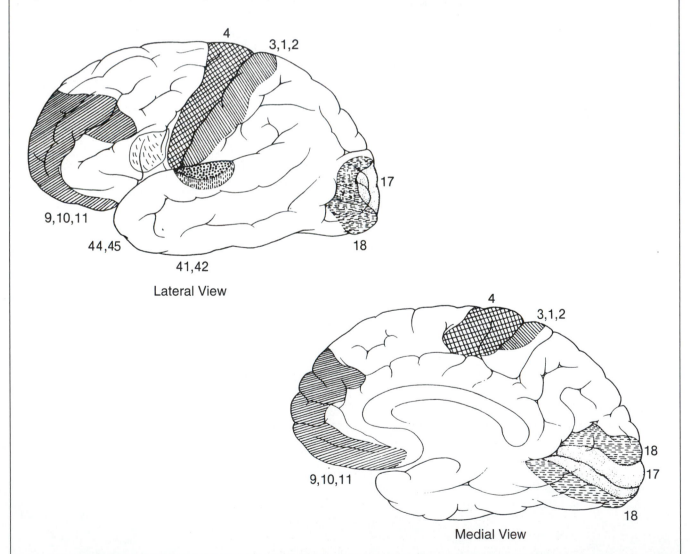

Lateral View

Medial View

C. HOMUNCULI

Much of the general sensory information and primary motor control is organized on the precentral and postcentral gyri and paracentral lobule according to specific body parts. For instance, the cell bodies that receive general sensory information from the right foot will be found in the paracentral lobule of the left cerebral hemisphere.

A *homunculus* (little man) is drawn when illustrations of body parts are placed on the cortex where that body part is represented. Figure 27-2 is a coronal section of the brain cut through the postcentral gyrus; therefore, the sensory homunculus is what you see. (If the section were through the precentral gyrus, it would be a motor homunculus, illustrated in Exercise 27.)

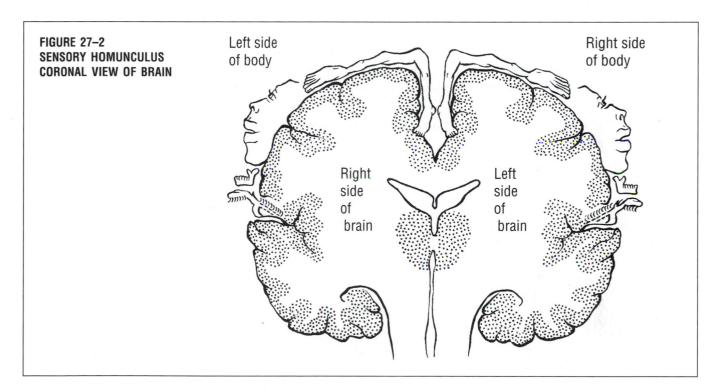

FIGURE 27–2
SENSORY HOMUNCULUS
CORONAL VIEW OF BRAIN

Left side of body

Right side of body

Right side of brain

Left side of brain

■ **Student Activities**

1. Referring to Figure 27–2, what part (lobe or gyrus) of the brain is receiving the sensory information from the foot? _____ From the hand? _____

2. What Brodmann area is represented by the homunculus in Figure 27-2? _____

3. Use a yellow pencil to color the position of CSF.

4. In Figure 27–1, use pink to color Brodmann area 3,1,2; use light green to color Brodmann area 4; use different colors to color the other Brodmann areas.

   With the same pink pencil, color Brodmann area 3,1,2 in Figure 27–3; it is the postcentral gyrus in the illustration on the upper right and the cerebral cortex of parietal lobe in the illustration on the upper left.

   With the same green pencil, color the Brodmann area 4 in Figure 27–3; it is the precentral gyrus in the brain on the lower right and the cerebral cortex of the frontal lobe in the brain on the left. (Don't forget to color the small portions of 3,1,2 and 4 in the paracentral lobule of the brain in the center and right and in both homunculi.)

1. Combining information from Figures 26–5, 27–1, and 27–3, answer the following:
   a. If the posterior cerebral artery is lost, what sensation might be affected? _____

   b. If the right middle cerebral artery is lost, what part of the body would lose sensations? _____ Motor control? _____
   c. If the left anterior cerebral artery is lost, what part of the body would be affected?
   d. In Figure 27–3, why would the hand occupy a larger area of the cortex than the entire trunk? _____

2. In Figure 27–3, put an X on the cells that will be stimulated when you step on a rock. Notice that you need to look at the medial view of the brain to see the label for foot. What is the name of the brain structure there? _____

3. In Figure 27-3, put an O on cells that are active as you write this answer. What brain part did you mark? _____

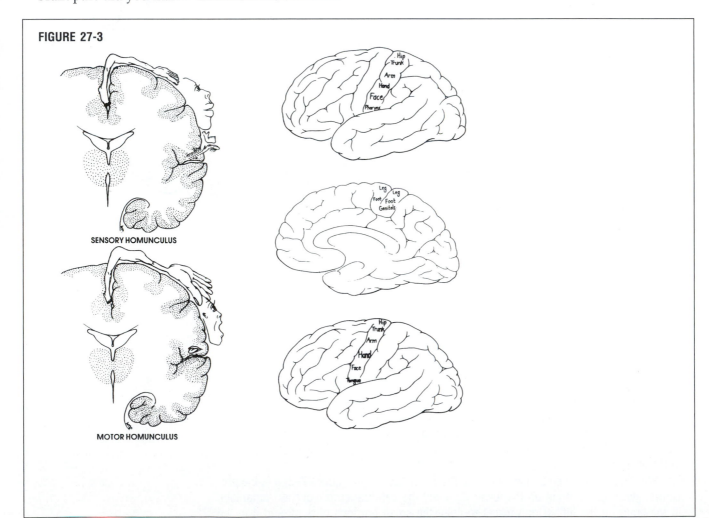

FIGURE 27-3

SENSORY HOMUNCULUS

MOTOR HOMUNCULUS

Lesson 28

Spinal Cord and Tracts

To understand how the brain communicates with the periphery we must look at the other component of the CNS, the spinal cord. Cranial nerves emerge directly from the brain; spinal nerves communicate with the brain by way of the spinal cord.

■ OBJECTIVES

1. Identify the structures in a transverse section of spinal cord.
2. Describe the meninges of the spinal cord.
3. Identify the position of the major afferent and efferent tracts.
4. State the name and function of selected afferent and efferent tracts.

■ METHODS

1. Perform the suggested activities as you study this exercise.
2. Observe the spinal cords available in the lab.

A. THE SPINAL CORD

The relationships of structures in the caudal end of the original neural tube change very little as the spinal cord develops. The gray matter, nerve cell bodies, remain in the center; white matter, nerve cell processes, are organized as bundles called *tracts* or *fasiculi.* These surround the gray matter (Figure 8–5).

At birth the spinal cord extends from foramen magnum to vertebra L3. The vertebral column grows faster than the cord, so in the adult the cord ends at the lower part of the first lumbar vertebra.

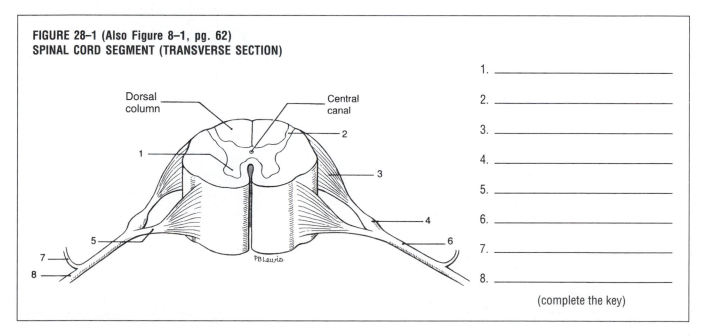

FIGURE 28–1 (Also Figure 8–1, pg. 62)
SPINAL CORD SEGMENT (TRANSVERSE SECTION)

Dorsal column

Central canal

PB Lewis

1. _____
2. _____
3. _____
4. _____
5. _____
6. _____
7. _____
8. _____

(complete the key)

185

FIGURE 28–2
SPINAL CORD (POSTERIOR VIEW, WITH POSTERIOR SACRUM CUT)

1. **Cervical enlargement,** for nerves of the brachial plexus.

2. **Dorsal median sulcus;** dorsal lateral sulci are seen on each side.

3. **Dura mater,** a single layer around the cord. It is shown cut open and lined with arachnoid. These two meningeal layers terminate at the second sacral vertebra.

4. **Lumbar enlargement,** for nerves of lumbosacral plexus.

5. Lamina of first lumbar vertebra.

6. **Conus medullaris**—the termination of the cord.

7. **Filum terminale**—a fibrous strand that extends from conus medullaris to S2. Distal to S2 it becomes a part of the coccygeal ligament, a ligament that helps anchor the spinal cord to the coccyx.

8. **Cauda equina**—the bundle of nerves that pass through the canal until they reach their foramina of exit.

9. Termination of dura and arachnoid at level of S2.

■ CLINICAL COMMENTS

In a **spinal tap** cerebrospinal fluid is withdrawn from the subarachnoid space by inserting a needle between vertebrae L3 and L4. The CSF is withdrawn when symptoms such as severe headaches or back pain indicate that there may be an infection in the CNS. By examining the fluid for bacteria, viruses, metabolic waste, or cell debris, the cause of the infection can often be diagnosed.

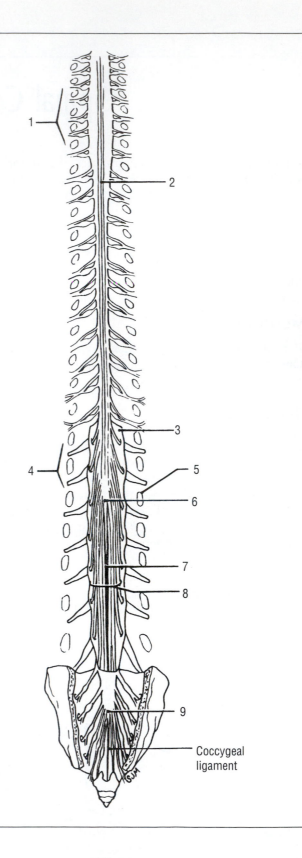

Coccygeal ligament

FIGURE 28–3
MENINGES OF SPINAL CORD

1. **Pia mater**—corresponds to pia on the brain. It adheres directly to the nervous tissue and blends with the spinal and cranial nerve sheaths. *Color it green.*

2. **Arachnoid mater**—separated from the pia by subarachnoid space in which CSF is found. *Color it red.*

3. **Dura mater**—directly continuous with the meningeal dura of the brain. It is separated from the arachnoid by the subdural (potential) space, and it is continuous with the membranous coverings of the nerves. *Color it blue. Complete the key.*

4. _____

5. _____

6. _____

7. _____

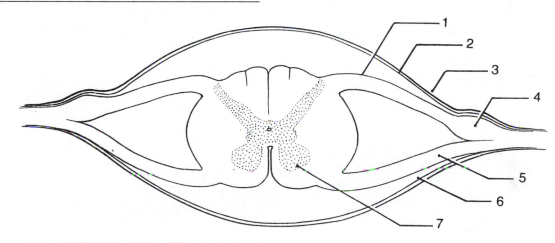

B. SPINAL NERVES

These were introduced in Figure 8–1 and included, in part, with the lumbosacral and brachial plexuses. There are 31 pairs of these nerves:

Cervical = 8 pairs	C1 emerges between occipital bone and atlas.
	C2–7 emerge from intervertebral foramina above the vertebra for which it is named.
	C8 emerges between vertebrae C7 and T1
Thoracic = 12 pairs	Emerge from intervertebral foramina below the thoracic vertebra for which they are named.
Lumbar = 5 pairs	Named for vertebra above the nerve.
Sacral = 5 pairs	Named for vertebra above the nerve.
Coccygeal = 1 pair	

C. TRACTS OF THE SPINAL CORD

Ascending pathways, sensory tracts, and descending pathways, motor tracts, occupy most of the white matter of the spinal cord. In this introductory course we will only describe a few of these tracts. Look at the simplified cross section (Figure 28–4). On the right, sensory tracts are labeled and indicated with shading; on the left, motor tracts are labeled and indicated with shading.

> ■ **Student Activities**
>
> Color the labeled sensory tracts blue on both right and left sides of the cord; color motor tracts red on both sides of the cord.

FIGURE 28–4
TRACTS OF THE SPINAL CORD

1. Lateral corticospinal tract

2. Fasciculus gracilis

3. Fasciculus cuneatus

4. Dorsal spinocerebellar tract

5. Lateral spinothalamic tract

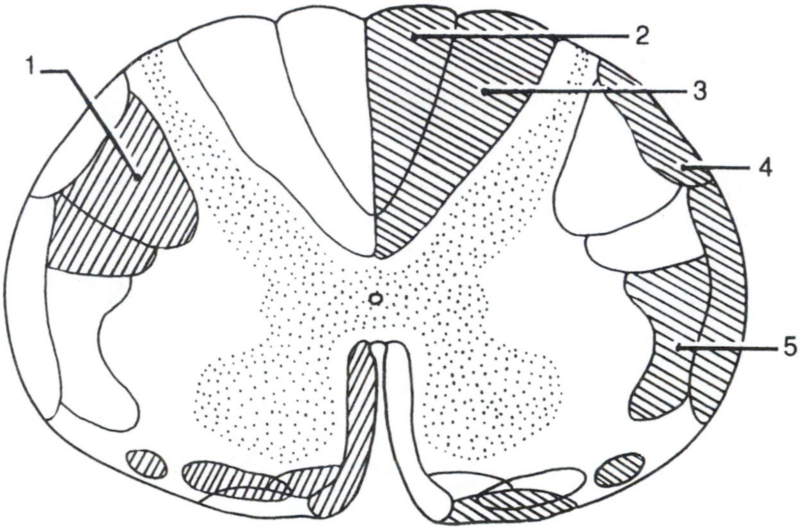

There are three things to know about each tract, both sensory and motor.

1. Its name.
2. Where it crosses over (recall the contralateral brain).
3. What type of information it carries.

1. SENSORY TRACTS

These ascending pathways bring sensations from the periphery to the brain (or brainstem). The type of information being carried by the tract determines its destination. Most sensory tracts require three neurons to get the information from the periphery to its location on the brain. There are some generalizations concerning these three neurons that will help you:

a. The cell body of the primary neuron, $1°$, is always in the dorsal root ganglion.
b. The secondary neuron, $2°$, will be the one that crosses over.
c. If present, the cell body of the tertiary neuron, $3°$, will always be in the thalamus.

The **dorsal column system** consists of two tracts that occupy the dorsal columns of the cord (Figure 28–5). These carry *general sensory information* (except pain and temperature) from the body to the **postcentral gyrus.**

FIGURE 28–5
DORSAL COLUMN SYSTEM

In this schematic representation, the spinal cord and medulla are shown in cross section, and the brain and brainstem are coronal sections. To simplify, each tract was drawn on one side only.

1. **Fasciculus gracilis** carries general sensory information from the lower limb and the lower half of the trunk. *Color it green.*

2. **Fasciculus cuneatus** carries general sensory information from the upper trunk and the upper limbs. *Color it yellow.*

   Compare the site of termination of these tracts with the body parts on the homunculus.

   Number, with 1°, 2°, or 3°, the cell body of each of the three neurons as it brings sensory information in from the periphery.

   1°, in dorsal root ganglion with a process synapsing in the nucleus underlying either the gracile or the cuneate tubercle.

   2°, its process is crossing in the brainstem.

   3°, with the cell body in the thalamus and the process taking information to the appropriate area of the cortex.

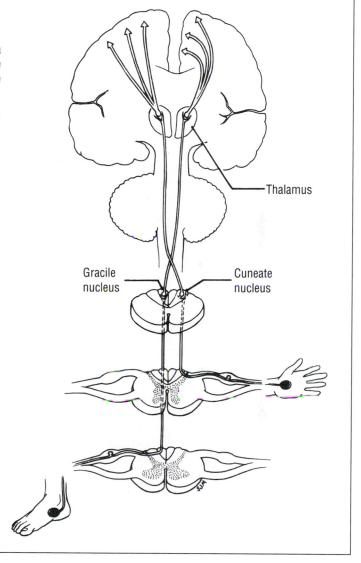

Thalamus

Gracile nucleus

Cuneate nucleus

■ **CLINICAL COMMENTS**

A **stroke,** or cerebrovascular accident **(CVA),** results in loss of blood to an area of the brain due to a blood clot or hemorrhage of a vessel. This ischemia results in damaged nerve cells, and the position of the injured vessel can often be determined by the symptoms of the patient. The middle cerebral artery is the vessel most frequently affected. If the CVA involves the right middle cerebral artery, symptoms might include motor and sensory deficits of the left upper limb.

The **lateral spinothalamic tract** is another sensory tract. It carries *pain and temperature* to the cortex so that it can be localized.

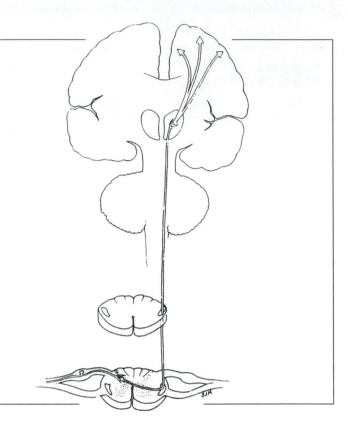

FIGURE 28–6
LATERAL SPINOTHALAMIC TRACT

Schematic representation shows information from the right side of the body arriving on the left side of the brain on the cortex of the postcentral gyrus.

Number the cell bodies of the three neurons involved.

1°, as with all sensory information, the cell body is in the dorsal root ganglion. *Color it blue.*

2°, the body in the dorsal horn has its process crossing over within one or two spinal cord segments. The process travels to the thalamus where the noxious element of pain is realized but not localized. *Color it yellow.*

3°, body in the thalamus, process going on to the cerebral cortex where the origin of the pain and temperature is localized. *Color it pink.*

The **dorsal spinocerebellar tract** is the last sensory tract we will discuss. It differs from the others in several ways. It does not reach the conscious level, it has only two neurons, and it does not cross over. This tract is necessary because *position sense* (proprioception) must arrive in the cerebellum to facilitate coordination of motor activity.

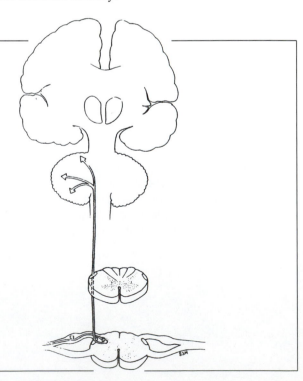

FIGURE 28–7
DORSAL SPINOCEREBELLAR TRACT

1°, sensory information comes from muscles in the periphery via dorsal root ganglion.
2°, travels on the same side to the termination of the tract on the cerebellar cortex.

2. MOTOR TRACTS (EFFERENT PATHWAYS)

Motor tracts are composed of fibers that leave the brain to go out to the periphery. These are often called **pyramidal tracts** if they originate in the cortex, and **extrapyramidal** if they originate in other structures such as nuclei. In our introductory study we will look at only one, a pyramidal tract. Motor pathways will not have a three-neuron path.

The **lateral corticospinal tract** originates in the cortex in Brodmann area 4. The cells of origin look like pyramids; they are referred to as **upper motor neurons** (UMN) because they originate in the brain. The UMN processes (axons) travel together to form this tract. The processes synapse on neurons in the gray matter of the cord. The cells that have their bodies in the cord and their processes in peripheral nerves are called **lower motor neurons** (LMN).

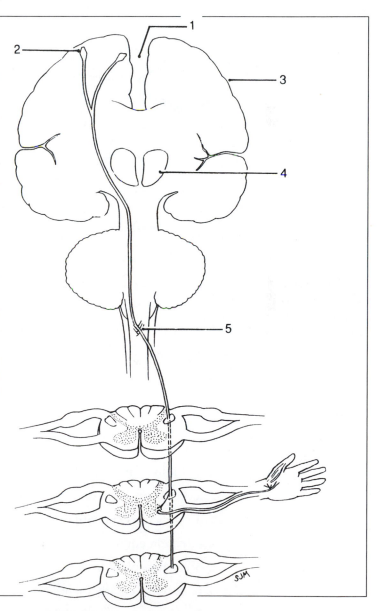

FIGURE 28–8
LATERAL CORTICOSPINAL TRACT

The tract passes through the cerebral peduncles and then the pyramids of the medulla. It carries fine motor control.

1. _____

2. **Pyramidal cells** (of Betz)

3. Cortex of precentral gyrus

4. _____

5. **Pyramidal decussation**—the crossing over of fibers in the tract. *Remember: opposite side control*

■ CLINICAL COMMENTS

When the upper motor neuron (either the body in cerebral cortex or the process in brainstem and spinal cord) is interrupted, there is no brain control of muscles and **spastic paralysis** may occur. The reflex arc through the spinal cord (LMN) is still intact to maintain tonus in the muscles.

If the lower motor neuron (either the cell body the in cord or process in peripheral nerve) is interrupted, **flaccid paralysis** occurs. No nerve impulse reaches the muscle and the muscle will atrophy.

■ Student Activities

Label the upper motor neuron with UMN and color it green; label the lower motor neuron with LMN and color it yellow. Complete the key.

Exercise Twenty-Eight

Name _____

1. On the spinal cord below:

   a. Using the following colors, color the meninges: green = pia mater; red = arachnoid; blue = dura mater.
   b. With yellow, draw in some motor cell bodies; with brown, draw in some sensory cell bodies.
   c. Fill in the key.

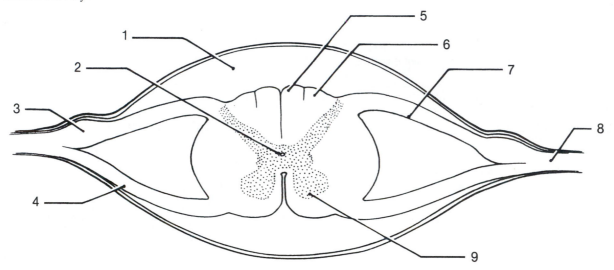

1. _____   6. _____

2. _____   7. _____

3. _____   8. _____

4. _____   9. _____

5. _____

2. Matching exercise: Use each letter only once.

   _____ 1. filum terminale   a. brachial plexus area

   _____ 2. conus medullaris   b. fine motor control

   _____ 3. fasciculus cuneatus   c. meninges

   _____ 4. cauda equina   d. below conscious level

   _____ 5. corticospinal tract   e. end of spinal cord

   _____ 6. cervical enlargement   f. lower motor neurons

   _____ 7. dorsal spinocerebellar   g. sensory tract for hand

   _____ 8. anterior horn   h. bundle of spinal
                                                    nerves

3. In the illustration on the right:

   a. Name the tract that is pictured:

   _____

   It is carrying the sense of:

   _____

   b. Draw in red the tract bringing the sense of touch from the right thumb. It is called the:

   _____

   c. Draw in blue the tract bringing in the sense of pressure from the left foot. It is called the:

   _____

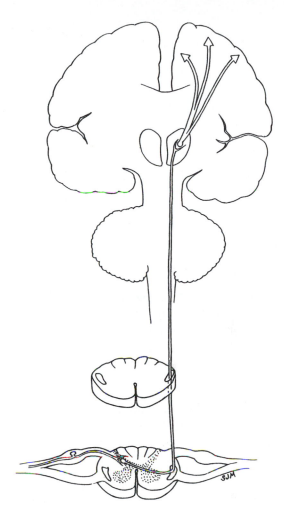

4. Answer the following questions.

   a. If your patient lost his corticospinal tract in the right cerebral peduncle, his motor deficit would be seen where?

   _____

   b. If your patient was shot in the spinal cord at the level of T_{11} and the bullet injured his dorsal column white matter on the left side, what deficits might you expect to see? Be sure to include which side is affected.

   _____

■ **CLINICAL COMMENTS**

Polio is a disease in which the cell bodies of motor neurons in the anterior horn are destroyed by a virus. Muscles innervated by these neurons will become paralyzed and eventually atrophy. If the motor cells in the medulla are affected, the patient may die of respiratory failure or cardiac arrest. The Salk and Sabin vaccines have almost eliminated this disease.

5. What kind of paralysis would a polio victim have, spastic or flaccid?

   _____

Cranial Nerves

The cranial nerves (CN) have already been identified on the brain, and the foramina through which the nerves are transmitted have been identified on the skull. This exercise is to help you understand the significance of the anatomical relationships and the association of the nerves with other anatomical structures.

■ OBJECTIVES

1. For each cranial nerve, be able to describe:
   a. Its position on the brain; other brain structures involved in its function.
   b. The foramen (or foramina) through which it passes.
2. State the function (motor, sensory, or both) of each cranial n.
3. Describe the distribution of each cranial n.

■ METHODS

1. Complete the activities suggested as you study this text.
2. Use the brains and/or models in the lab to identify each nerve.

CRANIAL NERVES

Cranial nerves provide for the head the same functions spinal nerves provide for the rest of the body. They bring general sensations to the cortex and send motor impulses to skeletal muscle. However, cranial nerves also do much more; they have special functions related to viscera and to the organs of special sense.

In some texts you will read that there is no such thing as a purely motor nerve. This is because there must be a sensory fiber for the tonus reflex within all motor nerves. If the only sensory fiber in a cranial nerve is the reflex component, we will consider it motor only. With that in mind, as you study the exercise, *complete the chart on the following page by listing the 12 pairs of cranial nerves based on their functional components.*

■ **Student Activities**

As you study this lesson, list each of the 12 pairs of cranial nerves in the appropriate column.

Sensory	Motor	Mixed
_____	_____	_____
_____	_____	_____
_____	_____	_____
	_____	
	_____	

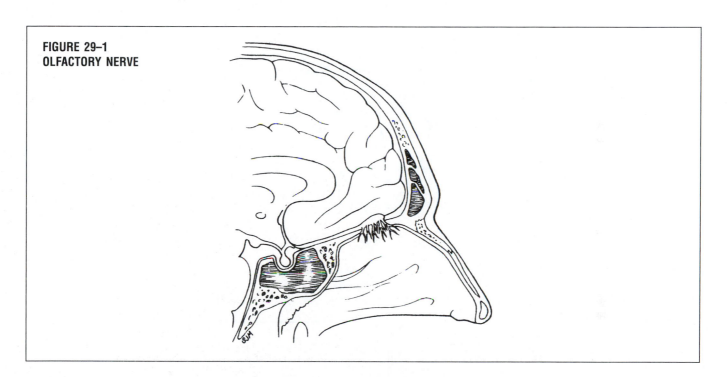

FIGURE 29–1
OLFACTORY NERVE

1. **CN I—olfactory nerve** (Figure 29–1)
   a. Olfactory cell bodies in the tissue lining the upper part of the nasal cavity are stimulated by gasses. Impulses travel on processes that enter the skull via the cribriform plate.
   b. Cells in the olfactory bulb receive the impulses, and the tract carries them to the primary olfactory cortex in the medial part of the temporal lobe. This is the only sensation that is not relayed through the thalamus.
   c. **Sensory only,** for the **special sense** of smell.

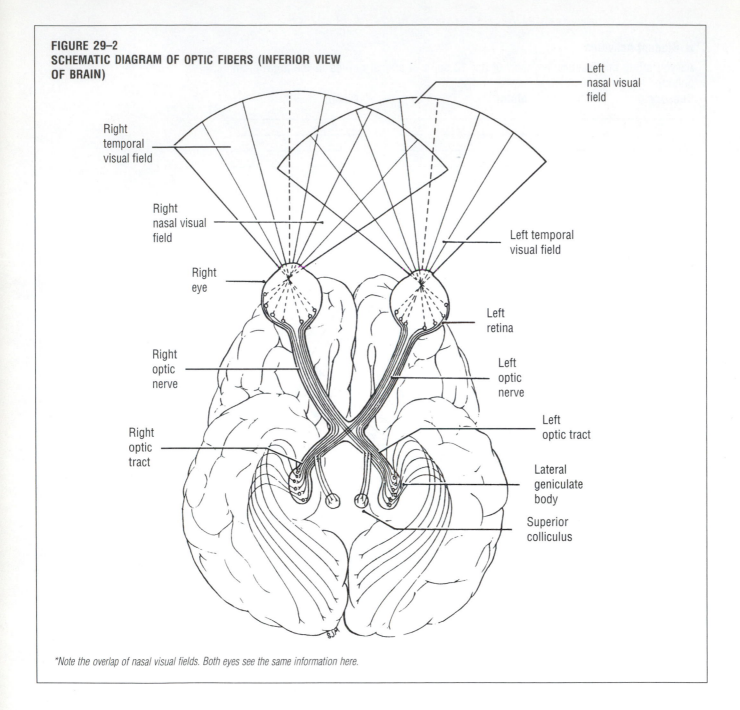

FIGURE 29–2
SCHEMATIC DIAGRAM OF OPTIC FIBERS (INFERIOR VIEW OF BRAIN)

Left nasal visual field

Right temporal visual field

Right nasal visual field

Left temporal visual field

Right eye

Left retina

Right optic nerve

Left optic nerve

Right optic tract

Left optic tract

Lateral geniculate body

Superior colliculus

Note the overlap of nasal visual fields. Both eyes see the same information here.

2. **CN II—optic nerve** (Figure 29–2)
   a. Cell bodies in the retina of the eye are stimulated by light. The processes of these cells form the optic n. It carries the impulses through the optic foramen.
   b. Fibers carrying light impulses from the periphery (temporal visual fields) cross over in the optic chiasma. This means the right optic tract carries the information coming from the left half of the visual fields of both eyes; thus left-side information goes to the right side of the brain. Right-side information goes to the left brain.

   The tracts synapse in the thalamic nuclei called the **lateral geniculate bodies.** Optic fibers then pass to the occipital cortex (area 17) for sight.

   Visual information is also relayed to the superior colliculus for reflex control of pupil and lens.
   c. **Sensory only,** carries the special sense of sight.

■ **Student Activities**

As you study the pathway of the optic fibers (see Figure 29–2), color (yellow) the temporal visual field of the right eye and the nasal visual field of the left eye. With the same color, color the portion of the retina where this visual stimulation would initiate the nerve impulse. Still using yellow, color the fibers onto the left cerebral hemisphere. You should have colored the fibers of the left optic tract.

■ CLINICAL COMMENTS

The temporal visual field is seen on the nasal retina. Because this is the information that crosses in the chiasma, a **pituitary tumor** or other obstruction of the chiasma would cause deficits of peripheral vision.

3. **CN III—oculomotor nerve** (see eye muscles, Lesson 30)
   a. Emerging from the interpeduncular fossa on the midbrain, this nerve leaves the skull by way of the superior orbital fissure.
   b. Composed of efferent fibers, it innervates most of the muscles of the eye.
   c. **Motor only,** to muscles of the eye (see page 205 for details). Contains parasympathetic fibers for smooth muscles.

4. **CN IV—trochlear nerve**
   a. Only nerve to emerge from the dorsal brainstem; it then wraps around the midbrain to enter the orbit by way of the superior orbital fissure.
   b. Motor fibers enter the superior oblique muscle.
   c. **Motor only,** to one muscle, the superior oblique (Lesson 30).

**FIGURE 29–3
TRIGEMINAL NERVE**

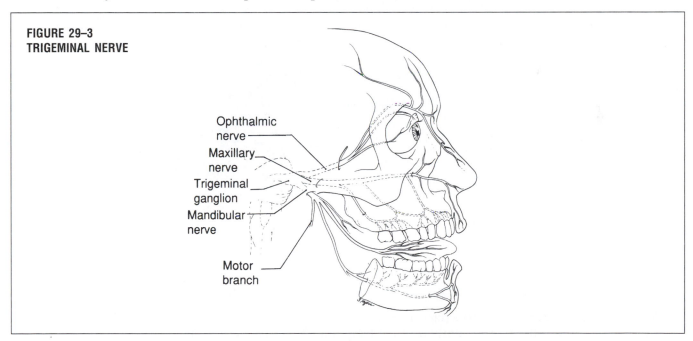

Ophthalmic nerve

Maxillary nerve

Trigeminal ganglion

Mandibular nerve

Motor branch

5. **CN V—trigeminal nerve** (Figure 29–3)
   a. Found on the side of the pons, it has three divisions.
   b. **CN V$_1$ or ophthalmic n.** enters the skull through the superior orbital fissure. It is **purely sensory,** bringing general sensory information from the upper face and eye region.
      CN V$_2$ or maxillary n. enters the skull through foramen rotundum. It is **purely sensory** to the face around the nose and from all the upper teeth.
      CN V$_3$ or mandibular n. is transmitted through foramen ovale. It is **both motor** (muscles of mastication) and **sensory,** bringing general sensations from the lower face, the tongue, and all the lower teeth.
   c. **Mixed nerve,** sensory to face; motor to muscles of mastication (Lesson 31).

6. **CN VI—abducens nerve**
   a. Emerges between pons and medulla on ventral brainstem.
   b. Leaves skull via the superior orbital fissure to enter the orbit and innervate only the lateral rectus muscle, which **abducts** the eye (Lesson 30).
   c. **Motor only.**

7. **CN VII—facial nerve**
   a. Emerges between pons and medulla lateral to abducens and is transmitted through the internal acoustic meatus. The component that is motor to muscles of facial expression continues through the temporal bone to emerge from the stylomastoid foramen onto the face.
   b. Sensory neurons with receptors in the taste buds of the anterior 2/3 of the tongue join the motor division in the petrous portion of the temporal bone.
   c. **A mixed nerve,** it is motor to muscles of facial expression and carries the special sense of taste from the anterior 2/3 of the tongue. Contains parasympathetic fibers.

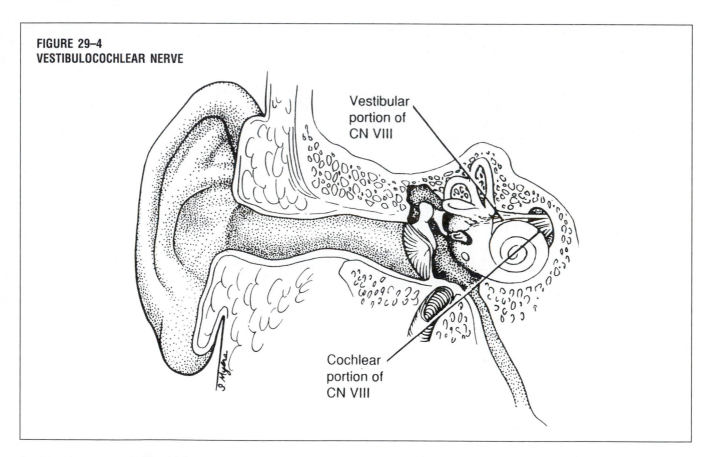

FIGURE 29–4
VESTIBULOCOCHLEAR NERVE

Vestibular portion of CN VIII

Cochlear portion of CN VIII

8. **CN VIII—vestibulocochlear nerve** (Figure 29–4)
   a. Originates within the petrous portion of the temporal bone. The *semicircular canals* stimulate cells of the vestibular portion of CN VIII for *equilibrium.*
      Cells in the *cochlea* are stimulated by sound waves and form the cochlear portion for *hearing.* This nerve passes through the internal acoustic meatus to enter the cranial vault.
   b. The impulses for hearing are relayed through the medial geniculate body of the thalamus and the inferior colliculus. The temporal lobe, area 41, receives the stimulus.
   c. **Sensory only, special senses** of hearing and equilibrium.

**FIGURE 29–5
TONGUE**

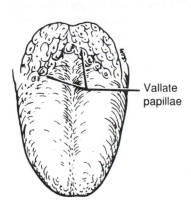

Vallate
papillae

9. **CN IX—glossopharyngeal nerve**
   a. Receptors, located in taste buds of the posterior 1/3 of the tongue, the portion behind the vallate papillae, initiate the **special sense of taste;** receptors for **general sensations** are also located in the posterior 1/3 of the tongue. This information enters the skull via the jugular foramen to go to the side of the medulla just inferior to CN VIII.
   b. Also traveling in CN IX are motor fibers that exit via jugular foramen to innervate one pharyngeal muscle.
   c. A **mixed nerve,** the motor fibers are to the pharynx. **General sensations** and the **special sense of taste** from the posterior 1/3 of the tongue are carried by this nerve. Contains parasympathetic fibers.

**FIGURE 29–6
VAGUS NERVE**

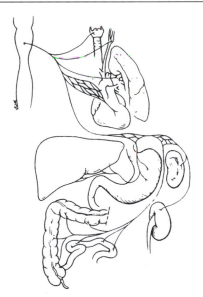

10. **CN X—vagus nerve** (Figure 29–6)
    a. On the lateral medulla below CN IX, this nerve is transmitted through the jugular foramen.
    b. With the widest distribution of any cranial nerve, Lesson 32, it innervates smooth muscle of the neck, thorax, and abdomen. It also carries general sensory information from all these areas. Because of its importance in the thorax and abdomen, it will be discussed in more detail in Unit IV.
    c. A **mixed nerve,** most widespread of all cranial nerves. Contains parasympathetic fibers.

11. **CN XI—accessory nerve**
   a. From many rootlets on the side of the medulla and the spinal cord. The spinal cord rootlets enter the skull via foramen magnum and join the medullary rootlets to form CN IX. It exits the skull via the jugular foramen.
   b. The cranial portion innervates muscles of the larynx and pharynx, and the spinal portion innervates sternocleidomastoid and trapezius muscles (Lessons 18 and 31).
   c. **Motor only.**

12. **CN XII—hypoglossal nerve**
   a. Rootlets emerge from the medulla, between the pyramids and the olive. It exits the skull via the hypoglossal canal to travel to the tongue.
   b. Innervates all tongue muscles, both intrinsic and extrinsic (Lesson 31).
   c. **Motor only,** to tongue.

Note: Cranial nerves that are sensory have ganglia within the skull. They are equivalent to the dorsal root ganglia of spinal nerves.

Exercise Twenty-Nine

Name _____

1. In Figure 29–1, label the following: frontal sinus, nasal bone, inferior nasal concha, sphenoid sinus, olfactory bulb.

2. The illustration on the right shows the cutaneous distribution of nerves to the face. The nerves that fit the letters are:

   a. _____

   b. _____

   c. _____

   Color each region a different color.

3. In Figures 29–1, 29–3, and 29–4 color each nerve yellow.

■ CLINICAL COMMENTS

In **Bell's palsy** the muscles of one side of the face are paralyzed and taste is lost from the anterior 2/3 of the tongue. Apparently a virus causes this condition and, after a few weeks, it usually heals itself.

4. What cranial nerve is affected by this virus? _____

5. On the illustration below:
   a. Use the label line to write one function of the nerve.
   b. Put a star by it if it innervates only one muscle.
   c. Color it green if it is motor only.
   d. Color it yellow if it is sensory only.

Caution: Labels are not in correct numerical order.

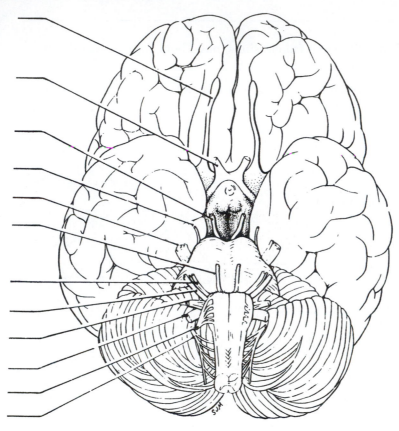

Lesson 30

Organs of Special Sense

■ **OBJECTIVES**

1. Identify the major structures of the nose, eye, tongue, and ear.
2. State the special sense related to each organ and the nerve that carries the impulses.
3. Name the area of the brain associated with each special sense.

■ **METHODS**

1. Perform the activities indicated in this unit. Each blank space should be filled with the appropriate cranial nerve, bone, bone marking, or brain structure.
2. Identify the gross anatomical structures on the models in the lab.

A. THE NOSE (SEE FIGURE 29–1)

Olfactory (smell receptors), sensitive to chemicals in solution, are located in the tissue lining the upper part of the nasal cavity above the superior nasal conchae. When the airborne chemicals enter the nose, they are dissolved in the mucous layer that lines the nasal cavity. The impulse is then carried by CN _____ through the _____ of the _____ bone.

B. THE EYE

Light striking the retina, site of sensory receptor cells, stimulates the impulses for vision. These impulses travel in the _____ n. through the _____ to enter the cranial vault.

■ **CLINICAL COMMENTS**

A **cataract** is a lens that has lost its transparency. Cataracts are the leading cause of blindness. Aging, ultraviolet rays, smoking, and disease are among the causes. Usually the lens can be replaced surgically. **Glaucoma** results when the aqueous humor cannot drain. When pressure of this accumulating fluid builds, it can damage the optic nerve. The condition can be treated with drugs and laser surgery.

FIGURE 30–1
THE RIGHT EYE (SUPERIOR VIEW OF TRANSVERSE SECTION)

1. **Pupil**—opening through which light enters.

2. **Iris**—circular, pigmented structure containing smooth muscles. It controls the size of the pupil and, therefore, the amount of light which passes through the **lens.**

3. **Ciliary body**—muscle that surrounds the lens. When it contracts, the pressure on the suspensory ligaments is decreased and the lens becomes more rounded for accommodation.

4. **Lens**—focuses the light rays.

5. **Choroid**—the middle layer of the eye. This vascular layer is continuous with the ciliary body and iris anteriorly.

6. **Sclera**—outer connective tissue layer; muscles attach here. *Color it pink.*

7. **Retina**—innermost layer, nervous tissue of the eye. *Color it yellow.*

8. **Optic n.**—processes of nerve cell bodies that are in the retina. *Color it yellow.*

9. **Cornea**—transparent continuation of the sclera.

10. **Aqueous humor**—watery filling of space anterior to the lens.

11. **Conjunctiva**—mucous membrane reflected from the eye onto the inside of the eyelids.

12. **Vitreous body**—gelatinous body helps maintain the shape of the eye.

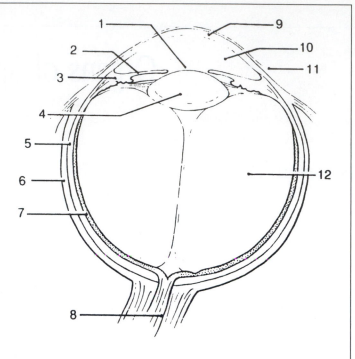

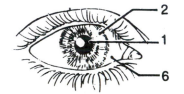

FIGURE 30–2
LACRIMAL APPARATUS: RIGHT EYE

1. **Lacrimal gland**—produces tears, which flow across the eye to lubricate it. *Color it yellow.*

2. **Nasolacrimal duct**—passes through the nasolacrimal canal and into the nasal cavity under the inferior nasal concha. *Color the nasolacrimal canal yellow; label the inferior nasal concha.*

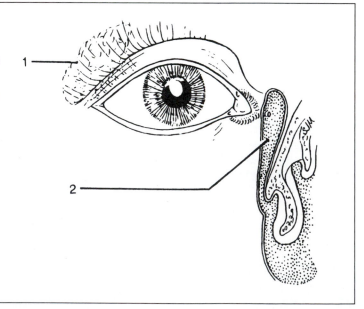

FIGURE 30–3
MUSCLES OF THE RIGHT EYE

1. **Levator palpebrae superioris**—continues into the upper eyelid and opens the eye. *Color it pink.*

2. **Lateral rectus muscle**—inserts into the sclera and moves the eye laterally, abducts it. *Color it blue.*

3. **Inferior rectus m.**—causes the eye to focus downward, depresses it. *Color it pink.*

4. **Superior oblique m.**—from the posterior orbit; it hooks around a trochlea and inserts superiorly. It helps rotate the eye. *Color it green.*

5. **Superior rectus muscle**—elevates eye, causes it to focus upward. *Color it pink.*

6. **Inferior oblique m.**—from medial origin to insertion laterally; helps rotate the eye. *Color it pink.*

7. **Medial rectus muscle**—moves eye medially; adducts it. *Color it pink.*

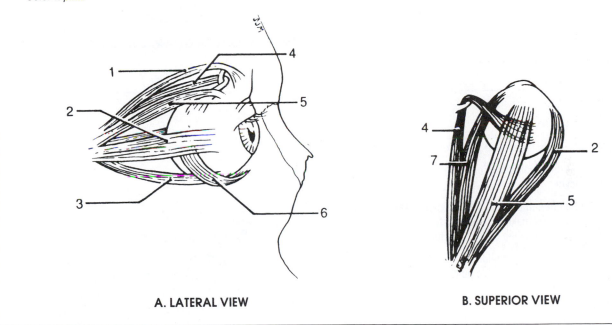

A. LATERAL VIEW   **B. SUPERIOR VIEW**

INNERVATION

CN III, oculomotor n. for all extraocular muscles *except:*

1. Superior oblique m.; innervated by trochlear n., it passes through a trochlea.
2. Lateral rectus muscle; innervated by abducens n., it abducts the eye.

Note: You colored all CN III innervation muscles pink; trochlear n. green, and abducens n. blue.

C. THE TONGUE

The taste buds of the tongue are the site of origin of the special sense of taste. The stimulation is from dissolved chemicals. The anterior 2/3 and posterior 1/3 have a different embryological origin and therefore are innervated by different nerves.

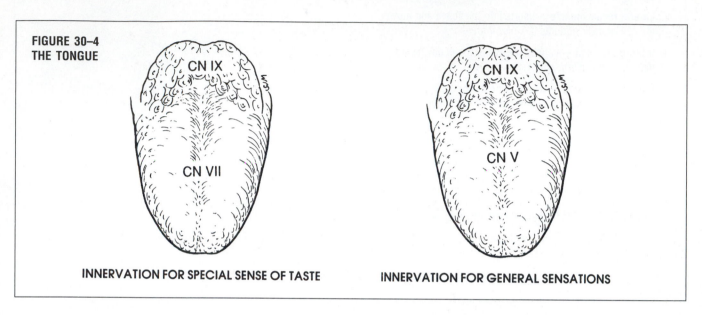

FIGURE 30–4
THE TONGUE

INNERVATION FOR SPECIAL SENSE OF TASTE   INNERVATION FOR GENERAL SENSATIONS

FIGURE 30–5
MUSCLES OF THE TONGUE

1. **Styloglossus**—pulls the tongue posteriorly.

2. **Hyoglossus**—from hyoid bone into tongue, this muscle pulls the tongue down.

3. **Body of the tongue**—made up of intrinsic **muscles** that run in different directions making it possible to curl and perform other movements within the body of the tongue.

4. **Genioglossus**—from the genoid tubercle to the glossus (tongue). This fan-shaped muscle pulls the tongue out of the mouth.

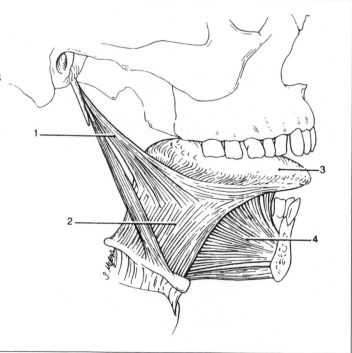

INNERVATION OF ALL TONGUE MUSCLES

Hypoglossal n., CN XII

■ **Student Activities**
Color the three extrinsic tongue muscles pink.

D. THE EAR

Within the petrous ridge of the temporal bone, structures of the inner ear serve as receptors for the special senses of hearing and equilibrium. The external and middle ear are also important in hearing. Study the structures in Figure 30–6.

FIGURE 30–6
THE RIGHT EAR (CORONAL SECTION THROUGH THE TEMPORAL BONE)

1. **Auricle**—helps to direct sound waves into auditory canal.

2. **External auditory canal**—passage through the bone that directs sound waves to the tympanic membrane.

3. **Lobe**

4. **Tympanic membrane** (ear drum)—vibrates when sound waves enter the canal. Separates external ear from middle ear.

5. **Malleus**—one of three small bones called *ossicles.* This one is connected to the tympanic membrane and moves when sound waves strike the membrane. *Color it green.*

6. **Incus**—the ossicle attached to the malleus. *Color it green.*

7. **Stapes** *(color it green)*—the ossicle attached to the incus. It fits into the oval window leading to the inner ear. When it is set into motion it causes the fluid in the cochlea to move. The movement stimulates hair cells, which send impulses through the cochlear nerve. (Two small muscles, tensor tympani and stapedius, decrease movement of the bones to prevent damage by loud sound.)

8. **Semicircular canals**—a fluid-filled inner ear structure that is arranged to detect movement of the head in all directions.

9. **Vestibular n.**—originates in the semicircular canals and conducts stimuli for equilibrium. *Color it yellow.*

10. **Cochlear n.**—originates in the cochlea and conducts impulses for the sense of sound. *Color it yellow.*

11. **Cochlea**—the fluid-filled compartment housing the apparatus for sound. It is an inner ear structure.

12. **Round window**—membrane covered, allows fluid to move in the closed system.

13. **Middle ear**—an air-filled chamber in which the ossicles are located. *Color it pink.*

14. **Auditory tube**—a cartilaginous tube leading from the pharynx (space behind the nose) to the middle ear. It allows air into the middle ear to equalize internal and external pressure across the tympanic membrane. *Color it pink.*

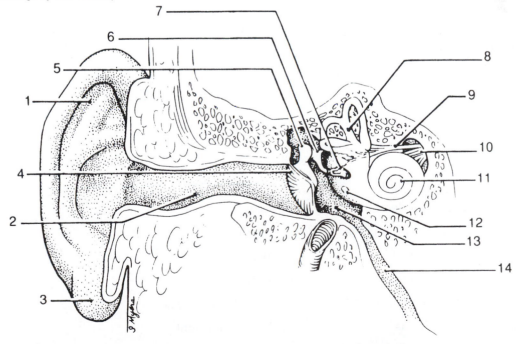

30

Name _____

1. Name in order all the cranial nerves that carry a *special sense,* name the sensation, the foramen through which the nerve passes, and, where indicated, name the lobe of the brain involved.

Nerve	Sensation	Foramen	Brain Structure
a.			——
b.			
c.			——
d.			——
e.			
f.			——

2. In the space provided, write the name of the nerve that innervates each muscle.

   a. styloglossus _____

   b. superior oblique _____

   c. intrinsic tongue _____

   d. inferior rectus _____

   e. lateral rectus _____

   f. genioglossus _____

3. Name the ossicles. _____, _____, _____

4. How many nerves are involved in innervation of the tongue? _____
   List them:

5. Matching exercise.

   _____ 1. pupil   a. nervous tissue

   _____ 2. sclera   b. accommodation

   _____ 3. conjunctiva   c. muscle attachment

   _____ 4. lens   d. focus light rays

   _____ 5. retina   e. controls amount of light

   _____ 6. choroid   f. covering membrane

   _____ 7. iris   g. opening for light

   _____ 8. ciliary body   h. vascular layer

Muscles and Vessels of the Head and Neck

I. MUSCLES OF THE HEAD AND NECK

The muscles of the head and neck are skeletal muscles. They are controlled voluntarily to produce facial expressions, to move the mandible for chewing, to move the head, and to help in swallowing and talking. The major muscles are included here.

■ OBJECTIVES

1. Describe the scalp.
2. Name the muscles of mastication; identify masseter and temporalis.
3. Identify selected muscles of facial expression and of the neck.
4. State the actions and innervations of the muscles of facial expression and mastication.

■ METHODS

1. Perform the activities indicated in the lesson.
2. Observe demonstrations of muscles and vessels indicated.
3. Study material and models provided in the lab.

A. THE SCALP

Deep to the skin of the scalp lies a fibromuscular sheet, **galea aponeurotica,** which extends from the superior nuchal lines to the eyebrows. The **aponeurosis** provides attachment for **frontalis m.** and **occipitalis m.**

B. MUSCLES OF THE FACE

These are either muscles of facial expression or of mastication.

MUSCLES OF FACIAL EXPRESSION

These are often called "mimetic" because they attach to subcutaneous fascia and move only skin. Their actions: smiling, frowning, puckering lips, or squinting eyes. Most are very thin; all are innervated by CN VII, the facial n.

There are many of these muscles. Identify those described in the key to Figure 31–1.

FIGURE 31-1
THE HEAD AND NECK: SUPERFICIAL DISSECTION (LATERAL VIEW)

1. **Occipitalis**—attaches from occipital bone into the galea aponeurotica.

2. **Galea aponeurotica**—fascial sheet for muscle attachment.

3. **Frontalis**—attaches from the galea aponeurotica to superficial fascia and muscles around the eye. It raises the eyebrows; wrinkles the forehead.

4. **Orbicularis oculi**—a sphincter muscle; surrounds and closes the eye.

5. **Buccinator**—a thicker muscle. Horizontally directed fibers form much of the cheek and are important in guiding food between the teeth and holding the cheeks to the teeth.

6. **Orbicularis oris**—surrounds the mouth, causes lips to pucker.

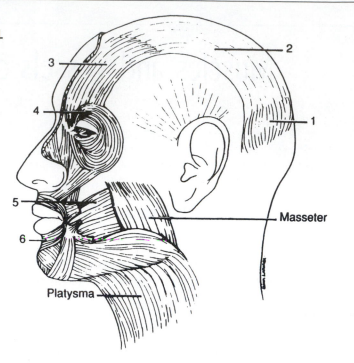

MUSCLES OF MASTICATION (CHEWING)

These differ from muscles of facial expression in two important ways. Attachments are from bone to bone and move the temporomandibular joint; and, the four muscles of mastication are innervated by the mandibular n., CN V_3.

FIGURE 31-2
MUSCLES OF MASTICATION

1. **Temporalis m.**

   Origin: temporal fossa

   Insertion: coronoid process of mandible after passing deep to zygomatic arch

   Action: closes and retracts mandible

2. **Masseter m.**
   Origin: zygomatic arch
   Insertion: lateral surface of angle of mandible
   Action: closes mandible

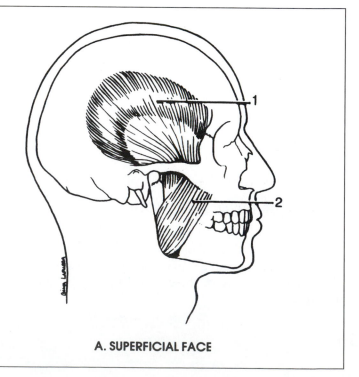

A. SUPERFICIAL FACE

FIGURE 31–2
MUSCLES OF MASTICATION (CONTINUED)

3. **Lateral pterygoid m.**
   Origin: lateral side of the lateral pterygoid plate
   Insertion: (region of) the condyle of the mandible
   Action: opens the mandible and moves it to the side

4. **Medial pterygoid m.**
   Origin: medial side of the lateral pterygoid plate
   Insertion: medial surface of the angle of the mandible
   With the masseter, forms a sling around the mandible
   Action: closes the mandible

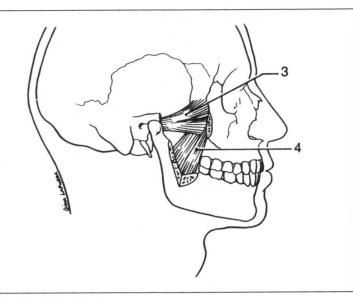

C. MUSCLES OF THE NECK

Platysma is a very thin sheet of muscle in the superficial fascia lying over the anterior thorax and shoulder. It extends to the area around the mouth, and covers the sternocleidomastoid. See Figure 31-1. Innervation: CN VII.

The **Posterior Triangle of the Neck** is bounded by the sternocleidomastoid m., trapezius m., and the middle third of the clavicle. The muscular floor of the triangle includes the semispinalis capitis, splenius capitis, levator scapulae, and the *middle scalene*. The major contents are the subclavian artery, external jugular vein, and brachial plexus. The roots of the brachial plexus enter the posterior triangle between the *middle* and *anterior scalene* muscles. (The anterior scalene m. is deep to sternocleidomastoid, and the *posterior scalene* m. may be absent or blended with the middle.) The **anterior triangle,** from the anterior border of the sternocleidomastoid to the midline of the neck, is further subdivided to make location of structures easier. It will not be discussed in detail here.

FIGURE 31–3
SUPERFICIAL, LATERAL NECK

1. **Trapezius** forms the contour of the posterior neck.
   Innervation: CN XI (details in Unit II)

2. **Sternocleidomastoid** (sternomastoid) is named for each of its attachments:
   Origin: sternum and medial clavicle
   Insertion: mastoid process of the temporal bone
   Action: turns face to the opposite side. When contracted it can easily be felt. Try it!
   Innervation: CN XI

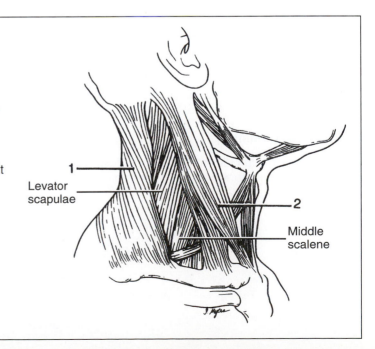

Levator scapulae

Middle scalene

SUPRAHYOID AND INFRAHYOID MUSCLES

There are four neck muscles above (suprahyoids) and four below (infrahyoids) the hyoid bone. These muscles elevate, depress, protract, and retract the hyoid bone and are important in swallowing and talking. (Innervation of these muscles: CN V, VII, XII and C1,2,3.) *Be sure you can identify the muscles with asterisks.*

FIGURE 31–4
SUPRAHYOID AND INFRAHYOID MUSCLES

(The mouth is tipped up to show the floor)
Suprahyoid Muscles (1 through 4)

1. **Mylohyoid m.***—these two muscles meet in a midline fascial strip that extends from the genoid tubercle to the hyoid bone. The origin is on the inner surface of the mandible.

2a. **Digastric, anterior belly***
    Origin: genoid tubercle
    Insertion: joins anterior belly at hyoid bone

2b. **Digastric, posterior belly***
    Origin: mastoid process
    Insertion: joins anterior belly at hyoid bone

3. **Stylohyoid**—splits around the posterior belly of the digastric m.
    Origin: styloid process of the temporal bone
    Insertion: hyoid bone

4. **Geniohyoid** —deep to the mylohyoid

Infrahyoid Muscles (5 through 8)

5. **Sternohyoid***—extends from sternum to hyoid bone

6. **Omohyoid**—superior and inferior bellies are held to the clavicle by way of a fascial sling. Extends from scapula to hyoid bone.

7. **Sternothyroid**—from the sternum to the thyroid cartilage; this muscle lies under the sternohyoid.

8. **Thyrohyoid**—direct continuation from the sternothyroid; this muscle also lies under the sternohyoid. It extends from the thyroid cartilage to the hyoid bone.

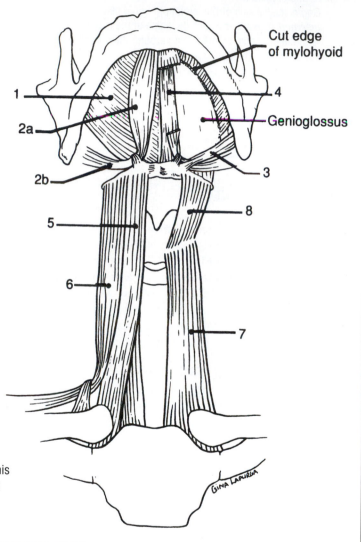

Cut edge of mylohyoid

Genioglossus

■ **CLINICAL COMMENT**

If the **posterior triangle** suffers a major trauma, death might occur as a result of hemorrhage of the sub-clavian artery. Serious damage can also be done to the brachial plexus in this location.

II. VESSELS OF HEAD AND NECK

The major blood supply to the head and neck is by way of the vertebral arteries and the common carotid arteries. Because the vertebral and internal carotid arteries supply structures within the skull, they were included in Lesson 26. The external carotid artery will be emphasized in this lesson.

■ OBJECTIVES

1. Describe the circulation of blood to the neck and head.
2. Identify the major arteries and veins of the head and neck.
3. State the purpose of the carotid sinuses and carotid bodies.

■ METHODS

1. Complete the activities described in this lesson.
2. Observe demonstrations of head and neck vessels.
3. Study the models and materials provided in the lab.

A. MAJOR ARTERIES OF THE HEAD AND NECK

There are two major pairs of arteries that ascend through the neck to supply blood to the head and neck:

1. **Common carotid arteries**—each vessel bifurcates into:

   a. Internal carotid artery—supplies internal skull structures

   b. External carotid artery—for neck and external head

2. **Vertebral arteries**—pass through the transverse foramina of the cervical vertebrae to enter the skull.

FIGURE 31–5
MAJOR BRANCHES FROM THE AORTA

1. **Arch of aorta**

2. **Brachiocephalic trunk**—leaves the arch and bifurcates to become the common carotid and subclavian arteries. (This is the pattern on the right only)

3. _____

4. _____

5. **Left common carotid a.**—directly from the arch of the aorta

6. **Vertebral a.**—both right and left, leave the subclavian arteries

7. **Left subclavian a.**—directly off the arch of the aorta

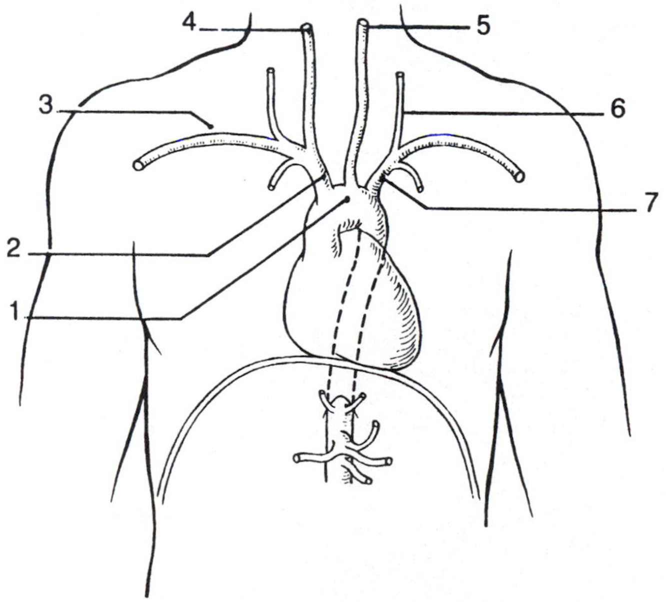

FIGURE 31-6
ARTERIES OF HEAD AND NECK (LATERAL VIEW OF RIGHT SIDE)

1. **Brachiocephalic trunk** exists only on the right side

2. **Subclavian a.**—will come off the arch of the aorta on the left

3. **Vertebral a.**—enters the skull through foramen magnum

4. **Common carotid a.**—lies in a neurovascular bundle with vagus n. and is often used to determine pulse in emergencies. It bifurcates at the superior border of the thyroid cartilage.

5. **Internal carotid a.**—more posterior branch from common carotid; will enter the skull at the carotid canal

6. **External carotid a.**—will provide the branches to supply much of the neck and the external head. Be familiar with the names of the unlabeled branches:

   superior thyroid a.

   lingual a.

   occipital a.

   posterior auricular a.

   ascending pharyngeal a.

   facial a.—you can palpate (feel) it as it crosses the midpoint of the inferior edge of the mandible. Try it!

7. **Maxillary a.**—a large terminal branch that lies in the infratemporal fossa and supplies the upper and lower jaws, teeth, muscles of mastication, and most of the nose.

8. **Superficial temporal a.**—the other terminal branch

Note: Additional branches from the subclavian help supply the neck.

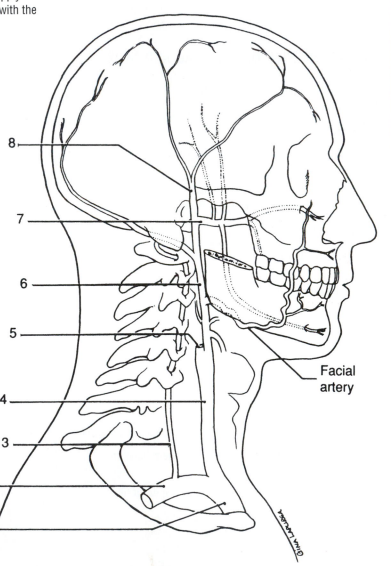

Facial artery

B. CAROTID SINUS AND CAROTID BODY

These very important structures are located near the bifurcation of the common carotid a. They will not be seen grossly.

1. **Carotid body,** a chemoreceptor, is a group of specialized cells that detect the concentration of oxygen in the blood. If the oxygen concentration is not high enough, a nerve impulse is sent to the medulla oblongata of the brain and the respiration rate increases.

2. **Carotid sinus,** a baroreceptor, is a group of special nerve receptors that determine the blood pressure. The message is sent to the medulla to either slow or increase the heart rate.

C. MAJOR VEINS OF THE HEAD AND NECK

There are two major pairs of veins through which the return blood flows:

1. **Internal jugular v.**—returns blood from inside the skull.

2. **External jugular v.**—formed as the external face, head, and neck veins anastomose.

FIGURE 31–7
VEINS FROM HEAD AND NECK

1. **Internal jugular v.**—forms at base of the skull and receives all blood from inside the skull.

2. **External jugular v.**—lies between platysma and sternocleidomastoid m. It is the vein you see standing out when someone is angry. Returns the blood delivered by the external carotid a.

3. **Subclavian v.**—returns blood from the upper extremity.

4. **Brachiocephalic v.**—formed on both the right and left when the internal jugular joins the subclavian v.

5. **Superior vena cava**—formed when the right and left brachiocephalic veins join. It returns all head and neck, upper extremity, and chest blood to the right atrium.

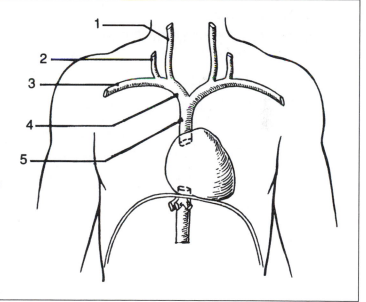

Exercise Thirty-One

Name _____

1. In Figure 31–1, color the muscles of facial expression and of the scalp pink; of mastication, blue.

2. List below the name of the muscles innervated by the nerve indicated. Exclude the suprahyoids and infrahyoids.

   CN VII, facial n.　　　**CN V$_3$, mandibular n.**　　　**CN XI, accessory n.**

   a. _____　　g. _____　　k. _____

   b. _____　　h. _____　　l. _____

   c. _____　　i. _____

   d. _____　　j. _____

   e. _____

   f. _____

3. List below the suprahyoid and infrahyoid muscles.

   Suprahyoid　　　　　　**Infrahyoid**

   a. _____　　e. _____

   b. _____　　f. _____

   c. _____　　g. _____

   d. _____　　h. _____

4. Muscles of mastication that can be seen in a superficial dissection are:

   a. _____ and b. _____

5. In Figure 31–5, color red the path of blood from the left ventricle into both the right and left common carotid a.

6. In Figure 31–7, color blue the path of blood from the external face to the right atrium.

7. Name the muscles pictured on the right. Write the name of the nerve that innervates each muscle.

   Muscle   **Nerve**

   a. _____   _____

   b. _____   _____

   c. _____   _____

   d. _____   _____

   e. _____   _____

   f. _____   _____

   g. _____   _____

   h. _____   _____

8. In the correct spaces below, list the vessels through which blood flows to get from
   (a) to the last structure listed.

   a. Heart   a. Masseter muscle

   b. _____   b. _____

   c. _____   c. _____

   d. Right common carotid a.   d. _____

                                         e. _____

                                         f. _____

                                         g. Right atrium

9. In the space below, define carotid sinus and carotid body.

Lesson **32**

The Autonomic Nervous System

The autonomic nervous system consists of **efferent fibers** that stimulate smooth muscles in structures such as blood vessels, bronchial tubes, and the digestive tract. Autonomics also control glandular secretions and regulate the rate of the heartbeat. This **involuntary system** has one major anatomical difference from that of the regular body (somatic) system. In the somatic system only one neuron is needed to get information from the central nervous system (CNS) to the effector organ, a skeletal muscle. In the autonomic nervous system (ANS) two neurons are needed between the CNS and the effector organ, a smooth muscle or gland.

The autonomic nervous system is involuntary, but it is controlled by the brain. The control is centered mainly in the **hypothalamus.** Reflex centers for actions such as coughing, vomiting, breathing, and pulse rate are in the **medulla.**

■ **OBJECTIVES**

1. State the major differences in the ANS and the regular somatic system.
2. Describe the origins of sympathetic and parasympathetic nerves.
3. State the major differences in function and distribution of the two autonomic divisions.
4. Identify the sympathetic trunk within the thorax.

■ **METHOD**

Perform the activities as you study the information in this lesson.

A. THE SYMPATHETIC NERVOUS SYSTEM

This is more widespread and is the system that usually speeds or stimulates body functions. The cell body of origin is in the spinal cord between the first thoracic level and the second lumbar level. The second cell body in this two-neuron pathway is either in the ganglia along the **sympathetic trunk** or in a **collateral ganglion** on the front of the aorta.

FIGURE 32–1
SYMPATHETIC CHAIN (VENTRO-LATERAL VIEW)

1. **Ganglion:** Contains cell bodies of the second neuron in the path of sympathetic innervation.

2. **Sympathetic trunk:** Formed of both pre- and postganglionic fibers, which may travel to different cord levels before exiting.

The chain extends from the cervical to the coccygeal level (Figure 32–3).

3. **Rami communicantes:** The bundles of preganglionic and postganglionic fibers going to and from the spinal nerves.

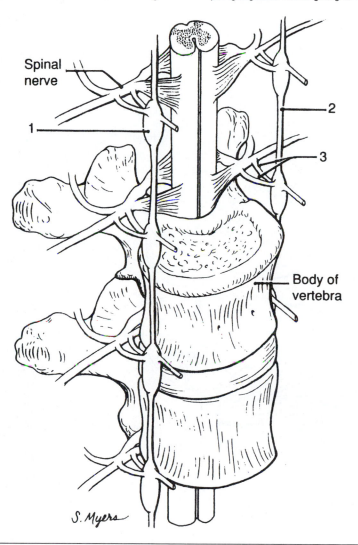

■ **CLINICAL COMMENTS**

Drug therapy is often used to change or mimic the effect of autonomic nerves. Autonomic responses occur when neurotransmitters stimulate receptors on postganglionic autonomic cells or on cells of the target organs. Since most of these receptors are stimulated only by specific neurotransmitters, drugs that block the receptor inhibit the response or activity of the effector organ. For example, if the desire is to reduce the heart rate, the drug propranolol can be used to attach to specific receptors in cardiac muscle in order to block the effect of sympathetic stimulation. Other drugs may stimulate the receptor and increase the activity of the effector organ.

There are three ways sympathetic fibers may get from the spinal cord to the effector organ. Each path must include the axon, **preganglionic fiber,** of the cell of origin and the axon of the second cell, a **postganglionic** fiber. Figure 32–2 is a schematic diagram to be used as a work sheet to draw the three pathways. A description of each path follows the diagram.

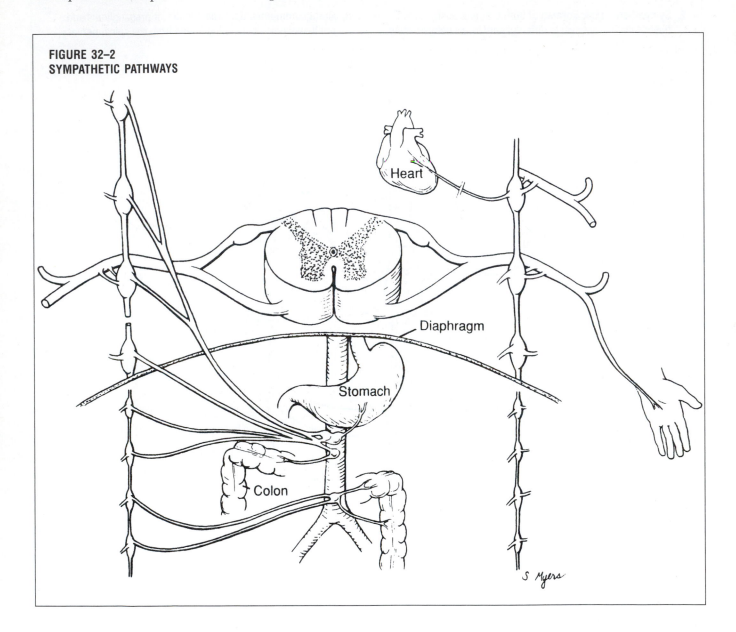

**FIGURE 32–2
SYMPATHETIC PATHWAYS**

1. **Cell bodies of origin** for the sympathetic nerves are always in the lateral horn of gray matter between cord levels T1 and L2. *(On the right side of your diagram, make a dot in the lateral horn with a red pencil; this will represent the original nerve cell bodies of the first pathway.)* The preganglionic processes (fibers) of this first pathway leave the spinal nerve by way of a ramus to enter a ganglion of the chain. *(Place a red dot in the ganglion; this is the site of the second nerve cell bodies.)* From these cells the postganglionic fibers enter the spinal nerve and travel as part of the spinal nerve to the periphery (represented by the hand). In the periphery they provide sympathetic innervation to the peripheral vessels, sweat and sebaceous glands, and erector pili muscles. *(With red, draw the fibers of this pathway.)*

2. Now, add **cell bodies of origin** of the second type of pathway. *(On the same side of the illustration, place a blue dot to represent the first, preganglionic, cells of the path.)* The preganglionic fibers leave by way of the ramus to enter the chain ganglion where they may travel up or down in the cord before they synapse. *(Draw the blue line up to the top ganglion and have it synapse on another blue cell.)* They do not reenter the spinal nerve. *(Draw the postganglionic fibers out the nerve directly to the heart.)*

3. **Cell bodies of origin** of the third pathway are also in the lateral horn, but we will use the left side now so it can be more easily seen. *(Draw a green dot and take the fibers out the ventral root and into a ganglion.)* The preganglionic fibers enter the chain by way of a ramus, but they do not synapse. They leave in bundles with other preganglionic fibers. These bundles are called **sympathetic splanchnic nerves.** They will pass through the diaphragm to reach the **abdomen.** They will then go to collateral ganglia that are anterior to the aorta. *(Draw the green, preganglionic fibers through the splanchnic n. to a ganglion just inferior to the stomach.)* There they will synapse with the second cell bodies *(place a green dot in the ganglion)*, and the postganglionic fibers will travel on blood vessels to innervate abdominal viscera. *(Color this green pathway to the segment of colon.)*

DIVISIONS OF THE AUTONOMIC NERVOUS SYSTEM

The two divisions of the autonomic nervous system are often antagonistic. Table 32–1 compares the divisions.

TABLE 32–1 DIVISIONS OF THE AUTONOMIC NERVOUS SYSTEM

	Sympathetic	Parasympathetic
Position of cell body of origin	Lateral horns of spinal cord from levels T1–L2	Nuclei of cranial nerves III, VII, IX, and X, and spinal cord levels S2–4
Position of second nerve cell body	1. Sympathetic trunk 2. Collateral ganglia found near the aorta	Ganglia on or near the organ innervated
General effect	To speed body functions for "fight or flight"	To stabilize body for functions at rest
*Specific effect on: a. Heart	Increases rate	Decreases rate
b. Blood pressure	Increases	Decreases
c. Peripheral vessels	Constrict	No effect
d. Sweat glands	Stimulated	No effect
e. Pupils	Dilate	Constrict
f. Digestion	Inhibited	Stimulated
g. Bronchioles	Dilate	Constrict

*Many functions have not been mentioned here.

FIGURE 32–3
ANATOMY OF THE AUTONOMIC NERVOUS SYSTEM:
SCHEMATIC REPRESENTATION

The solid lines represent preganglionic fibers; dashed lines are
postganglionic.

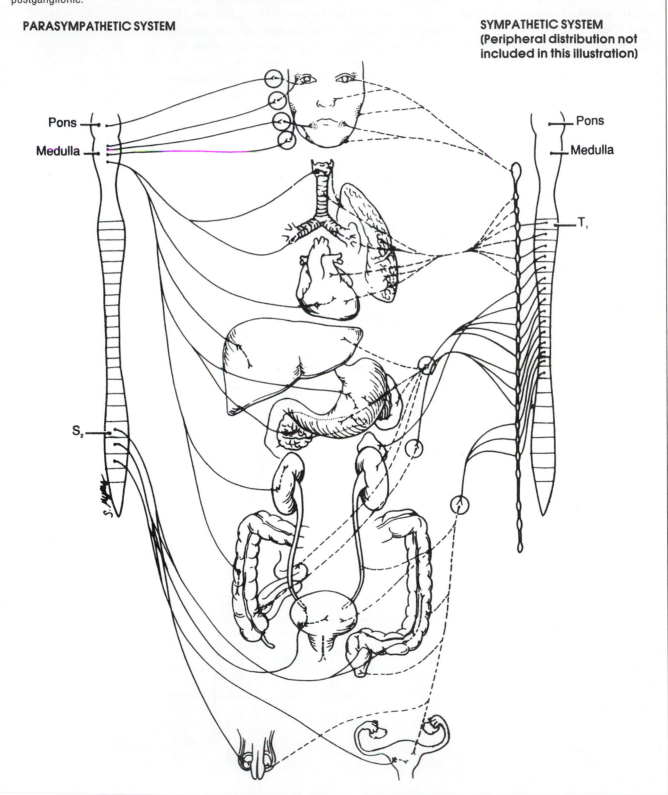

PARASYMPATHETIC SYSTEM

SYMPATHETIC SYSTEM
**(Peripheral distribution not
included in this illustration)**

Pons

Medulla

Pons

Medulla

T₁

S₂

B. THE PARASYMPATHETIC SYSTEM

This is often called the craniosacral system because of the position of its cell body of origin (see Table 32–1). This is the system that usually is inhibitory or restorative. There is no chain of ganglia in this system. The second nerve cell body of this pathway is located in a ganglion either near or on the effector organ. Details of all these ganglia will not be presented here.

The pathway of the parasympathetic fibers can be seen in the schematic representation of Figure 32–3. Study this illustration to understand the general distribution of the autonomic nerves. (The peripheral sympathetics are not pictured; there are no peripheral parasympathetics.) For more specific distribution of these fibers, see a reference text.

C. VISCERAL SENSORY INFORMATION

Since the visceral sensory fibers enter the spinal cord at the same cord levels as regular somatic sensory fibers, pain may radiate to the body part served by that spinal cord level. This phenomenon is called *referred pain.* One example of this is the pain felt in the left arm when visceral afferents from the heart are stimulated.

■ **Student Activities**

1. A nerve that is composed of preganglionic autonomic fibers is called a _____ n.
2. In Figure 32–3, color red the segments of the spinal cord that have sympathetic cells of origin; color green the segments that contain cells of origin of parasympathetic fibers.
3. List the cranial nerves that have parasympathetic fibers that supply head and neck only: _____, _____, and _____.
   Which has parasympathetics in the thorax and abdomen? _____
4. Using the spinal cord segment below, label all structures that relate to the autonomic nervous system only. (You should have four.)

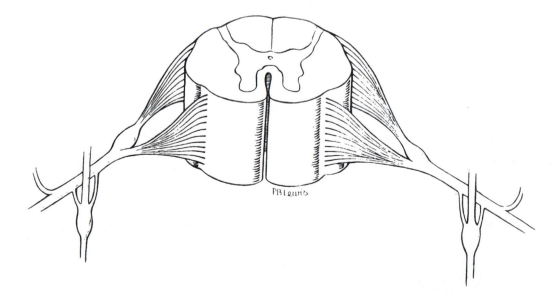

PB Lennis

Review of Unit III

You should study the unit, all reports and activities, then try to answer all questions
in this review without referring to the text.

I. Name the eight bones of the cranial vault.

_____

_____ (2)

_____

_____

_____ (2)

_____

II. Label each structure.

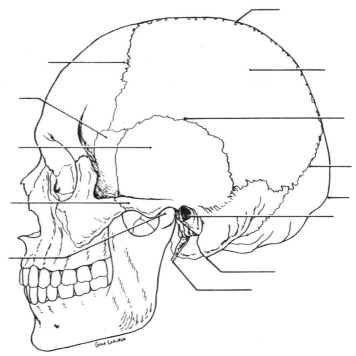

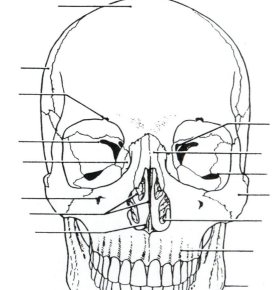

III. For each pair of cranial nerves:
   a. Draw it on the skull and label it on the brain.
   b. In the spaces provided, state: its name, whether it's mixed, motor, or sensory, its major distribution (what it innervates), and what sensation it carries, if sensory.

Number	Name	Mixed, Motor, Sensory	Distribution	Sensation
I	_____	_____	_____	_____
II	_____	_____	_____	_____
III	_____	_____	_____	_____
IV	_____	_____	_____	_____
V	_____	_____	_____	_____
VI	_____	_____	_____	_____
VII	_____	_____	_____	_____
VIII	_____	_____	_____	_____
IX	_____	_____	_____	_____
X	_____	_____	_____	_____
XI	_____	_____	_____	_____
XII	_____	_____	_____	_____

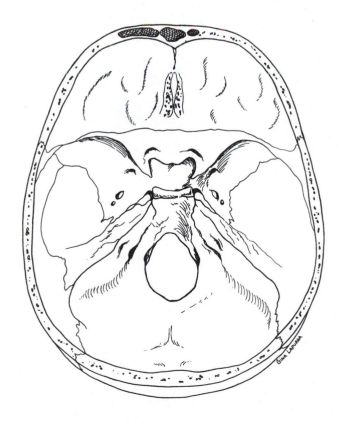

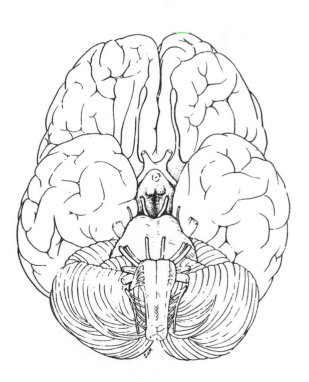

IV. On the illustrations, label the structures listed and state their functions.

View A

a. precentral gyrus
b. central sulcus
c. frontal lobe
d. lateral fissure
e. temporal lobe
f. pons
g. medulla oblongata
h. postcentral gyrus
i. parietal lobe
j. occipital lobe
k. cerebellum
l. olive of medulla
m. spinal cord

View B

a. corpus callosum
b. septum pellucidum
c. massa intermedia
d. interventricular foramen
e. mammillary body
f. optic chiasma
g. hypophysis
h. temporal lobe
i. cerebral peduncle
j. cerebral aqueduct
k. pons
l. central sulcus
m. paracentral lobule
n. parieto-occipital sulcus
o. choroid plexus of third ventricle
p. calcarine fissure
q. superior colliculus
r. arbor vita
s. choroid plexus in fourth ventricle
t. medulla oblongata
u. central canal of cord

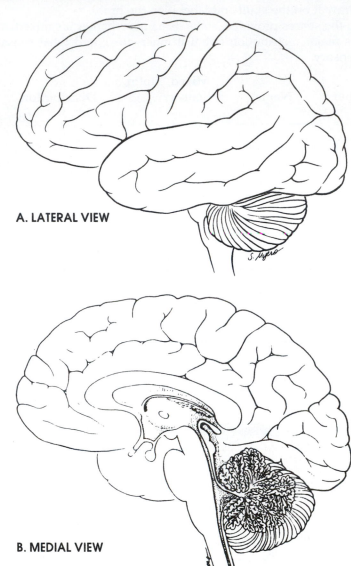

A. LATERAL VIEW

B. MEDIAL VIEW

V. On the illustrations, label all muscles of mastication. Color muscles of facial expression pink.

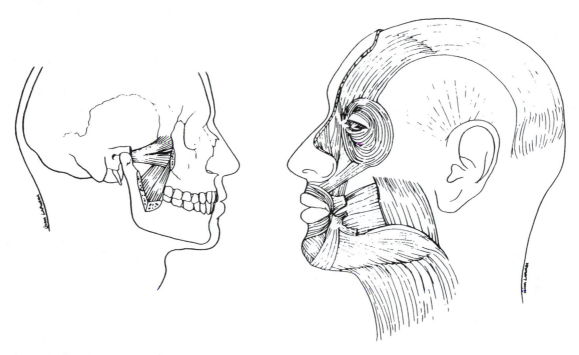

VI. Give answers for the following blanks or questions.
1. List the blood vessels needed to get the blood from the left ventricle to the right buccinator muscle.
2. Name three specific facial muscles.
3. Name four muscles of mastication.
4. Cerebrospinal fluid (CSF) is produced by _____ _____.
5. Name three functions of CSF.
6. List the pathway of CSF from the time it is produced in the lateral ventricle until it is released into the superior sagittal sinus.
7. What is a suture of the skull? Name four.
8. Name the three meningeal layers from superficial to deep. _____, _____, _____
9. Name two structures that are made of double folds of meningeal dura. _____, _____
10. What is the purpose of the dural sinuses? _____
11. What vessel receives all the used blood from the inside of the skull? _____
12. What are paranasal sinuses? What do they contain? Name four.
13. If the trigeminal nerve is injured, does it affect your ability to smile? Why?
14. If calcium deposits decrease the opening of foramen ovale and squeeze the nerve found there, what kind of problem might you have?
15. Name the components of the nasal septum. _____, _____
16. Name the foramina necessary for the internal carotid a. to get to the brain. _____, _____

17. What bone of the skull is movable? Name the joint.
18. Name the brain structure most closely related to each of the levels of the cranial vault:

    anterior cranial fossa _____

    middle cranial fossa _____

    posterior cranial fossa _____
19. What cranial nerve is most important in helping you smile? _____
20. Explain the actions of the supra- and infrahyoid muscles. What two functions are made possible by these actions? _____, _____
21. What are the two muscles most important in forming the contour of the neck? _____ and _____. They are both innervated by the _____ nerve.
22. What is the significance of the carotid body? The carotid sinus? Where is their approximate location?
23. What branch of the external carotid artery is so important for the blood supply of the nose and upper jaw?
24. Draw the pattern of vessels that get blood from the external and internal head to the right atrium. Include the subclavian v.
25. Draw the circle of Willis. Include the major pairs of vessels that bring the blood into the skull. Those pairs are: _____ and _____.
26. What is the significance of Brodmann numbers? Area 4? Area 3,1,2?
27. What is a homunculus?
28. On what gyrus would pressure from your little finger arrive? What is the blood supply to these cells?
29. If the left anterior cerebral artery is occluded, what body part will lose its motor function?
30. What tract would be involved in carrying the information from question 29?
31. If the lateral spinothalamic tract on the right side is cut in the spinal cord, what might you lose on your hand? Right hand or left hand?
32. What type of communicating fibers connect the two hemispheres of the brain? What type are in the fasiculus gracilis?
33. What is meant by the term *contralateral brain control?*
34. In the brain, where are nerve cell bodies located? In the spinal cord?
35. Where does the spinal cord end in the adult? What is the name of the end of the cord? What is the filum terminale?
36. What do the terms *upper motor neuron* and *lower motor neuron* mean?
37. Name two locations of intrinsic eye muscles and name the function of each.

38. Choose the appropriate illustration and label the structures on the sense organs shown below. In the illustration of the ear, color the auditory tube and the space within the middle ear yellow; color the inner ear structures pink. Beside the illustration, list the structures of the middle ear and the inner ear.

   a. pupil
   b. stapes
   c. cochlea
   d. retina
   e. auditory tube
   f. sclera
   g. tympanic membrane
   h. ciliary body
   i. semicircular canal
   j. external auditory canal
   k. incus
   l. cornea
   m. vestibulocochlear n.
   n. optic n.
   o. cochlear n.
   p. lateral rectus m.
   q. iris

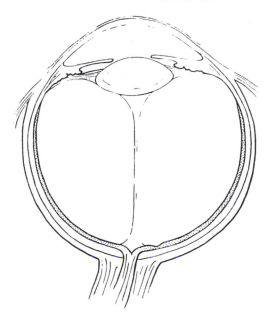

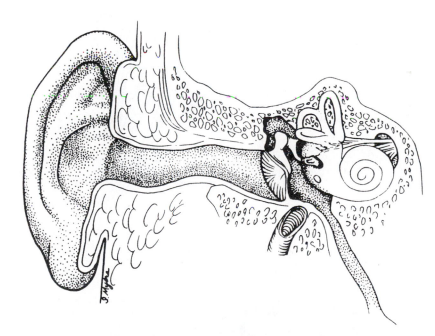

39. Name the four cranial nerves that contain autonomic fibers.
40. What are the two divisions of the autonomic nervous system?
41. Name four specific functions of each autonomic nervous system division.
42. What two brain structures are most involved with autonomic function?

VII. In the correct position on the tongues: place the names of the cranial nerves
responsible for taste on the left; those responsible for general sensation on the
right.

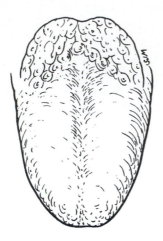 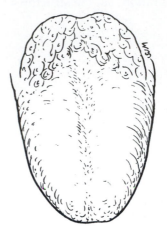

VIII. Label the illustrations below.

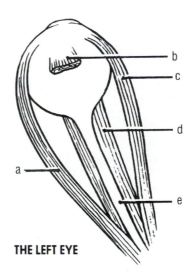

THE LEFT EYE

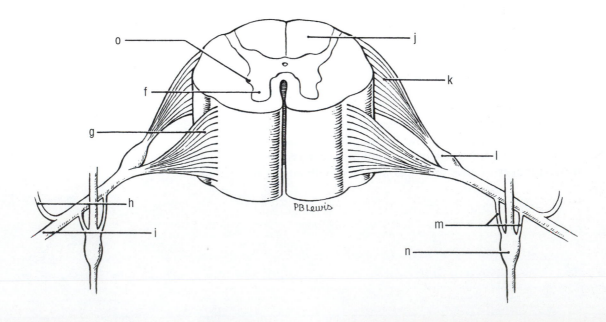

The Abdomen, Pelvis, and Thorax

With:

· Digestive System
· Urinary System
· Reproductive System
· Endocrine System
· Respiratory System
· Lymphatic System

Muscles of the Abdomen and Pelvis

Because the abdominal cavity has no bony cage, as does the thorax, the muscles serve to hold the abdominal viscera (organs) in place and aid in the functioning of some of the viscera.

■ OBJECTIVES

1. Identify the four muscles of the abdominal wall.
2. List the functions of the abdominal muscles.
3. Name the aponeurotic structures related to the abdominal muscles.
4. Describe the innervation of the abdominal muscles.
5. Describe the position and function of the pelvic diaphragm.

■ METHODS

1. Study the information presented in this unit; perform the student activities.
2. Observe demonstrations of the muscles and fascial structures.
3. Review lab material until you can find all structures easily.

ORIENTATION TO THE ABDOMINAL REGION

The abdominopelvic cavity extends from the thoracic diaphragm superiorly to the pelvic diaphragm, which closes the opening of the inferior pelvis. The separation from abdomen to pelvis is not distinct. The wall of the abdomen extends from the ribs down to the iliac crests laterally and the **inguinal ligaments** anteriorly. This large cavity contains the major viscera of digestive, urinary, and reproductive systems.

■ CLINICAL COMMENTS

A **hernia** results when a body organ protrudes through a body tissue, usually one where there is a weakness in tissue separating two areas. The most common type (particularly in the male) is the **inguinal hernia.** When pressure is exerted in the abdomen, intestinal organs are pushed into the inguinal canal along the path of the spermatic cord. When a diaphragmatic hernia occurs, abdominal contents are forced through the thoracic diaphragm into the thorax.

A. MUSCLES OF THE ABDOMINAL WALL

These muscles can be seen in Figures 34–1 and 34–2. They compress abdominal viscera to aid in forced expiration, defecation, urination, vomiting, and childbirth. They also help in twisting of the trunk.

Attachments (general): to external surfaces of ribs, thoracolumbar fascia, iliac crest, and linea alba.
Innervation: ventral rami of T7–L2.

FIGURE 34–1
MUSCLES OF ABDOMINAL WALL: SUPERFICIAL DISSECTION

1. **Rectus abdominis**—deep to the anterior rectus sheath on the right side of the body. Fibers are oriented vertically.

2. **External abdominal oblique**—the most extensive lateral muscle. Note the fiber direction.

3. **Linea alba**—fascia that extends from the xiphoid process to the pubic symphysis. The aponeurosis from muscles of the lateral wall is continuous with this.

4. **Tendinous intersection**—strips of fascia interrupt muscle segments.

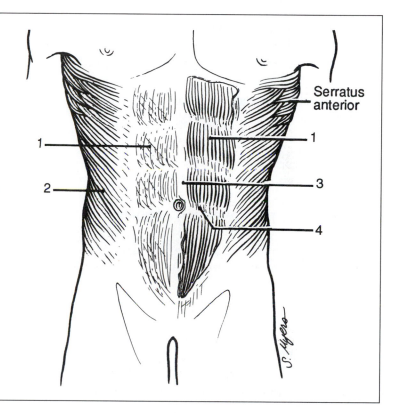

FIGURE 34–2
MUSCLES OF ABDOMINAL WALL: DEEP DISSECTION

1. **Internal abdominal oblique** just deep to the external muscle and with fibers perpendicular to it.

2. **Transverse abdominis**—deepest abdominal muscle. Nerve fibers lie between internal oblique and transverse m.

3. **Posterior rectus sheath**—seen when rectus abdominis is removed.

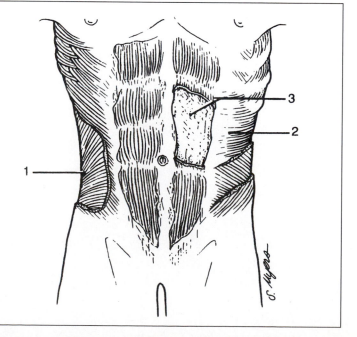

FIGURE 34-3
INGUINAL REGION

1. **Aponeurosis** of external abdominal oblique m.

2. **Inguinal ligament,** formed by the rolled-under, inferior portion of the external abdominal oblique aponeurosis; attaches from the anterior superior iliac spine to the pubic tubercle.

3. **Inguinal canal,** passageway leading from the outside of the abdominal wall into the abdominal cavity. It contains the spermatic cord in the male and the round ligament of the uterus in the female.

4. **Deep inguinal ring,** the opening from the inguinal canal into the abdominal cavity.

5. **Superficial inguinal ring,** an opening in the abdominal fascia.

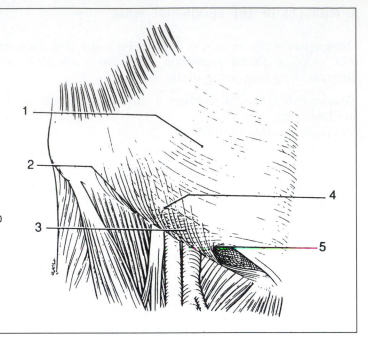

B. MUSCLES OF THE POSTERIOR ABDOMEN

Psoas major and minor lie in the posterior abdomen but are considered lower limb muscles. The **quadratus lumborum m.** is the only other muscle of the posterior abdomen.

FIGURE 34-4
QUADRATUS LUMBORUM

Attachments: from iliac crest to the inferior border of rib 12 and transverse processes of the first four lumbar vertebrae.

Action: lateral flexion of lumbar vertebral column.

Innervation: from lumbar plexus

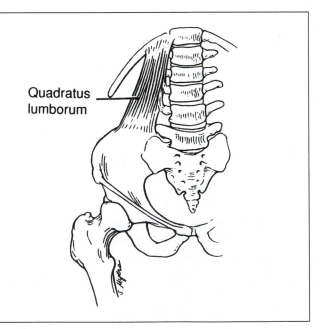

Quadratus lumborum

C. MUSCLES OF THE PELVIS

Obturator internus m. and piriformis m., studied in Lesson 6, help close the lateral pelvic opening. The major structure closing the remainder of the inferior pelvis is the **pelvic diaphragm.** The pelvic diaphragm accommodates the passage of the urethra and anal canal and, in the female, also the vagina.

FIGURE 34–5
PELVIC DIAPHRAGM: LEVATOR ANI AND COCCYGEUS* (SUPERIOR VIEW)

Attachments: between pubis and coccyx and to fascia of the lateral pelvic wall.

Action: supports and raises pelvic floor; assists in support of abdominopelvic viscera.

Innervation: fibers from lower sacral spinal nerves.

*For details of these muscles and others related to the anal and urogenital regions, see an anatomy textbook.

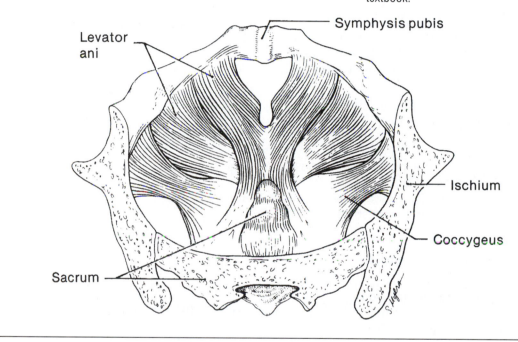

Levator ani

Symphysis pubis

Ischium

Coccygeus

Sacrum

■ **Student Activities and Exercise 34**

1. In Figure 34–1, color fibers of rectus abdominis and external abdominal oblique pink. Be sure to leave the linea alba and tendinous intersections uncolored.
2. In Figure 34–2, color fibers of internal abdominal oblique red and those of transverse abdominis pink.
3. In Figure 34–3, color the inguinal ligament and the superficial and deep inguinal ring yellow.
4. In Figure 34–4, color the quadratus lumborum pink. Number the lumbar vertebrae.
5. In Figure 34–5, color the pelvic diaphragm pink.
6. Answer the following questions:
   a. What is the innervation of the muscles of the abdominal wall? _____
   b. Are they autonomic or somatic? _____
   c. Name the structures you would find going from superficial to deep if you entered the body just lateral to rectus abdominis: skin, fascia, _____ m., _____ m., and _____ m.
   d. What three structures would you encounter if you dissected deep to the skin just lateral to the linea alba? _____, _____ m., and _____.
      (**Hint:** The first and the last are fascial layers.)

Digestive System and Peritoneum

A large portion of the abdomen is filled with structures of the digestive system. Food is changed both physically and chemically by this system to provide nutrients for proper functioning of all body cells.

■ OBJECTIVES

1. State the general purpose of the digestive system.
2. Name, identify, and state the major function of each part of the alimentary canal.
3. Describe the general histology of the digestive tube.
4. Name, identify, and state the anatomic position and function of the accessory digestive organs found in the abdomen.
5. Define peritoneum; state its two major functions.
6. Describe the mesenteries related to each organ.

■ METHODS

1. Observe the demonstration of each abdominal muscle and organ.
2. Observe the peritoneal structures presented.
3. After the demonstrations, find each structure on other material in the lab.
4. Complete the student activities as you study the lesson.

FUNCTIONS OF THE DIGESTIVE SYSTEM

1. **Ingestion**—taking the food into the body.
2. **Digestion**—changing the food product both physically and chemically so that it is broken down into molecules.
3. **Absorption**—taking the molecules (nutrients) and most of the fluid into the blood stream.
4. **Elimination**—removal of the solid waste.

A. DIVISIONS OF THE ABDOMEN

Dividing the abdomen into four quadrants is one method used to describe the location of abdominal viscera. Fill in the key below as you study the organs that are located in each quadrant.

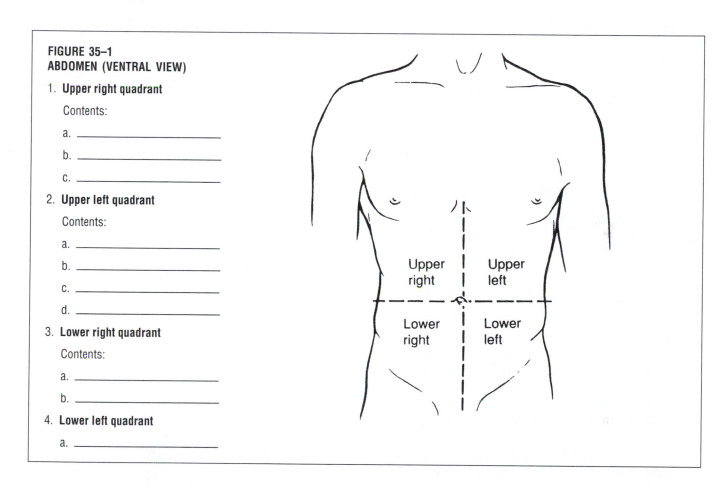

FIGURE 35–1
ABDOMEN (VENTRAL VIEW)

1. **Upper right quadrant**

   Contents:

   a. _____

   b. _____

   c. _____

2. **Upper left quadrant**

   Contents:

   a. _____

   b. _____

   c. _____

   d. _____

3. **Lower right quadrant**

   Contents:

   a. _____

   b. _____

4. **Lower left quadrant**

   a. _____

Upper
right

Upper
left

Lower
right

Lower
left

■ CLINICAL COMMENTS

 Appendicitis, an inflammation of the appendix, often causes sharp pain that is localized in the lower right quadrant of the abdomen. Initially, the infection may produce toxins that cause nausea and vomiting. Appendicitis often requires surgical removal of the appendix.

B. THE ALIMENTARY CANAL

This is the passageway from the mouth to the anus. In the mouth, the teeth begin the physical breakdown of food; saliva, produced by **salivary glands,** initiates the digestion of carbohydrates. The food, now called a **bolus,** passes into the **pharynx,** the beginning of the mucous membrane–lined alimentary canal, or gastrointestinal (GI) tract. This lining produces mucus to lubricate the bolus for passage through the digestive tract.

FIGURE 35–2
DIGESTIVE TUBE

1. **Pharynx**—shared passageway of respiratory and digestive systems.

2. **Esophagus**—the direct continuation of the pharynx. This muscular tube collapses unless a bolus of food is being squeezed through by **peristalsis,** the action of the longitudinal and circular muscles located in the wall. The esophagus passes through the thorax and pierces the diaphragm.

3. **Stomach**—located largely in the upper left quadrant of the abdomen. Important in storage of food (holds about 1 liter). Some chemical change occurs here. Protein digestion begins.

4. **Small intestine**—approx. 16 feet of convoluted tube. This is the site of most of the chemical change as well as absorption of nutrients and liquid by capillaries.

    The **duodenum,** about 10 in. long, is the shortest and most fixed segment. The accessory organs empty their digestive juices into this segment of the tube.

    Next, is the **jejunum,** approximately 2/5 of the tube. The **ileum,** the remaining 3/5, terminates at the ileocecal junction.

5. **Large intestine,** or colon. Although some absorption of fluid occurs here, mostly solid waste remains in this portion of the tube. (See Figure 35-8.)

6. **Anal canal,** passage for the elimination of solid waste.

Note: The three accessory digestive organs within the abdomen, *liver, gall bladder,* and *pancreas,* can also be seen in this figure.

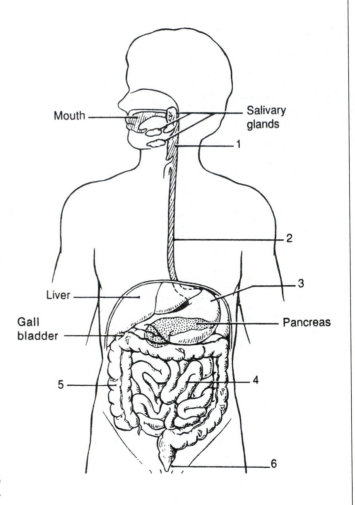

Mouth — Salivary glands — 1 — 2 — 3 — Liver — Gall bladder — Pancreas — 5 — 4 — 6

C. THE PERITONEUM

This is a serous sac similar to the pleura and pericardium. The peritoneum provides the serous fluid to lubricate the organs within the abdominopelvic cavity. All abdominal organs lie outside this sac but project inward, carrying peritoneum with them. Double folds, or reflections, of peritoneum connect the organs to the body wall or to each other and often provide passageway for vessels, nerves, and lymphatics. The serous fluid produced by this membrane is important for two reasons: (1) it allows organs to move against each other without causing friction, and (2) it prevents fusion of these organs to each other or the body wall.

Organs that do not need to move as they function are not surrounded by this membrane. They lie behind the peritoneal sac and are, therefore, referred to as **retroperitoneal.**

The *spleen* is covered by peritoneum and is seen in the upper left quadrant near the fundus of the stomach. It is not a digestive organ, however. It is a lymphatic structure.

FIGURE 35-3
SCHEMATIC REPRESENTATION OF PERITONEUM:
TRANSVERSE SECTION OF ABDOMEN (INFERIOR VIEW)

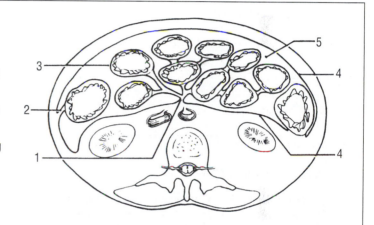

1. **Mesentery (proper)**—double fold of peritoneum that holds the small intestine to the posterior abdominal wall.

2. **Mesocolon**—double fold of peritoneum. Holds colon to the abdominal wall.

3. **Visceral peritoneum**—the layer of peritoneum surrounding the organ.

4. **Parietal peritoneum**—lines the abdominal wall. Retroperitoneal organs, kidney, adrenal glands, and aorta, can be seen posterior to this lining. Other retroperitoneal organs include the pancreas and most of the duodenum as well as portions of the colon.

5. **Peritoneal cavity,** or **potential space** inside the peritoneal sac and extending from the diaphragm to the pelvic floor. Although space does not actually exist because the organs fill it, the visceral peritoneum surrounding each organ would allow the organs to be easily separated by injected fluid.

■ CLINICAL COMMENTS

In addition to x-rays, technology now includes other noninvasive ways to view the body. Magnetic resonance imaging **(MRI)** and computerized tomography **(CT scans)** have changed the way cross sections are viewed. (The old orientation can be viewed in the lower limb, Figures 6–4 and 7–1.) We now look at the inferior view with the posterior body at the bottom of the picture. The right side of the body is on the left side of the picture. Figures 35–3, 36–1, and 41–3 are in this new orientation.

FIGURE 35–4
PERITONEUM (LATERAL VIEW)

1. **Coronary ligament**—attaches liver to diaphragm.

2. **Lesser omentum**—double fold of peritoneum between lesser curvature of stomach and liver.

3. **Visceral peritoneum**

4. **Parietal peritoneum**

5. **Greater omentum**—reflection of peritoneum hanging from greater curvature of stomach. This is often called the omental apron.

6. **Mesentery (proper)** holding the small intestine to the posterior body wall.

7. **Mesocolon**

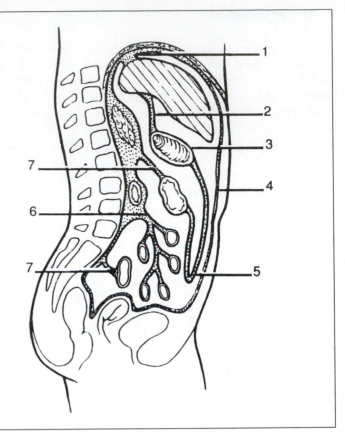

■ CLINICAL COMMENTS

Peritonitis, an inflammation of the peritoneum, can affect all the organs within the abdomen and result in death if the peritoneal structures do not succeed in sealing off the infected area and/or massive doses of antibiotics are not effective. Some causes of peritonitis are ruptured appendix, perforated ulcer, and piercing wounds of the abdomen. As you look at the extent of the peritoneal sac, you can see that any infection has the potential to affect many organs.

■ Student Activity

With a colored pencil, trace the extent of the peritoneal sac beginning with the #4 label line on the parietal peritoneum.

D. ORGANS OF DIGESTION

Each organ of the digestive system has a specific function in the conversion of food. The general histology of the alimentary canal is the same throughout, but there are differences in each region depending on its function. The histology of a typical digestive tube segment consists of:

mucosa—the lining of the lumen

submucosa—may contain mucous glands, vessels

muscularis—longitudinal and circular layers of smooth muscle that help propel food product

serosa or *adventitia*—the outer covering of most of the tube within the peritoneum; or the connective tissue if not covered by the serous membrane

---

FIGURE 35–5
THE STOMACH AND DUODENUM

1. **Fundus,** pouches up and to the left.

2. **Cardia,** area of entrance to the stomach. Contains a sphincter muscle to help prevent backflow of **chyme,** partially digested, semiliquid form of food.

3. **Lesser curvature**

4. Muscular layer, **muscularis**—consists of 3 layers (longitudinal, circular and oblique).

5. **Greater curvature**

6. **Rugae,** folds within the stomach body covered by the mucosal lining layer, **mucosa.**

7. **Pylorus,** last portion of stomach. Contains a sphincter muscle.

8. **Duodenal papilla,** at entrance of ducts for accessory digestive organs. The duodenum receives the enzymes and bile to be mixed with the chyme as it continues in the small intestine.

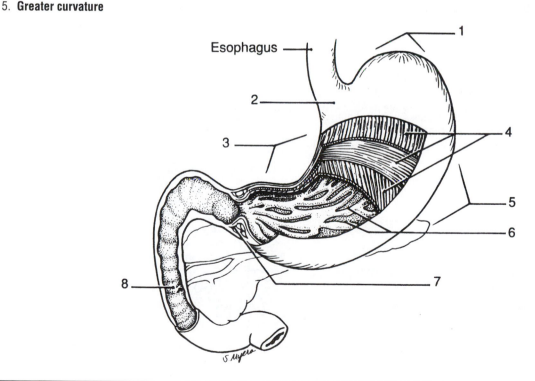

FIGURE 35–6
TRANSVERSE SECTION OF SMALL INTESTINE

Because most chemical digestion occurs in the small intestine, the histology is very important here.

1. **Mesentery (proper)**—the double fold of peritoneum that holds the small intestine to the body wall.

2. **Serosa**—visceral peritoneum (not on esophagus)

3. **Muscularis**—muscle layer composed of inner circular fibers to narrow the lumen and longitudinal outer fibers to shorten the tube. (A third, oblique layer exists in the stomach.)

4. **Submucosa**—layer of connective tissue where blood vessels, nerves, and glands are located.

5. **Mucosa**—innermost layer of the tract. It is composed of a superficial epithelium and glandular cells that secrete mucus and digestive juices. (Only mucus is secreted by the esophagus and colon.)

6. **Plicae circulares**—folds of mucosa and submucosa that increase the surface area of the small intestine for greater absorption. It is illustrated in Figure 35–7.

NOTE: The parasympathetic innervation of the small and large intestine is by way of the **vagus nerve** and the **pelvic splanchnic nerves,** sacral levels 2–4. The preganglionic processes of these nerves synapse on ganglia that are located within the walls of the digestive tube.

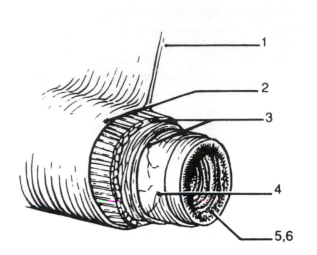

FIGURE 35–7
SECTION OF PLICA CIRCULARES

This section shows specializations of the mucosa layer that are needed to increase its surface area. This is important because of the digestive and absorptive functions of this portion of the tube.

The plicae circulares—large, permanent folds of the entire thickness of the mucosa—contain a core of submucosa.

1. **Serosa** (visceral peritoneum)

2. **Muscularis**

3. **Mucosa and submucosa**

4. **Villi,** finger-like projections of mucosa containing blood vessels and a lymphatic vessel.

5. **Microvilli** are projections from all the epithelial (lining) cells.

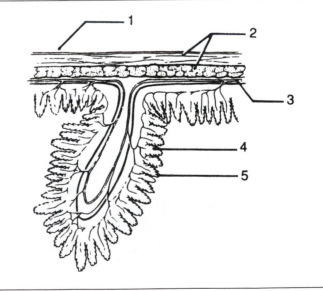

FIGURE 35–8
LARGE INTESTINE

1. **Vermiform appendix,** small tag of intestine extending from cecum in lower right quadrant

2. **Cecum,** pouch-like origin of the colon. Found in the lower right quadrant.

3. **Ascending colon**

4. **Hepatic flexure,** the bend in the colon near the liver (in the upper right quadrant)

5. **Traverse colon**

6. **Splenic flexure,** bend in colon near the spleen (in the upper left quadrant)

7. **Descending colon**

8. **Sigmoid colon,** where S-shape leads to rectum

9. **Rectum,** a pelvic organ, begins about the third sacral level

Three special characteristics of the colon are:

10. **Teniae coli,** continuous bands of muscle

11. **Epiploic appendage,** fat tags

   Haustra coli are are the sac-like pouches seen on the entire length of the large intestine. They are created because the *tenia coli* are shorter than the tube.

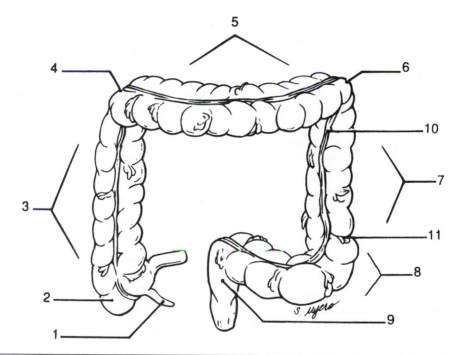

■ **Student Activities**

Color the teniae coli pink; the epiploic appendages yellow; choose one haustra coli from the transverse colon and color it blue.

ACCESSORY DIGESTIVE ORGANS

In the abdomen there are three accessory digestive organs. They are connected to the digestive tube by way of ducts that empty into the duodenum.

The liver, located in the upper right quadrant, is the largest internal organ. It produces bile that is needed to emulsify (break down into smaller droplets) fat.

The gall bladder lies on the inferior surface of the liver and its only function is to concentrate and store the excess bile produced by the liver.

The pancreas is located deep to the stomach in the upper left quadrant. The head of the pancreas lies in the crook of the duodenum (Figure 35–9); its body is deep to the stomach, and its tail is near the spleen (Figure 36–3). The pancreas is both an endocrine (no ducts) and exocrine gland. In the digestive system, it serves as an exocrine gland and produces digestive enzymes that are delivered to the duodenum by way of a duct system. These pancreatic enzymes digest fats (lipases), carbohydrates (carbohydrases) and proteins (proteases, peptidases).

FIGURE 35–9
DUCT SYSTEM FOR ACCESSORY DIGESTIVE ORGANS

1. **Left hepatic duct**—because the right and left lobes of the liver function independently, bile is carried by two ducts.

2. **Right hepatic duct**

3. **Common hepatic duct**—formed when the right and left hepatic ducts join.

4. **Cystic duct**—connects gall bladder to bile ducts.

5. **Common bile duct**—carries bile from liver or gall bladder to the duodenum. Formed when cystic and common hepatic ducts join.

6. **Duodenal papilla**—site of sphincter muscle and common entrance of ducts.

7. **Pancreatic duct**—carries digestive enzymes produced by the pancreas to the duodenum.

8. **Tail of pancreas**—located near the spleen.

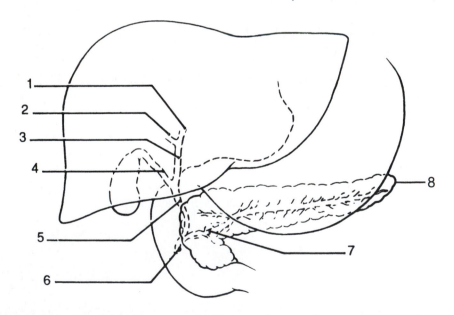

■ **Student Activities**
Color green the gall bladder and all ducts that carry bile. Color the pancreatic duct yellow.

FIGURE 35–10
THE LIVER (ANTERIOR VIEW)

With peritoneal reflections and related structures

1. **Coronary ligament** is a reflection of the peritoneum onto the inferior diaphragm. The anterior and posterior reflections leave a portion of the superior liver uncovered by serous membrane. This portion of the liver is called the **"bare area"** and it fuses to the diaphragm.

2. **Falciform ligament** holds liver to the anterior abdominal wall and divides the liver into right and left lobes.

3. **Left lobe** covered with visceral peritoneum.

4. **Right lobe** covered with visceral peritoneum.

5. **Ligamentum teres hepatis** is the remnant of the fetal umbilical vein.

6. **Gall bladder**

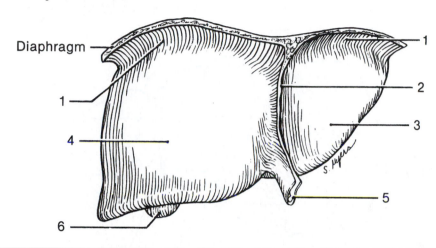

FIGURE 35–11
THE LIVER (SUPERIOR VIEW)

If you free the liver from the diaphragm and tip it toward you, you see this view.

1. **Bare area.** Bare of peritoneum, this was fused to the diaphragm.

2. **Inferior vena cava** indents the posterior liver

3. **Hepatic veins** will enter IVC (see Figure 36–6)

4. **Falciform ligament**

5. **Coronary ligament** serves to attach the liver to the diaphragm

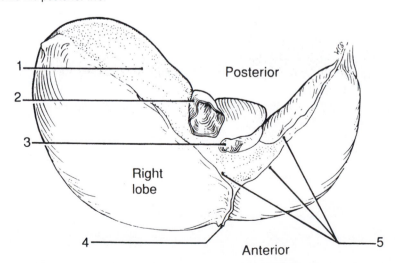

FIGURE 35–12
THE LIVER (INFERIOR VIEW)

With the liver tipped up, you see this view.

1. **Gall bladder.** The fundus can be seen from the anterior view. If the liver is tipped up so that the inferior view is seen, the entire gall bladder with the duct system can be seen.

2. _____

3. **Portal vein** enters at the porta. It brings in blood rich in nutrients from the intestines and with toxic substances from the spleen.

4. **Inferior vena cava (IVC)**—the liver lies against the posterior body wall and therefore against the IVC, which causes an indentation.

5. **Ligamentum teres hepatis**

6. **Proper hepatic a.** can be seen entering this area of the liver called the **porta,** or entrance.

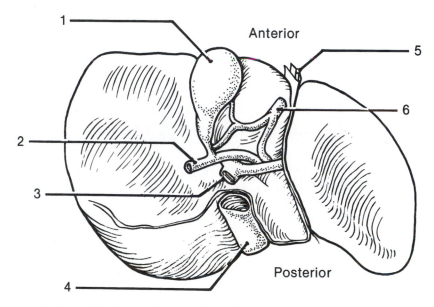

Schematic illustration of the histology of the liver is shown in Figure 36–7.

■ Student Activities

1. Be sure you have filled in the content lines for Figure 35–1. Lightly sketch those organs in the correct location.

2. In Figure 35–2, color each named segment of the alimentary canal a different color. (Use the same color for jejunum and ileum.)

3. In Figure 35–3, place the letters **R, L, A,** and **P** to indicate right, left, anterior, and posterior positions on the illustration.

4. In Figure 35–12, complete the key. Color the arteries red; the veins blue; the ducts green.

Exercise Thirty-Five

Name _____

1. Label each structure in the illustration at the right.

   a. _____

   b. _____

   c. _____

   d. _____

   e. _____

   f. _____

   g. _____

   h. _____

2. Fill the blank with a letter from the column on the right. Use each letter only once.

   _____ 1. liver   a. lower left quadrant

   _____ 2. spleen   b. food storage

   _____ 3. pancreas   c. retroperitoneal

   _____ 4. cecum   d. bile storage

   _____ 5. sigmoid colon e. lower right quadrant

   _____ 6. jejunum   f. thoracic structure

   _____ 7. stomach   g. largest organ in body

   _____ 8. gall bladder   h. pelvic organ

   _____ 9. rectum   i. lymphatic organ

   _____ 10. esophagus   j. chemical digestion

3. Name three distinguishing characteristics of the large intestine.

a. _____

b. _____

c. _____

4. Fill in the blank with the appropriate peritoneal structure.

_____ a. holds small intestine to the posterior body wall.

_____ b. covers most digestive organs as well as the spleen.

_____ c. hangs from the greater curvature of the stomach.

_____ d. attachment between liver and anterior abdominal wall.

_____ e. found between the lesser curvature of the stomach and the liver.

_____ f. attaches from colon to body wall.

_____ g. lines the wall of the abdomen.

_____ h. attaches liver to diaphragm.

5. Name one ligament related to the liver that is not a peritoneal structure. _____ What is it? _____

6. In the process of digestion several things must occur. Fill in the chart below to indicate the site of each named function. (Choose from the following: mouth, esophagus, stomach, small intestine, large intestine, anus.)

Functions of the Digestive Organs	Organ(s) Where Specific Function Occurs
1. Ingestion (taking food into the body)	a. _____
2. Peristalsis	b. _____ c. _____ d. _____ e. _____
3. Mechanical breakdown	f. _____ g. _____
4. Chemical breakdown (digestive juices added)	h. _____ i. _____ j. _____
5. Absorption of nutrients (major site)	k. _____
6. Elimination of wastes	l. _____

Vessels and Nerves of the Abdomen and Pelvis

The blood supply and the innervation of the parietal abdomen are different from that of the abdominal viscera. We will consider the parietal (walls) abdomen first; it will provide a "room" in which we can place the organs.

■ OBJECTIVES

1. Name the major blood vessels of the walls of the abdomen.
2. Name paired vessels that supply the abdominal and pelvic viscera.
3. Describe the three major midline arterial trunks and list the organs supplied by each.
4. List the tributaries of the inferior vena cava (IVC).
5. Describe the anatomy and major purpose of the hepatic portal system.
6. State the general distribution of the autonomic nerves to the abdominal and pelvic viscera.

■ METHODS

1. Study the information presented and perform the indicated activities.
2. Observe the demonstrations of vessels.
3. Name each vessel seen on the models in the lab.
4. Sketch the aorta and all its major branches, indicating the distribution of each.
5. Sketch the hepatic portal system.

Innervation of the parietal abdomen is the same as of abdominal muscles; regular somatic nerves, T7–L2, provide both the motor and sensory innervation to the walls. You will be able to complete the chart below as you study this unit.

TABLE 36–1. BLOOD SUPPLY AND INNERVATION OF THE ABDOMEN

	Parietal supply	Visceral supply
Vessels		
Nerves	Ventral rami T7–L2	

A. MAJOR ARTERIES OF THE ABDOMEN

The major blood supply to the parietal abdomen includes a ventral source of blood from the superior and inferior epigastric arteries and a dorsal source of blood from the aorta. Branches from these vessels travel through the abdominal wall and anastomose.

FIGURE 36–1
TRANSVERSE SECTION OF ABDOMEN (INFERIOR VIEW)

1. **Abdominal aorta**—extends from diaphragm to the fourth lumbar vertebra, where it bifurcates.

2. **Lumbar a.**—four pairs leave postero-lateral aorta. (Accompanied by lumbar v.)

3. **Inferior epigastric a.**—a branch from external iliac a. The superior epigastric a. is in this position if the section is more superior. These vessels travel between rectus abdominis m. and the posterior rectus sheath.

4. **Lumbar vein**

5. **Inferior vena cava**

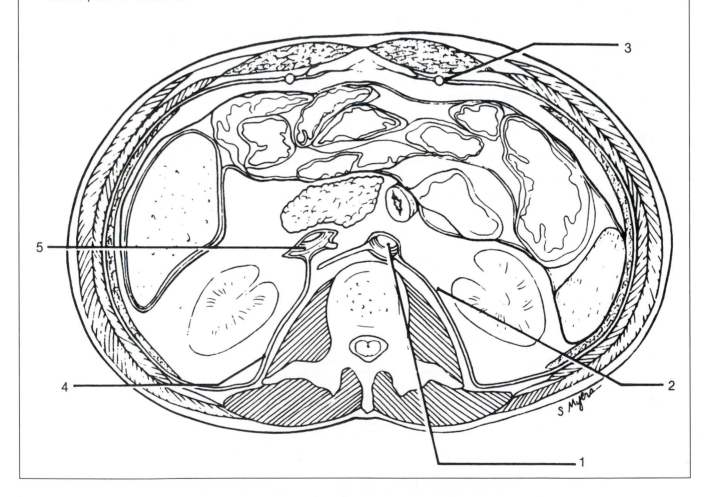

■ **Student Activities**

In Figure 36–1, color the labeled arteries with red and the labeled veins blue.

Place the letters **R, L, A,** and **P** to indicate right, left, anterior, and posterior positions on the illustration.

FIGURE 36–2
ABDOMINAL AORTA

1. **Internal thoracic a.**—this branch of the subclavian a. bifurcates to become the **musculophrenic a.** to help supply the diaphragm and the **superior epigastric a.** to help supply the anterior abdominal wall.

2. **Inferior phrenic a.**—helps supply diaphragm.

3. **Lumbar a.**

4. **Median sacral a.**—from the posterior aorta. This small vessel and branches from the internal iliac a. supply the pelvic wall and pelvic diaphragm.

5. **Inferior epigastric a.**

6. **Internal iliac a.**

7. **Celiac trunk**—single trunk with three major branches (details in Figure 36–3)

8. **Superior mesenteric a.**—single vessel that travels in the mesentery (Figure 36–4)

9. **Renal a.**—paired vessels that supply the kidneys

10. **Gonadal a.**—paired vessels that supply the testes or ovaries

11. **Inferior mesenteric a.**—single trunk (Figure 36–4)

Note: Nos. 1–5 are parietal; 6–11 are visceral.

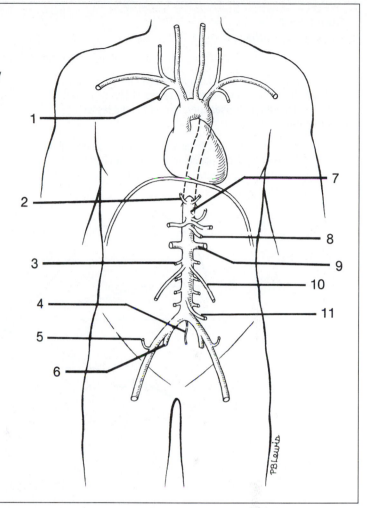

■ CLINICAL COMMENTS

The aorta is a common site for the occurrence of an **aneurysm,** a weak area in the wall of an artery that causes it to bulge out like a balloon. Atherosclerosis, trauma, and congenital weakness of vessel walls are some of the causes. Aneurysms may interfere with blood supply, damage tissue nearby by pressing against it, or burst. In the brain, an aneurysm can cause a stroke.

FIGURE 36–3
THE CELIAC TRUNK

1. **Celiac trunk**—comes off the aorta just below the diaphragm.

2. **Left gastric a.**—smallest branch. Runs up to the left, where it supplies some esophagus and cardia of stomach; it then branches onto the lesser curvature within the lesser omentum.

3. **Splenic a.**—largest branch; very tortuous as it passes along the upper border of the pancreas. Sends branches to spleen, pancreas, greater curvature of the stomach.

4. **Common hepatic a.**—bifurcates to:
   a. **Gastroduodenal a.** to stomach and duodenum.

   b. **Proper hepatic a.** divides to become

      · left hepatic a. to left lobe of liver

      · right hepatic a. to right lobe of liver and its branch, the

   c. **cystic a.** (c.) to the gall bladder

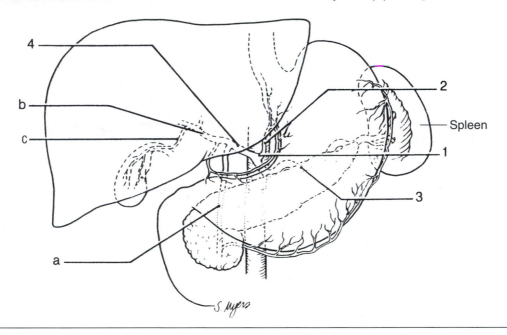

■ CLINICAL COMMENTS

Cirrhosis is a liver disease in which functional liver cells (hepatocytes) are destroyed and replaced with connective tissue. It can be caused by viral infection or exposure to chemicals such as alcohol. Cirrhosis can be a fatal disease because the liver is a vital organ.

Liver functions: include production of bile, pickup and storage of nutrients, detoxification of ingested substances such as drugs and alcohol, metabolism of proteins, and production of blood clotting factors.

FIGURE 36–4
SUPERIOR AND INFERIOR MESENTERIC ARTERIES

1. **Superior mesenteric a.**—comes off the aorta about 1 cm below the celiac trunk. It supplies all the small intestine except upper part of the duodenum. It also supplies the cecum, ascending colon, and about 2/3 of the transverse colon.

2. **Ileocolic a.**—branch that runs toward the ileocecal junction.

3. **Right colic a.**—branches toward ascending colon.

4. **Middle colic a.**—branches toward transverse colon.

5. **Branches of superior mesenteric a.**—to all the jejunum and ileum. *These branches travel in the mesentery and form many arching, anastomosing branches. This is very important to provide an adequate supply of vessels to absorb fluids and nutrients.*

6. **Inferior mesenteric a.**—arises about 3 cm above the bifurcation of aorta. Supplies the left third of the transverse colon, the descending colon, the sigmoid colon, and the superior part of the rectum.

7. **Left colic a.**—branches anastomose with those of the middle colic.

8. **Sigmoid branches**

9. **Superior rectal a.**—terminal branch

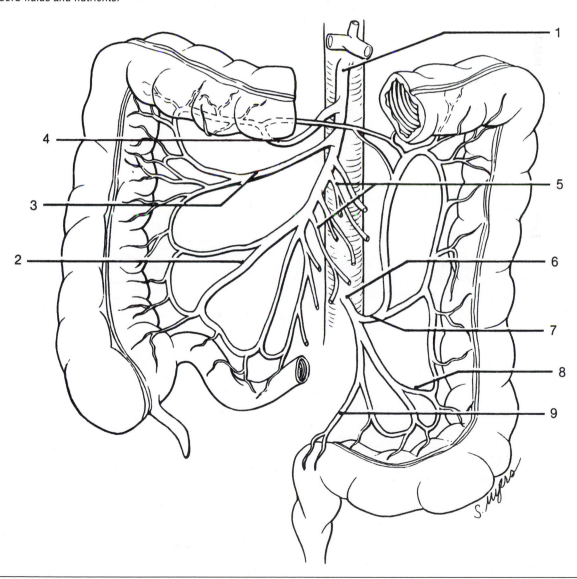

B. INNERVATION OF THE ABDOMINAL VISCERA

The innervation of the abdominal viscera is included before we consider the venous return of the blood. This is done because the autonomic fibers that provide sympathetic and parasympathetic innervation for these viscera travel on arteries. Therefore, if you have learned the distribution of vessels, it helps you understand the nerve supply. (Review Lesson 32.)

1. **Sympathetic nerve supply**—collateral ganglia for synapse of the thoracic and lumbar splanchnic nerves are: (a) celiac ganglia; (b) superior mesenteric ganglia; and (c) inferior mesenteric ganglia. The postsynaptic fibers leave these ganglia and travel to the effector organs on the arteries supplying the viscera.
2. **Parasympathetic nerve supply** is by way of the:
   a. **Vagus n.** passes into the abdomen as a plexus on the esophagus. It reaches the celiac trunk and superior mesenteric arteries and is distributed to the organs supplied by them. **Remember:** These are presynaptic fibers that will not synapse until they reach the walls of the organs.
   b. **Sacral parasympathetics** are distributed to the organs supplied by the inferior mesenteric artery.

C. MAJOR VEINS OF THE ABDOMEN

These are almost all tributaries of the inferior vena cava. A very important exception involves the hepatic portal system.

FIGURE 36–5
INFERIOR VENA CAVA: WITH MAJOR TRIBUTARIES

1. **Common iliac. v.**

2. **Median sacral v.**

3. **Inferior vena cava**—formed when the common iliac veins join. It lies just to the right of the aorta and in front of the vertebral column. It carries all the blood below the diaphragm back to the right atrium.

4. **Gonadal v.**—notice that the left gonadal v. empties its blood into the left renal v. because it is a more direct route.

5. **Lumbar veins**—from parietal abdomen.

6. **Renal v.**—bringing blood from the kidneys.

7. **Hepatic vs.**—very short since the liver lies against the IVC.

■ **Student Activities**

In Figure 36–5, color the veins blue; label the veins indicated by letters.

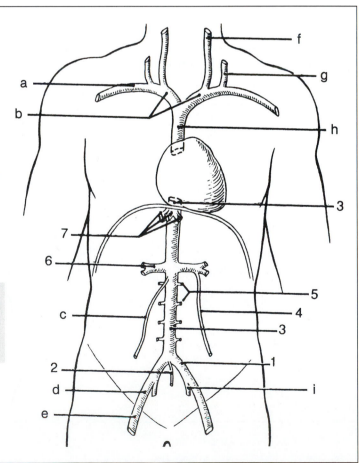

D. HEPATIC PORTAL SYSTEM

The tributaries of the IVC do not include any of the veins from the digestive organs or from the spleen. These veins are tributaries of the **portal vein.** The portal v. will take this blood to the liver to be filtered before it enters the IVC by way of the hepatic veins. Several functions of the liver make this necessary.

In addition to producing bile, the liver breaks down toxic substances from food products and from products of the spleen; it also stores vitamins and processes nutrients for storage and for use by the body.

FIGURE 36–6
THE PORTAL VEIN

1. **Portal v.**—formed when the superior mesenteric v. and the splenic v. join.

2. **Splenic v.**—contains products of blood cell destruction; the **bilirubin** from the breakdown of hemoglobin from red blood cells is an important component of bile.

3. **Superior mesenteric v.**—contains most of the nutrients produced by the digestive process and most of the liquid consumed.

4. **Inferior mesenteric v.**

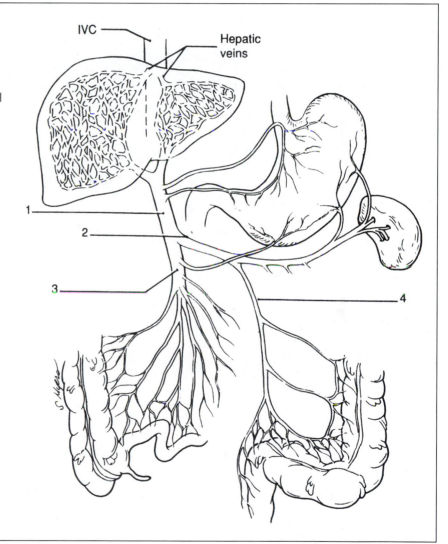

FIGURE 36–7
LIVER HISTOLOGY (SCHEMATIC)

This microscopic view shows two of the liver lobules; there are approximately 200,000 of these in the liver. A hepatic triad at each corner of each lobule (typically hexagonal) consists of a branch of the hepatic artery, a branch of the portal vein, and a bile ductule that collects bile being produced by liver cells. Blood from branches of both the hepatic arteries and the portal vein fills the sinusoids, capillary-like spaces that allow passage of materials into and out of hepatocytes. In the center of each lobule is a central vein that collects the blood from sinusoids and takes it to the hepatic veins. Hepatic vein blood enters the inferior vena cava.

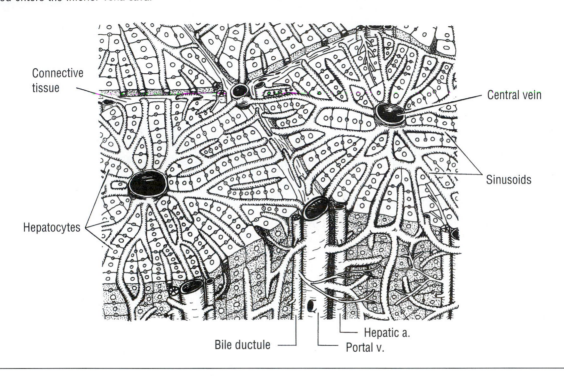

Connective tissue

Central vein

Sinusoids

Hepatocytes

Bile ductule

Hepatic a.

Portal v.

■ Student Activities

1. In Figure 36–2, use red to color the aorta from the heart to the bifurcation into common iliac arteries. Color all parietal arteries red. With a pink pencil, color all paired and single arteries that provide blood to viscera.

2. In Figure 36–3, color all arteries red; the liver and the spleen brown; the gall bladder green.

3. In Figure 36–4, color arteries red; label the celiac trunk.

4. In Figure 36–6, color the liver and the spleen brown. Color the splenic v., the superior mesenteric v., and the portal v. blue. The other veins of the digestive system feed into this system.

5. List the vessels that would be needed to take the blood from the heart to the small intestines and back to the heart.

6. In Figure 36–7, color arteries red, veins blue, and bile ductules green. Place arrows in liver sinusoids to show direction of blood flow.

Name _____

1. Matching exercise. Choose a vessel from the column on the right to supply the organ on the left. Use each letter only once.

_____ 1. stomach   a. superior rectal a.

_____ 2. liver   b. left colic a.

_____ 3. spleen   c. ileocolic a.

_____ 4. ascending colon   d. renal a.

_____ 5. descending colon   e. gonadal a.

_____ 6. gall bladder   f. cystic a.

_____ 7. rectum   g. proper hepatic a.

_____ 8. kidney   h. splenic a.

_____ 9. ovary   i. right colic a.

_____10. appendix   j. left gastric a.

2. a.   List four abdominal veins that are tributaries of the portal vein.

      1. _____   3. _____

      2. _____   4. _____

   b. Why is the portal vein so important?

3. Give the autonomic innervation for the following organs. For the sympathetic supply, name the ganglia where the splanchnic n. synapses. For the parasympathetic supply, choose either the vagus n. or the sacral level parasympathetics, S2–4.

	Sympathetic	Parasympathetic
a. stomach	_____	_____
b. small intestine	_____	_____
c. descending colon	_____	_____
d. ascending colon	_____	_____
e. duodenum	_____	_____
f. liver	_____	_____
g. rectum	_____	_____
h. transverse colon	_____	_____

4. **In Figure 36–8,** a schematic view of the abdominal vessels:

1) Color red all abdominal vessels with high O_2 content; color those with high CO_2 content blue.

2) **Label:** aorta, IVC, renal artery and veins, celiac trunk, gonadal artery and vein, common iliac artery and vein, common hepatic artery and right and left hepatic veins, superior and inferior mesenteric arteries. (Use Figures 36–2 and 36–5 if you need help.)

FIGURE 36–8

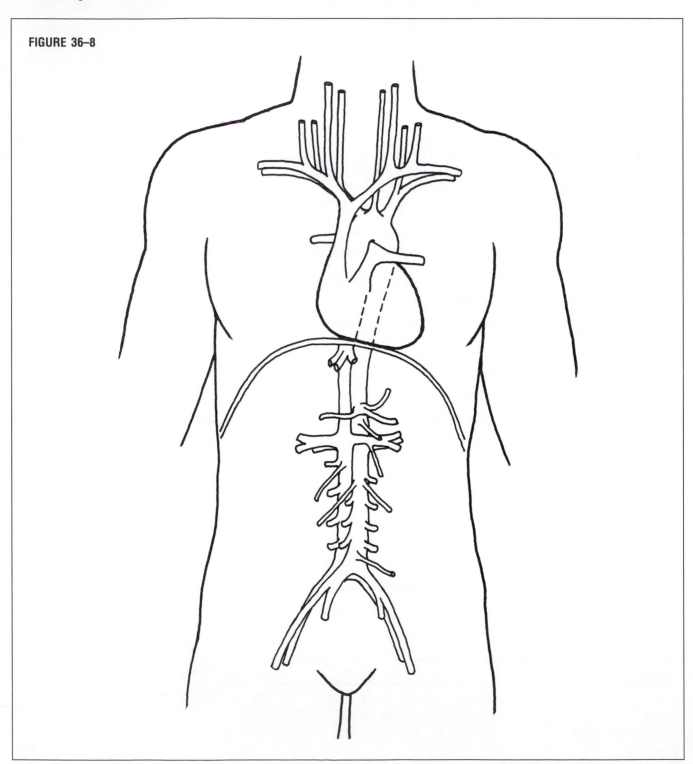

Lesson 37

The Urinary System

The blood picks up excess fluid (mainly from the intestines) and waste products of protein metabolism as it travels to all cells of the body. The urinary system serves a vital function in filtering the blood to rid the body of these substances.

■ OBJECTIVES

1. State the functions of the urinary system.
2. Name the organs of the urinary system and the major function of each.
3. Describe the gross anatomy of the kidney.
4. Identify each structure, in sequence, in the path of urine.
5. Describe the nephron.
6. Name each vessel needed to get the blood from the renal a., to the nephron, to the renal v.

■ METHODS

1. Study this unit, performing the indicated activities.
2. Observe each structure of the urinary system.
3. Identify each urinary structure visible on the x-rays.
4. Sketch a section of kidney. Include all structures visible grossly.

A. FUNCTIONS OF THE URINARY SYSTEM

1. Cleans blood of toxic waste of protein metabolism.
2. Converts waste into urine and eliminates it from the body.
3. Helps regulate fluid balance.
4. Helps maintain acid–base balance.

■ CLINICAL COMMENTS

If the kidneys are diseased and unable to function, **hemodialysis** (dialysis) may be used to remove the toxic wastes from the blood. This type of dialysis is performed by filtering blood through a machine.

B. ORGANS OF THE URINARY SYSTEM

These are shown in Figure 37–1.

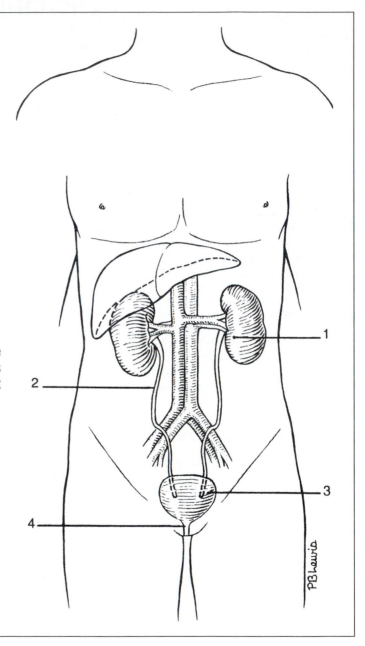

FIGURE 37–1
ORGANS OF THE URINARY SYSTEM

1. **Kidney**—paired, bean-shaped structures, reddish brown in color because of their vascularity. Located retroperitoneally between the 12th thoracic and third lumbar vertebrae, they are partially protected by ribs 11 and 12. The kidney on the right is slightly lower because of the space occupied by the liver.

2. **Ureter**—muscular tube (10–12 in.); propels urine to the urinary bladder.

3. **Urinary bladder**—a hollow muscular organ situated in the pelvis just behind the symphysis pubis. It is the storage vessel for urine before it is expelled from the body.

4. **Urethra**—tubular structure for the passage of urine from the bladder out of the body. Much shorter in the female than the male. (See Lesson 38.).

■ CLINICAL COMMENTS

Cystitis, an infection of the lining of the urinary bladder, may be caused by bacteria or chemicals. It is more frequent in females because the urethra is shorter, and bacteria can enter the tract more easily.

■ **Student Activities**
In Figure 37–1, color kidneys brown; arteries red; veins blue; ureter and urethra yellow.

FIGURE 37–2
KIDNEY: CORONAL SECTION

1. **Renal cortex**—the outer layer

2. **Renal medulla**—inner layer. It contains the cone-shaped renal pyramids. In this type of section they appear to be pyramids.

3. **Renal pyramid**—made up of many microscopic collecting ducts (see Figure 37–4).

4. **Renal papilla**—the tip of a pyramid. Urine passes out from this site.

5. **Minor calyx**—funnel-shaped connective tissue structure that slips over the tip of the pyramid to receive the urine from the papilla.

6. **Major calyx**—2 or 3 of these are formed when minor calyces join.

7. **Renal pelvis** is formed when the major calyces join. Urine collects here and then passes into the ureter.

8. **Ureter**

9. **Hilus**—the entrance into the medial, concave area. The tubes carrying urine, the nerves, lymph, and blood vessels enter and leave at this site.

10. **Renal sinus**—fat-filled space between the tissue of the kidney and the renal pelvis.

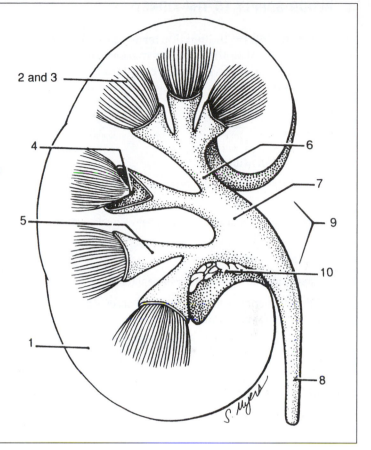

C. BLOOD SUPPLY TO THE KIDNEY

This is provided by the renal arteries, branches that come off the aorta about 1 cm below and lateral to the superior mesenteric a.

 The entire blood volume is circulated through the kidney about 60 times each day. (Autonomic nerves help regulate blood flow.)

FIGURE 37–3
KIDNEY CIRCULATION

1. **Renal a.**—enters the hilus between the vein and the renal pelvis

2. **Interlobar a.**—branches that pass between pyramids to reach the cortex

3. **Arcuate a.**—arch over pyramids

4. **Interlobular a.**—passes between nephrons

5. **Afferent arteriole**—the vessel that will become a capillary tuft called the **glomerulus**

6. **Interlobar v.**—formed when tiny venules join

7. **Renal v.**—takes blood to the inferior vena cava

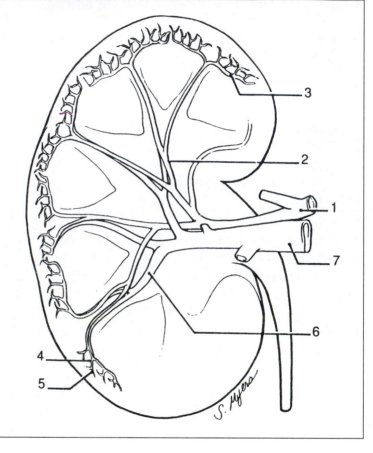

D. THE NEPHRON

The nephron, Figure 37–4, is the functional unit of the kidney. There are about 1 million of these microscopic units in the cortex of each kidney. The kidneys filter about 180 liters of fluid each day but conserve 99% of it. (The body contains only about 42 liters of fluid.) Each nephron consists of a long, thin tubule with a cup-shaped indentation in the closed end in which a capillary tuft is located. The open end empties into a collecting duct.

FIGURE 37–4
SCHEMATIC ILLUSTRATION OF THE NEPHRON

1. **Afferent arteriole**—brings blood to Bowman's capsule.

2. **Glomerulus**—capillary tuft. Fluid, ions, and some molecules pass through the capillary wall and then through the membrane of Bowman's capsule. Large proteins and formed elements in the blood do not pass through.

3. **Bowman's capsule**—the indented, closed end of the tubule. The glomerulus plus Bowman's capsule = a **renal corpuscle.**

4. **Efferent arteriole**—smaller than the afferent arteriole, continues as a network of capillaries surrounding the tubes of the nephron.

5. **Proximal convoluted tubule**—the tube is very long to allow the processing of the fluid as it becomes urine. Capillaries

surround the tube for fluid, nutrients, and certain ions to be reabsorbed by the circulatory system. The waste and excess fluid that is left is called *urine*.

6. **Descending limb of the loop** of the nephron may dip into medulla.

7. **Ascending limb of the loop**

8. **Distal convoluted tubule**—located near the afferent and efferent arterioles. (Special cells of these structures work together to control renal blood pressure.)

9. **Collecting duct**—receives urine from many nephrons. Many of these ducts are located together as the pyramid.

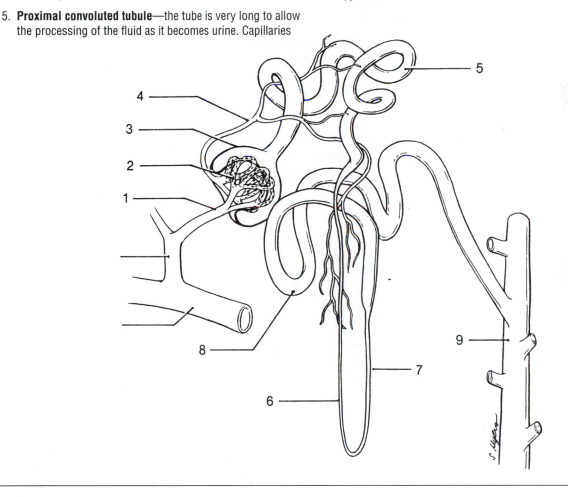

■ **Student Activities**

1. In Figure 37–2, color the minor calyces, major calyces, renal pelvis, and ureter yellow. Lightly shade the renal cortex pink.
2. In Figure 37–3, color the arteries red, the veins blue, and the renal pelvis and ureter yellow.
   Which structure is in the most posterior position? _____
   Anterior? _____
3. In Figure 37–4, color the arterioles and glomerulus red. Label the vessels that lead to the afferent arteriole.

Exercise Thirty-Seven

Name _____

1. Name the two structures that provide the contact between the urinary system and the circulatory system. a. _____ and b. _____

   Together these structures are called the c. _____

2. Provide the name of the appropriate structure in each blank.

   _____ a. storage organ for urine

   _____ b. carries urine between kidney and bladder

   _____ c. composed of many collecting ducts

   _____ d. expels urine from the body

   _____ e. functional unit of the kidney

   _____ f. formed when 2 or 3 major calyces join

   _____ g. site of entrance or exit of vessels, nerves, and tubular system to the kidney

3. In the illustrations below, name the indicated labeled structures.

   a. _____
   b. _____
   c. _____
   d. _____
   e. _____
   f. _____
   g. _____
   h. _____
   i. _____
   j. _____
   k. _____
   l. _____

The Male Reproductive System

The male reproductive system has two major functions: (1) to *produce the male germ cell*, the sperm, and introduce it into the female reproductive tract, and (2) to *produce hormones*, mainly *testosterone*. The hormones are important in development of the male sex organs, and in development of secondary sex characteristics such as development of body hair, enlargement of the larynx for a lower voice, and increased muscularity.

■ OBJECTIVES

1. State the major functions of the male reproductive system.
2. Identify the organs of the male reproductive system and state the general function of each.
3. List in order the structures through which sperm pass.
4. Describe the location of the spermatic cord and name its contents.

■ METHODS

1. Study this exercise, performing the student activities.
2. Observe the demonstration of the male reproductive structures.
3. Use the models to find all male reproductive organs.
4. Cover the keys to the illustrations and name all structures.

A. THE TESTES

The testes are paired oval organs and are the primary reproductive structures of the male. The site of sperm formation and hormone production, the testes are housed in a pouch called the **scrotum,** an evagination of the lower abdominal wall. The temperature within the scrotum is lower than that of the internal body. This is necessary for the viability of the sperm, over 200 million of which are produced daily.

FIGURE 38–1
THE TESTIS (LATERAL VIEW OF SAGITTAL SECTION)

1. **Tunica albuginea,** or white coat, is a tough fibrous covering that protects the testis.

2. **Seminiferous tubules**—the site of sperm production.

3. **Efferent ductules**

4. **Epididymis**—convoluted continuation of tubular system. Serves as a location for sperm maturation and storage.

5. **Ductus (vas) deferens**—tube that contains and propels sperm and fluid (sperm + fluid = semen). It leaves the scrotum within the spermatic cord, then passes through the inguinal canal to enter the abdomen via the deep inguinal ring. When it reaches the posterior bladder, it joins the duct of the seminal vesicle to form the ejaculatory duct.

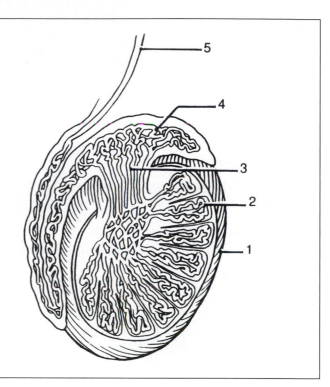

■ CLINICAL COMMENTS

Descent of the testes from the original position in the abdomen occurs during the seventh month of fetal development. They descend through the inguinal canals and into the scrotum. Frequently in premature births the testes have not descended, a condition called **cryptorchidism.** If they do not descend after birth, surgery may be needed.

B. ACCESSORY GLANDS

These provide additional fluid and nutritive elements for the sperm as they proceed through the tubular system and are released into the female reproductive system. They are the seminal vesicles, prostate gland, and bulbourethral glands.

FIGURE 38–2
ACCESSORY GLANDS OF THE MALE REPRODUCTIVE SYSTEM (POSTERIOR VIEW)

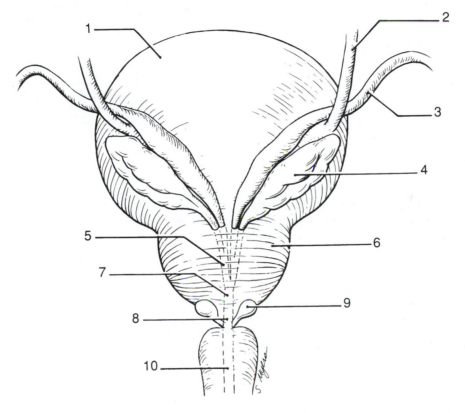

1. **Urinary bladder**

2. **Ureter**

3. **Ductus deferens**

4. **Seminal vesicle**—paired glands located posterior to and at the base of the urinary bladder. They produce an alkaline fluid containing nutrients.

5. **Ejaculatory duct**—the seminal fluid and the fluid containing the sperm join and pass through this duct into the prostatic urethra.

6. **Prostate gland**—this single gland is the largest accessory gland. It is located beneath the bladder and surrounds the urethra. It contracts to add its milky, alkaline fluid to the urethra through many small ducts.

7. **Prostatic urethra**

8. **Membranous urethra**—the segment that passes through the pelvic floor.

9. **Bulbourethral gland**—pea-size, paired glands found inferior to the prostate gland on each side of the membranous urethra. They add additional alkaline fluid to the semen. (The alkaline fluid that is added by these accessory organs is needed to neutralize the acidic fluid of the ductus deferens and the vaginal canal. Sperm need an almost neutral pH to be motile.)

10. **Penile urethra**—is the third and last segment of the male urethra. Sperm will leave the body through this section.

■ **Student Activities**

In Figure 38–2, color all accessory glands pink; color all tubes through which sperm pass, yellow.

C. THE PENIS

The penis consists of root, body, and glans. The root is the attached portion; the cylindrical body leads to the glans, an expanded portion at the end. This organ functions to place sperm in the vaginal canal of the female.

FIGURE 38–3
THE PENIS (TRANSVERSE SECTION)

1. **Corpora cavernosa penis**—two masses of erectile tissue filled with sinusoids.

2. **Corpus spongiosum.** A ventrally positioned mass of erectile tissue filled with sinusoids.

3. **Spongy (penile) urethra**

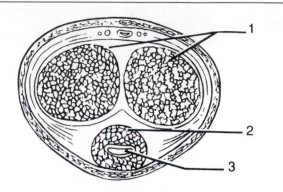

Parasympathetic innervation causes all three erectile bodies to be filled with blood to produce an erect penis. Sympathetic innervation stimulates the glands to emit secretions and the ducts to undergo peristalsis, which results in ejaculation.

■ **Student Activities**

1. In Figure 38–5 review the structures as you complete the key. Color the passage of sperm yellow; color the accessory glands pink; color the erectile tissue tan.
2. Name the parts of the reproductive tubes that are shared by the urinary system:

   a. _____   b. _____   c. _____

D. THE SPERMATIC CORD

This is a bundle of structures enclosed in a fascial sheath. It can be seen between the scrotum and the superficial inguinal ring. The cord travels through the abdominal wall by way of the inguinal canal. At the deep inguinal ring the contents are no longer enclosed in a sheath, so can be seen individually.

The contents of the spermatic cord are ductus (vas) deferens, testicular vessels, lymph vessels, and nerves.

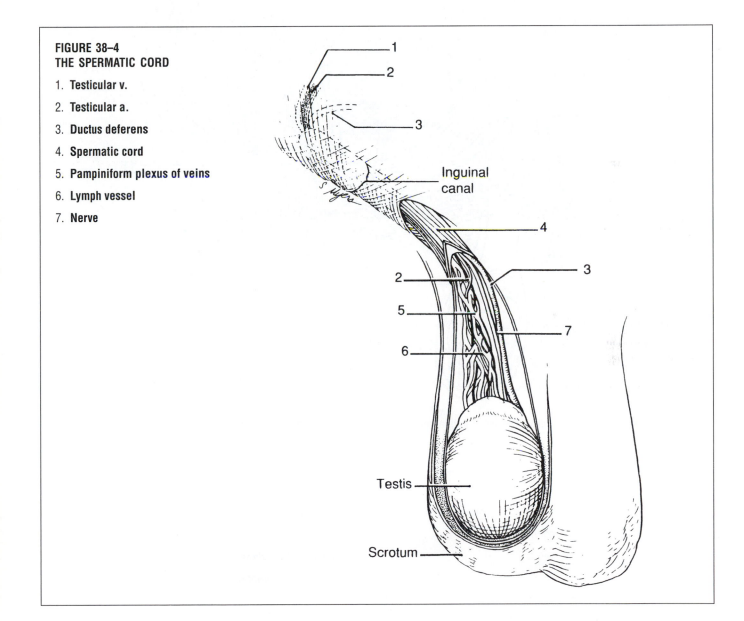

FIGURE 38–4
THE SPERMATIC CORD

1. Testicular v.
2. Testicular a.
3. Ductus deferens
4. Spermatic cord
5. Pampiniform plexus of veins
6. Lymph vessel
7. Nerve

Inguinal canal

Testis

Scrotum

FIGURE 38–5
MIDSAGITTAL SECTION THROUGH MALE PELVIS

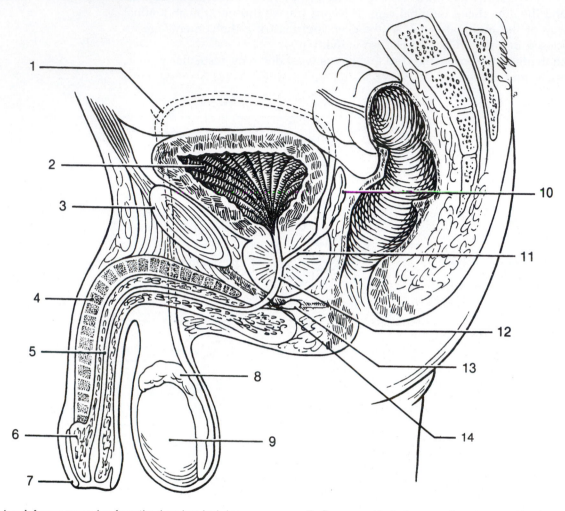

1. **Ductus deferens** emerging from the deep inguinal ring.
2. **Urinary bladder**
3. _____ _____
4. **Corpus cavernosum penis**
5. **Penile urethra** seen within corpus spongiosum penis.
6. **Glans penis,** expanded end of corpus spongiosum.

7. **Prepuce,** skin that covers glans; removed in circumcision.
8. _____
9. _____
10. _____
11. **Ejaculatory duct**
12. **Prostatic urethra**
13. **Bulbourethral gland**
14. **Membranous urethra**

Exercise Thirty-Eight

Name _____

1. What two structures join to form the ejaculatory duct?

   a. _____   b. _____

2. The primary reproductive structure of the male is the:

   _____

3. Name the three accessory glands of the male reproductive system.

   a. _____   b. _____

   c. _____

4. What are the two major functions of the testis?

   a. _____   b. _____

5. Name, in sequence, each structure in the path of the sperm.

   a. _____   e. _____

   b. _____   f. _____

   c. _____   g. _____

   d. _____   h. _____

6. Matching exercise. Use each letter only once.

   _____ 1. testosterone   a. within spermatic cord

   _____ 2. epididymis   b. surrounds urethra

   _____ 3. seminiferous tubules   c. fibrous covering

   _____ 4. bulbourethral gland   d. provides nutrients

   _____ 5. testicular a.   e. within testis

   _____ 6. corpus cavernosa penis   f. within pelvic diaphragm

   _____ 7. prostate gland   g. secondary sex characteristics

   _____ 8. tunica albuginea   h. evaginated wall of abdomen

   _____ 9. scrotum   i. erectile tissue

   _____ 10. seminal vesicle   j. sperm maturation

The Female Reproductive System

The female reproductive system serves three major functions: it *produces* the *germ cell* or *ovum*; it *produces hormones*; and it *houses and supports the development of the fetus.* **Estrogen** is the hormone responsible for initiating maturation of the ova and for development of the female sex organs and secondary sex characteristics such as hair and fat distribution, broad pelvis, and voice pitch; **progesterone** is the hormone that prepares the uterus for fetal development and the mammary glands (breasts) for lactation. The hormonal control of this system is very complex and is studied in physiology.

■ OBJECTIVES

1. State the major functions of the female reproductive system.
2. Identify the internal structures of female reproduction.
3. Describe the relationship of female reproductive organs to peritoneum.
4. Name the ligaments related to female reproductive structures.
5. Describe the external female genitalia.
6. List the structures of the female reproductive system with their homologues in the male.

■ METHODS

1. Study this unit, performing all indicated activities.
2. Observe the demonstration of female reproductive structures.
3. Find all reproductive structures on the models provided in the lab.
4. Sketch a midsagittal section of the female pelvis and include all reproductive structures and their relationships.

A. THE OVARIES

The ovaries produce the ova and female hormones and are the primary reproductive structures of the female. Testes and ovaries are **homologous** structures because they came from the same embryological tissue. They are **analogous** because they have the same function. The testis descended into the scrotum but the ovary remained in the posterosuperior pelvis and is covered by peritoneum.

The peritoneum fuses to the ovarian tissue and becomes its outer layer. Ovarian vessels and nerves reach the ovary from the lateral wall of the body through a double layer of peritoneum called the **suspensory ligament of the ovary.** This attaches the ovary to the body wall.

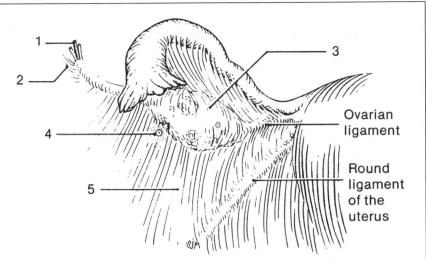

**FIGURE 39–1
THE OVARY**

1. **Ovarian a. and v.**

2. **Suspensory ligament of the ovary**

3. **Ovary**—about the size and shape of an almond in its shell

4. **Ovum**—released from the surface of the ovary into the peritoneal sac

5. **Broad ligament**—a double fold of peritoneum that hangs from the uterine tube, ovary, and ovarian ligament.

B. THE UTERUS AND UTERINE TUBES

The uterine tubes, also called Fallopian tubes or oviducts, are needed for transport of the ova. The uterus provides housing for the development of the fetus. Peritoneum covers the uterus and becomes its outer layer, the **perimetrium.** Peritoneum also collapses over the uterine tubes lateral to the uterus to become double folds called the **broad ligament.**

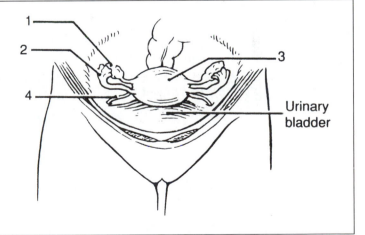

**FIGURE 39–2
RELATIVE POSITION OF FEMALE REPRODUCTIVE ORGANS**

1. **Ovary**

2. **Uterine tube (oviduct or Fallopian tube)**—muscular tube for passage of ova from the peritoneal cavity into the uterus.

3. **Uterus**—about 3 in. long, this is the hollow, muscular, pear-shaped organ that houses the developing fetus. During pregnancy the uterus is capable of enlarging 20 times its original size.

4. **Round ligament of the uterus**—the direct continuation of the ovarian ligament. It passes through the inguinal canal and fuses with the tissue of labia majora.

■ CLINICAL COMMENTS

Approximately 500,000 primary oocytes, the female germ cells, are in the female ovary when the baby is born. Of these, only about 400 will mature. Because these cells are aging from the time of the birth of the female, there is a greater chance that age or environmental hazards such as radiation and chemicals will cause genetic changes in this germ cell than in that of the male. Spermatozoa are constantly replenished by cell division.

FIGURE 39–3
UTERUS AND UTERINE TUBE (POSTERIOR VIEW)

1. **Fundus of the uterus**—the portion that is directed into the abdominal cavity. Covered by perimetrium, visceral peritoneum.

2. _____

3. _____

4. _____

Three segments of **uterine tube:**

(a) **isthmus**—narrow, nearest uterus

(b) **ampulla**—enlargement, site where fertilization (fusion of sperm and ovum) usually occurs

(c) **infundibulum**—wider termination of uterine tube. Fingerlike extensions called **fimbriae** surround the opening of the tube. Motion of the fimbriae help propel ova into the uterine tube. Peritoneum covering the uterine tube is reflected from the fimbriae into the opening of the tube and is continuous with the lining of the tube. There is, therefore, a direct continuity from the outside of the female body into the peritoneal cavity.

5. **Endometrium**—lining of the uterus, which proliferates during each hormonal cycle in preparation for pregnancy. This excess tissue sloughs off as menstrual flow if a pregnancy does not occur; it helps develop the placenta if fertilization does occur.

6. **Myometrium**—muscle of the uterus

7. **Cervix**—the neck of the uterus, which extends into the vagina. Provides an opening through which sperm can enter the uterus and menstrual flow can be eliminated from the body.

8. **Fornix**—recessed area between the cervix and the vaginal wall.

9. **Vagina**—mucous membrane-lined tube that leads to the outside of the female body.

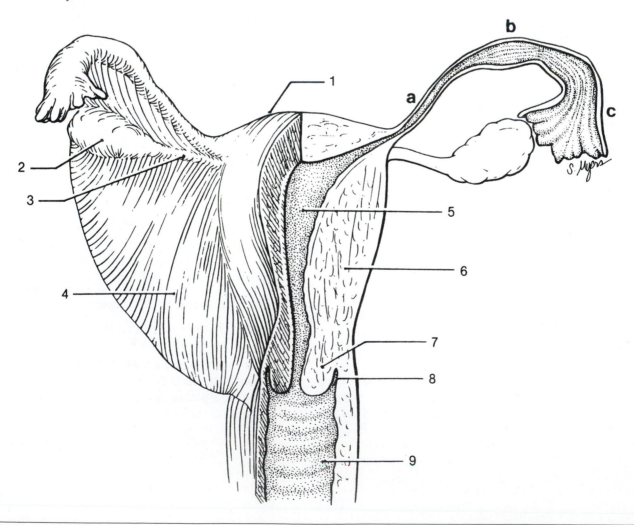

FIGURE 39–4
MIDSAGITTAL SECTION THROUGH FEMALE PELVIS

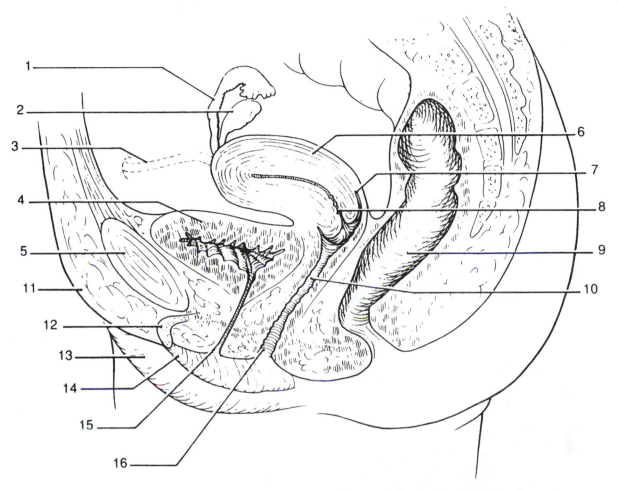

1. **Ampulla** of uterine tube

2. **Ovary**

3. **Round ligament of the uterus**

4. **Urinary bladder**

5. **Symphysis pubis**

6. **Myometrium** of body of uterus

7. **Fornix**

8. **Cervical canal,** passageway through cervix

9. **Rectum**

10. **Vaginal canal**

EXTERNAL GENITALIA (VULVA OR PUDENDUM)
OF THE FEMALE

11. **Mons pubis**—mound of fat over the symphysis pubis

12. **Clitoris**—erectile tissue, homologue of male penis

13. **Labia majora**—outer, larger fold or lip. This is the direct continuation of tissue from the mons pubis and is the homologue of the scrotum in the male. In female development, the tissue separates to provide openings for both the genital and urinary structures.

14. **Labia minora**—smaller, inner lip. The two folds come together ventrally at the clitoris.

15. **Urethral orifice**—anterior opening between lips of labia minora.

16. **Vaginal orifice**—posterior to the urethral opening.

C. PERINEUM

The **perineum** is the area of the pelvic outlet and it is bounded by the symphysis pubis anteriorly, the coccyx posteriorly, and the ischial tuberosities laterally. It is composed of the structures that are below the pelvic floor. A line drawn between the ischial tuberosities divides it into an anterior triangle, the urogenital (UG) triangle, and a posterior triangle, the anal triangle. The urethral and vaginal openings in the female and the urethral opening in the male are found in the anterior triangle. The anal triangle is similar in both sexes.

FIGURE 39–5

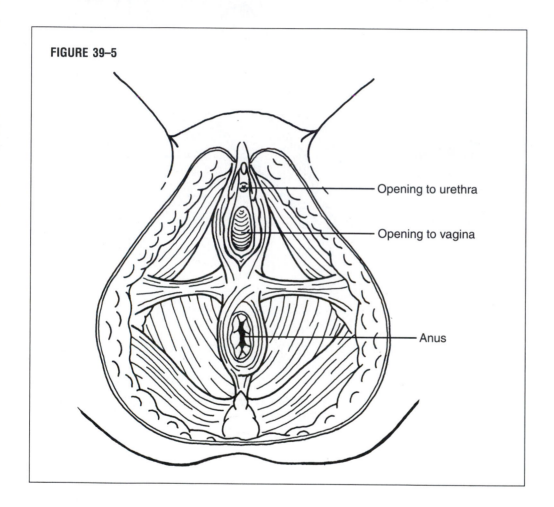

— Opening to urethra

— Opening to vagina

— Anus

■ CLINICAL COMMENTS

An **episiotomy,** a surgical incision through the perineum in a posterolateral direction from the vaginal opening, may be made during delivery of a baby. This is done to prevent the tissue from tearing. A tear is harder to repair than a surgical incision.

D. ACCESSORY REPRODUCTIVE ORGANS

Accessory reproductive organs of the female include the mammary glands or breasts. They lie over pectoralis major and serratus anterior muscles and are connected to them by fascia. The breasts have varying amounts of fat and contain glands that are responsible for lactation, the production and secretion of milk.

FIGURE 39–6
MAMMARY GLAND

1. **Areola**—pigmented area surrounding the nipple

2. **Nipple**—site of opening of lactiferous ducts

3. **Lobules**—containing milk-producing cells

4. **Mammary ducts**—carry milk from lobules

5. **Lactiferous sinus** receives milk

6. **Lactiferous ducts** excrete milk through nipple

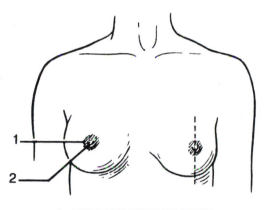

A. ANTERIOR VIEW OF CHEST

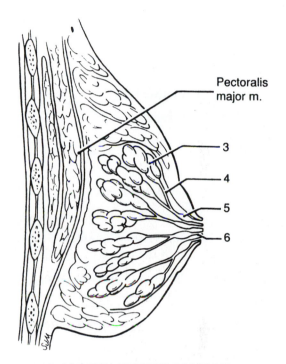

Pectoralis major m.

B. SAGITTAL SECTION OF BREAST

■ **Student Activities**

1. Place the following ligaments in the correct list: round ligament of the uterus, ovarian ligament, suspensory ligament of the ovary, broad ligament.

Peritoneal Structures	Solid Cords
a. _____	a. _____
b. _____	b. _____

2. Name the site of the ovum from the time it is ejected from the ovary until it is eliminated from the body if not fertilized.

   a. _____   e. _____

   b. Infundibulum of uterine tube   f. _____

   c. _____   g. _____

   d. _____

3. Complete the key for Figure 39–3.

Exercise Thirty-Nine

Name _____

1. Matching exercise. Use each letter only once.

   _____ 1. ovary   a. houses developing fetus

   _____ 2. uterus   b. structure of pudendum

   _____ 3. clitoris   c. extends into the vagina

   _____ 4. uterine tube   d. lactiferous structure

   _____ 5. cervix   e. erectile tissue

   _____ 6. mammary gland   f. primary reproductive structure

   _____ 7. ovum   g. anchors ovary to uterus

   _____ 8. labia majora   h. contain vessels of ovary

   _____ 9. ovarian ligament   i. germ cell

   _____ 10. suspensory ligament   j. usual site of fertilization
                  of the ovary

2. Complete the following chart comparing male and female structures.

   Homologous Structures

Male	*Female*
Scrotum	
	Ovary
Penis	

3. List the layers of the uterus from superficial to deep.

   a. _____

   b. _____

   c. _____

4. In the illustration at the right, label the structures related to the uterine tube.

   a. _____

   b. _____

   c. _____

   d. _____

Lesson 40

The Endocrine System

The endocrine system is one of two integrating systems of the body; the nervous system, discussed in Unit III, is the other. The nervous system works by sending electrical impulses directly to specific muscles and glands by way of nerve fibers. The endocrine system works by sending chemicals called hormones to many body tissues by way of the circulatory system.

■ OBJECTIVES

1. List the general functions of the endocrine system.
2. State the difference between endocrine and exocrine glands.
3. Name and give the location of all endocrine glands.

■ METHOD

Complete the indicated activities as you study the information presented in the lesson.

A. FUNCTIONS OF THE ENDOCRINE SYSTEM

These functions can generally be stated as:

1. Involvement in the general growth and development of the body
2. Involvement in most processes related to reproduction
3. Helping control the internal environment by regulating chemical composition
4. Responding to environmental conditions such as emotional stress, dehydration, starvation, hemorrhage, and extreme heat and cold

B. ORGANS OF THE ENDOCRINE SYSTEM

Endocrine glands produce hormones and secrete them directly into the bloodstream. **Exocrine glands,** such as the salivary glands or lacrimal glands, have a duct system through which their secretions travel to an epithelial surface—the skin or into a body cavity.

The ultimate control over the endocrine glands comes largely from the hypothalamus. Disorders of this system make apparent its complexity in both control and action. We will leave the details to physiology. Some basic information about specific hormones is included here for the interested student.

FIGURE 40–1
THE ENDOCRINE GLANDS

1. **Pineal gland**—in the brain in the roof of the third ventricle

2. **Pituitary gland**—found in the sella turcica of the sphenoid bone. It's posterior lobe, the neurohypophysis, is derived from nervous tissue of the **hypothalamus,** with which it is continuous.

3. **Thyroid gland**—just below the larynx

4. **Parathyroid glands**—behind the thyroid gland

5. **Thymus**—posterior to the sternum

6. **Adrenal glands** (suprarenal)—cap superior end of each kidney

7. **Pancreas**—in the abdomen, postero-inferior to the stomach

8. **Gonads**
   a. ovaries—in the true pelvis
   b. testes—in the scrotum

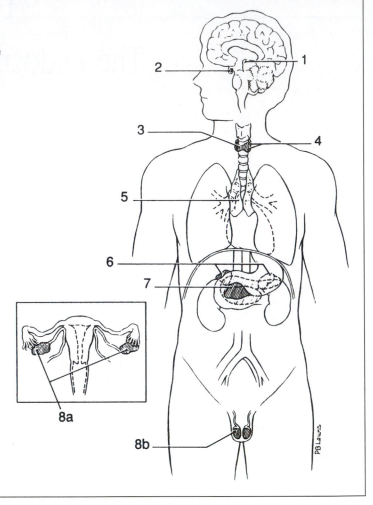

1. **Pituitary gland.** Found in the sella turcica of the sphenoid bone and divided into regions; secretes several hormones.
   a. **Adenohypophysis**—the anterior lobe; it is the glandular portion and secretes some hormones that stimulate functional activities of other hormones. For this reason, the pituitary gland is often called the "master gland" of the body. These hormones are:
      (1) Thyroid stimulating hormone (TSH)—it affects the thyroid gland.
      (2) Adrenocorticotrophic hormone (ACTH)—affects the adrenal cortex.
      (3) Follicle stimulating hormone (FSH)—acts on ovaries.
      (4) Interstitial cell stimulating hormone (ICSH)—acts on testes.
      (5) Luteotropic hormone (LH)—acts on ovaries and mammary glands.
      (6) Human growth hormone (HGH)—acts on the hard and soft tissues of the body to increase growth and maintain body size.
   b. **Neurohypophysis**—secretes **oxytocin,** which stimulates uterine contractions and the ejection of milk; and **antidiuretic hormone (ADH),** which promotes reabsorption of water by the kidney and so decreases urine output. Neurosecretory cells of the **hypothalamus** actually produce the two hormones released by the neurohypophysis.

2. **Thyroid gland.** Located just below the larynx with a lobe on each side of the trachea and an isthmus connecting the lobes at the region of the second and third tracheal rings. Secretes **thyroxin,** which increases metabolism, so the energy level rises; and **calcitonin,** which decreases the amount of calcium in the blood.

3. **Parathyroid glands.** These four glands secrete **parathormone,** which acts to increase the amount of calcium in the blood.

4. **Thymus.** Posterior to the sternum and *not* controlled by the pituitary gland, the thymus is actually an organ of the **lymphatic** system. It is often mentioned with the endocrine system because it secretes two peptide hormones, **thymosin** and **thymopoietin,** that are necessary in the development of the immune system.

5. **Adrenal glands.** Cap each kidney and considered as two structures.
   a. **Cortex**—produces **steroids** that aid in electrolyte balance and normal cell metabolism. Also produces small amounts of sex hormones.
   b. **Medulla**—produces **epinephrine** and **norepinephrine,** which simulate effects of the sympathetic nervous system (epinephrine = adrenalin).

6. **Pancreas.** Situated in the abdomen postero-inferior to the stomach. It functions as both exocrine (digestive) and endocrine. The endocrine function is to produce **insulin,** which decreases the blood sugar level, and **glucagon,** which increases blood sugar level.

7. **Gonads**
   a. **Ovaries**—produce female sex hormones, **estrogens** and **progesterone,** which work with secretions of the pituitary gland to regulate the menstrual cycle, maintain pregnancy, and prepare the mammary glands for lactation.
   b. **Testes**—found in the scrotum of the male. **Testosterone** is the major hormone, and it develops and maintains the male sex characteristics.

8. **Pineal gland.** Produces **melatonin,** a hormone that is related to sleep-wake cycles.

■ CLINICAL COMMENTS

Diabetes mellitus is a disease of the pancreas that results in hyperglycemia, an elevation of glucose (sugar) in the blood. There are different types of diabetes, but the most common (90%) is Type II or non-insulin-dependent diabetes. In this type, the pancreas usually produces insulin, but the tissue receptors do not allow the insulin to function in the uptake of glucose. When the body cells are not using the glucose, it builds up in the blood. This causes the kidney to produce too much urine (polyuria) trying to get rid of the excess glucose, and the patient is thirsty (polydipsia). Because the glucose is not being used properly, the patient is hungry (polyphasia).

■ Student Activities

1. Name the gland that is both endocrine and exocrine. _____
2. Name two glands (different from 1) that produce substances in addition to hormones.

   a. _____   b. _____

The Thorax

The thoracic (chest) cavity is one of the largest body cavities and contains major organs of both the circulatory system and the respiratory system. These important organs are protected by the bones of the thorax: the thoracic vertebrae, the ribs, and the sternum. Review Lesson 14 for details of the bones.

When studying the thorax it is helpful to consider the **parietal thorax,** the walls, and then look at the structures, **viscera,** housed within the cavity.

■ OBJECTIVES

1. Name the bony elements of the thorax.
2. List the muscles of the parietal thorax.
3. Describe the diaphragm and list the structures that pass through it.
4. Describe the nerves and the vessels of the parietal thorax.
5. Name the contents of the thorax.
6. Define mediastinum; identify the contents.

■ METHODS

1. Review the bones of the thorax in the laboratory.
2. Observe the demonstration of muscles and neurovascular structures on the lab material.
3. Complete the indicated activities in this lesson.

A. BONES OF THE THORAX

These are illustrated and described in Lesson 14.

1. Bodies of the 12 thoracic vertebrae, posterior attachment for ribs.
2. Twelve pairs of ribs with costal cartilages.
3. Sternum (breastbone), anterior attachment of ribs.

B. MUSCLES OF THE THORAX

In the spaces between ribs, **intercostal muscles** complete the "walls" of the thorax. For more detail of these and other small thoracic muscles, see a reference text. The "floor" is formed by the **diaphragm,** a musculotendinous sheet separating the thorax from the abdomen.

FIGURE 41–1
INTERCOSTAL MUSCLES (ANTERIOR VIEW OF THORAX)

1. **External intercostal muscles.** The fibers are oriented in an oblique direction and fill the intercostal spaces from the thoracic vertebrae posteriorly to an aponeurosis that lies over the costal cartilages.

2. **Internal intercostal muscles** lie deep to the external intercostals with fibers that are at a right angle to them. The internal intercostals extend from the sternum to an aponeurosis at the angle of the ribs.

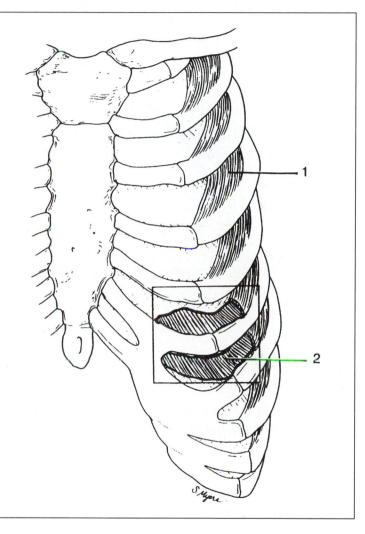

■ CLINICAL COMMENTS

Pulmonary ventilation is the moving of air into (inspiration) and out of (expiration) the lungs. This is accomplished by the contraction of the muscles of the diaphragm and the external and internal intercostal muscles.

FIGURE 41–2
THE DIAPHRAGM: (INFERIOR VIEW)

1. **Esophagus.** Passes through muscle fibers to reach abdomen.

2. **Aorta.** Taking blood to all of body below the diaphragm.

3. **Inferior vena cava.** Only structure piercing the central tendon; brings blood back to the heart.

4. **Central tendon.** Muscle fibers from the xiphoid process of the sternum—the lower six pairs of ribs—and the upper two lumbar vertebrae attach into this tendon. When the fibers contract, the tendon is pulled down and the size of the thoracic cavity increases.

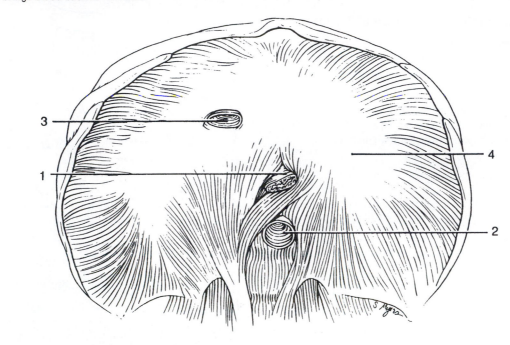

In addition to the structures shown, smaller vessels, nerves, and lymphatic structures must pass through or behind the diaphragm.

C. INNERVATION OF THE PARIETAL THORAX

The muscles found between ribs (voluntary, skeletal muscles) are innervated by corresponding intercostal nerves. Sensory fibers of these nerves provide innervation for the overlying skin. Intercostal nerves are the ventral rami of thoracic level spinal nerves, T1–T11. The last thoracic spinal nerve, T12, is called the subcostal n. These nerves are located in the costal grooves of the ribs. Intercostal nerves T7–T11 and the subcostal n. also send fibers into the abdominal wall. (**Remember:** Much of T1 becomes a part of the brachial plexus.)

The innervation of the thoracic floor, the diaphragm, is by way of the **phrenic nerve,** C3, 4, 5. Because of the folding of the embryo during development, this nerve can be seen lying in the mediastinum as it descends to the diaphragm.

D. BLOOD SUPPLY TO THE PARIETAL THORAX

Intercostal arteries and veins can be found in neurovascular bundles with the intercostal nerves. The **anterior intercostal arteries** are branches from the **internal thoracic a.;** the posterior intercostal arteries are primarily from the aorta.

The diaphragm receives most of its blood from:
Musculophrenic arteries, major terminal branches of the internal thoracic a. (Figure
41–4) and superior phrenic arteries from the aorta superiorly, and,
Inferior phrenic arteries, also from the aorta, inferiorly.

The **azygos vein** collects venous blood from the thorax and returns it to the
superior vena cava.

FIGURE 41–3
BLOOD SUPPLY TO THORACIC WALLS

1. **Posterior intercostal a.**—a branch from the aorta

2. **Anterior intercostal a.**—coming from the internal thoracic a.
   Notice the anastomosis with the posterior vessel.

3. **Internal thoracic a.**

4. **Internal thoracic v.**

5. **Azygos v.** empties into the superior vena cava.

6. **Posterior intercostal v.**

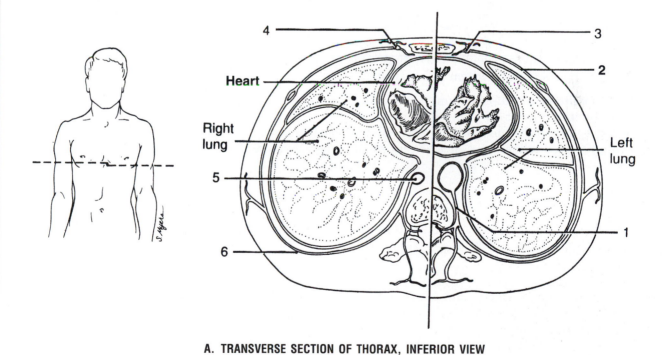

A. TRANSVERSE SECTION OF THORAX, INFERIOR VIEW

FIGURE 41–3
BLOOD SUPPLY TO THORACIC WALLS (CONTINUED)

1. **Posterior intercostal a.**—a branch from the aorta

5. **Azygos v.** empties into the superior vena cava.

6. **Posterior intercostal v.**

7. **Intercostal n.** is the most inferior structure in the intercostal space.

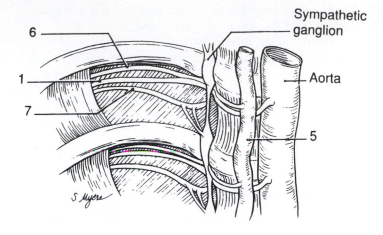

B. INTERCOSTAL SPACE IN POSTERIOR THORAX

E. CONTENTS OF THE THORAX

1. **Lungs and pleura.** The major organs of the respiratory system and their serous coverings, pleura, fill the lateral thorax. These organs will be considered in more detail with the respiratory system in Lesson 42.

2. **The mediastinum** (me'di-as-ti'num) is the space between the lungs. All structures in the thorax except the lungs and pleura are located here. The heart is the largest structure in the mediastinum and will be considered in detail in Lesson 43. All other mediastinal structures, except the thymus gland, are illustrated in Figure 41–5.

■ CLINICAL COMMENTS

Pleurisy is an inflammation of the serous membranes of the lungs. The two layers of pleura rub against each other and result in painful breathing.

FIGURE 41–4
THE THORAX

In this anterior view, the chest wall has been cut and opened to
permit a view of the inside of the anterior chest wall.

1. Left lung
2. Heart
3. Diaphragm
4. Internal thoracic v.
5. Body of sternum
6. Subclavian a.
7. Internal thoracic a.
8. Musculophrenic a.
9. Superior epigastric a.

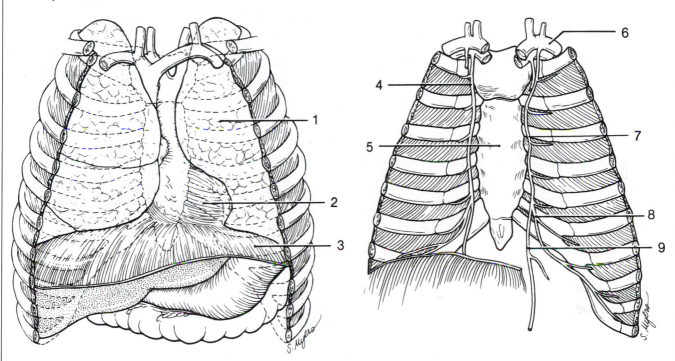

■ **Student Activities**

In Figure 41–4:

Color the arteries red and the veins blue.
Label the external intercostal and internal intercostal muscles.
Label the aorta and the common carotid arteries in the illustration on the left; label the
common carotid arteries on the right.

FIGURE 41–5
POSTERIOR THORAX

With the lungs and heart removed, the remaining structures of the mediastinum can be seen.

1. Superior vena cava
2. Phrenic n.
3. Intercostal vein, artery, and nerve
4. Sympathetic chain and rami communicantes
5. Sympathetic ganglion
6. Greater splanchnic n.
7. Trachea
8. Vagus n.
9. Aorta
10. Primary bronchus
11. Esophagus
12. Azygos v.
13. Thoracic duct

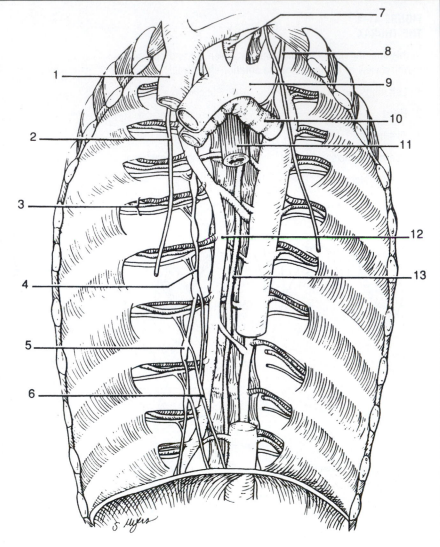

■ **Student Activities**

1. In Figure 41–1, color the external intercostal muscle pink; color the internal intercostal muscle red.
2. In Figure 41–2, color the muscle fibers pink; color the aorta red, the inferior venae cava blue, and the esophagus green.
3. In Figure 41–3, color the arteries red, the veins blue, and the nerves yellow.
4. In Figure 41–5, color all arteries red, all veins blue, and all nerves yellow. Color the thoracic duct brown and the esophagus green. What structure lies between the aortic arch and the esophagus? _____
5. In the middle of the thorax the aorta is _____ (anterior or posterior) to the esophagus?
6. The largest structure in the mediastinum is the _____.
7. The azygos vein is to the thorax what the _____ is to the abdomen.

The Respiratory System

The respiratory system provides oxygen from the atmosphere for the body cells; it returns to the atmosphere the carbon dioxide produced when the oxygen is used by the cells. While the circulatory system and other regulatory systems are needed in this process, the structures in this unit will provide the contact between the air and the circulatory system.

Because air enters by way of the nose, some review is included with additional head and neck structures involved in respiration.

■ OBJECTIVES

1. Identify structures and openings of the internal nose.
2. Describe the three regions of the pharynx and locate its continuation as the esophagus.
3. Identify the four laryngeal cartilages described in the text.
4. Distinguish between true and false vocal folds.
5. Trace the path of air from the nose to the alveoli.
6. Differentiate between right and left lungs.

■ METHODS

1. Observe the demonstration of head and neck structures as seen in a midsagittal head and neck.
2. Identify on models of sagittal heads each structure listed in the order in which air encounters them.
3. Sketch the pathway of air. Note the structures used by both respiration and digestion.
4. Perform the activities indicated in the text.

A. THE NOSE

The nose provides an entrance for air into the body.

FIGURE 42–1
EXTERNAL NOSE

1. **Alae,** winglike extensions that outline the openings.

2. **External nares** (nostrils) provide entrance for air.

3. **Nasal septum** divides the nasal cavity into right and left sides.

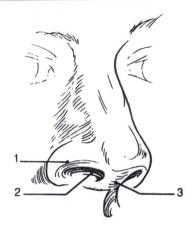

The *internal nose* is bounded above by the bones of the floor of the cranium and below by the hard and soft palate. The scroll-shaped conchae on the lateral wall cause turbulence of the air. This is important to:

1. Aid in warming the air by exposing it to the blood supply in the mucous membrane lining.
2. Clean the air of particles; these are caught in the cilia, the hairlike projections of the lining.

The spaces below the conchae are referred to as *meatuses.* The nasolacrimal duct and the paranasal sinuses (Lesson 24) open into the meatuses. The lining of the nose is continuous into these spaces.

FIGURE 42–2
INTERNAL NOSE

1. **Middle nasal concha**

2. **Inferior nasal concha**

3. **Superior nasal concha**

4. **Internal nares or choanae** are the openings from the nasal cavity into the pharynx. The arrow indicates its position at the posterior limit of the nasal septum, not shown here.

5. **Inferior meatus.** The opening for the nasolacrimal duct is found here.

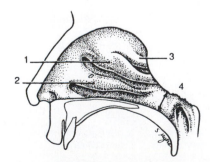

A. THE LATERAL WALL OF THE RIGHT SIDE OF THE NASAL CAVITY

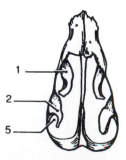

B. ANTERIOR VIEW OF THE BONES OF THE NOSE

B. THE PHARYNX (FAIR′INKS)

This is a fibromuscular tube that serves both the respiratory system and the digestive system. It is bounded above by the sphenoid bone and posteriorly by the bodies of the cervical vertebrae. This tube opens anteriorly into the nasal cavity, oral cavity, and larynx. Inferior to the level of the larynx, it continues as the **esophagus.** The pharynx is divided into three regions:

NASOPHARYNX

Goes from the base of the skull to the soft palate. This portion is respiratory only and contains:

a. **Pharyngeal tonsil** in its posterior wall (called **adenoids** if enlarged).
b. **Opening of auditory tube** protected by a mound of tissue called the **torus tubarius.**

OROPHARYNX

From the soft palate to the level of the hyoid bone. This region serves both the respiratory and digestive systems. It houses the **palatine tonsils** and the lingual tonsils.

LARYNGOPHARYNX

From the level of the hyoid bone to the lower border of the cricoid cartilage.

The pharyngeal constrictor muscles form the posterior wall of the pharynx and aid in swallowing. We will not study these in detail. (Find these muscles in Figure 42–4 and color them pink.) Notice that they are continuous with the esophagus.

Innervation: CN IX and X supply both sensory and motor fibers. Sympathetics are from cervical plexus fibers.

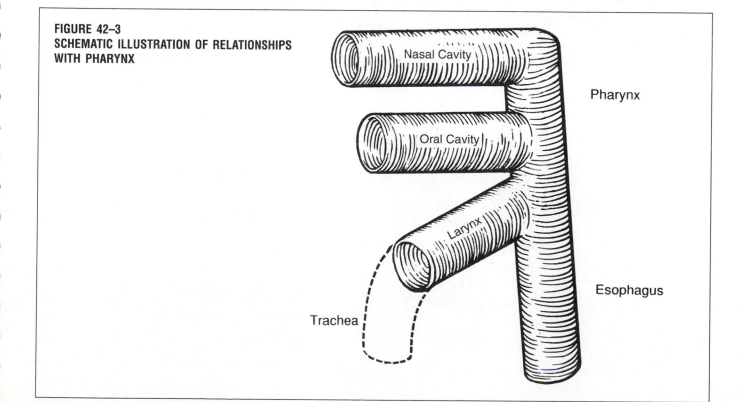

FIGURE 42–3
SCHEMATIC ILLUSTRATION OF RELATIONSHIPS WITH PHARYNX

Nasal Cavity

Pharynx

Oral Cavity

Larynx

Esophagus

Trachea

FIGURE 42–4
MIDSAGITTAL HEAD AND NECK

1. _____ _____
2. _____ _____
3. _____ _____ _____
4. Ala at external nares
5. Maxilla
6. Tongue
7. _____
8. _____

9. Mylohyoid m.
10. Hyoid bone
11. Thyroid cartilage
12. Cricoid cartilage
13. Tracheal cartilages
14. _____ _____
15. Pharyngeal tonsil
16. Torus tubarius (protects open-
    ing of auditory tube)

17. Soft palate
18. Uvula
19. Palatine tonsil
20. Epiglottis
21. Pharyngeal constrictor m.
22. False vocal fold
23. True vocal fold (vocal cord)
24. Esophagus

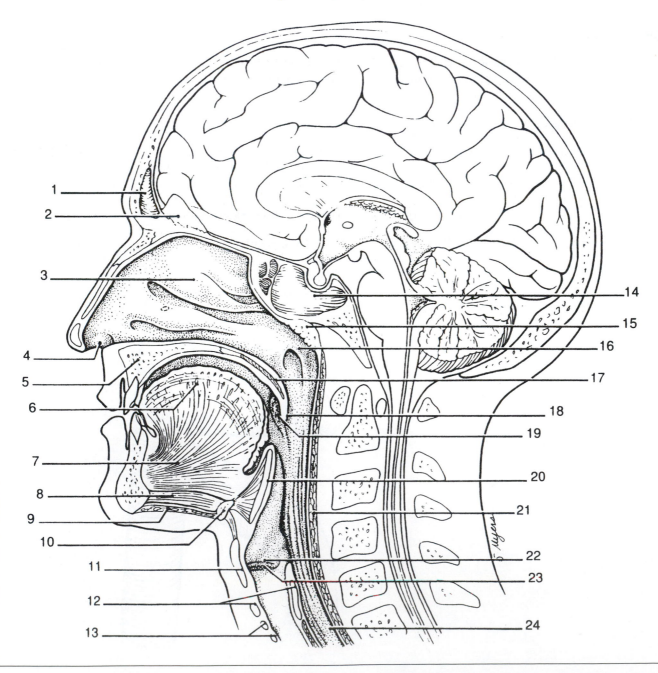

C. THE LARYNX (LAIR'INKS)

Commonly called the *voice box,* the larynx is formed from nine cartilages, three single and three pairs, which hold open a mucous membrane-lined space. Air passes through the laryngopharynx and moves forward into the larynx.

**FIGURE 42–5
CARTILAGES OF THE LARYNX**

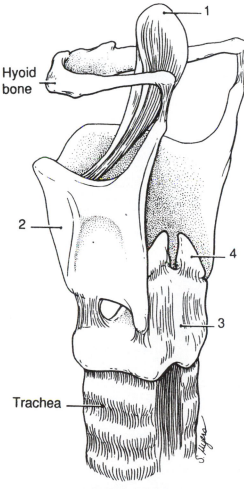

Hyoid bone

2

4

3

Trachea

A. POSTERO-LATERAL VIEW

1. **Epiglottis,** a single cartilage that attaches to the thyroid cartilage and extends behind the tongue. It helps protect the opening of the larynx by directing food toward the esophagus.

2. **Thyroid cartilage.** This is commonly called the "Adam's apple." In the male it is more prominent because it is formed from two plates that fuse anteriorly at a 90° angle. In the female the angle is 120°.

3. **Cricoid cartilage.** This is the only complete ring cartilage of the larynx. On its posterior extremity the two triangular-shaped *arytenoid cartilages* are located.

4. **Arytenoid cartilage**

5. **False (ventricular) vocal fold.** Created by the membranous lining covering the ligaments between cartilages listed above (as well as two very small, unpictured pairs, the *corniculates* and the *cuneiforms*).

6. **True vocal fold.** These folds, similar to those above, are also called **vocal cords.** Sound is produced when air is expelled and passes between the true folds. These folds can be tightened by the intrinsic laryngeal muscles that attach to the cartilages. The pitch of the voice is then higher.

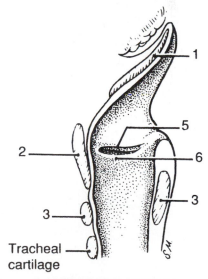

1

5

2

6

3

3

Tracheal cartilage

B. MIDSAGITTAL SECTION

MUSCLES OF THE LARYNX

a. **Extrinsic muscles** are the suprahyoid and infrahyoid muscles. These muscles help move the larynx in both talking and swallowing. They are included in Lesson 31.
b. **Intrinsic muscles** are those tiny muscles that attach to the laryngeal cartilages and change the shape and tension of the vocal folds. They are not covered individually in this text.

INNERVATION OF THE LARYNX

Cranial n. X supplies both intrinsic muscle and sensory innervation.

BLOOD SUPPLY OF THE LARYNX

Branches from the external carotid artery.

D. THE TRACHEA

The trachea is the direct continuation of the larynx and is held open by C-shaped cartilages. It lies anterior to the esophagus as it descends into the thorax.

FIGURE 42–6
LARYNX, TRACHEA, AND LUNGS (ANTERIOR VIEW)

1. _____ _____

2. _____ _____

3. **Trachea**

4. **Left primary bronchus**—smaller and less direct than the right primary bronchus. The primary bronchi result when the trachea bifurcates. They enter the root of the lung.

5. **Secondary bronchus**—three of these are on the right, one for each lobe. Only two are on the left. Each branches to form several numbered and predictable tertiary bronchi.

6. **Bronchial arteries**—provide blood to the bronchial tree.

7. Horizontal fissure to separate lobes; the oblique fissue is inferior. The fissures divide the right lung into three lobes.

8. Oblique fissue—the only fissure on the left because the left lung has only two lobes.

9. **Diaphragmatic surface**—the lungs are just superior to the diaphragm.

10. **Cardiac impression**—the heart indents the medial inferior surface of the left lung.

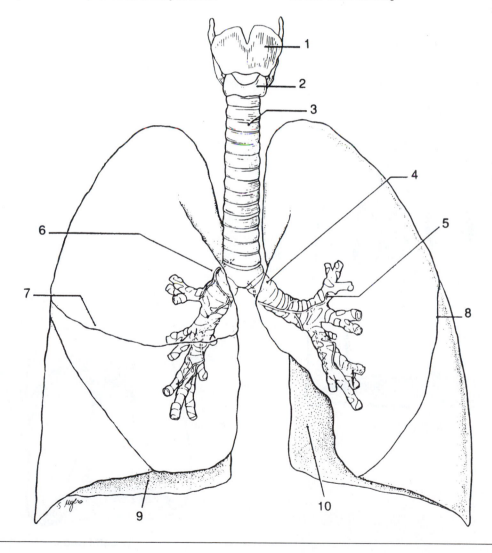

THE LUNGS

In the anterior view of the lungs (Figure 42–6), you can see the three lobes of the right lung and the two lobes of the left lung. Each lung is further divided into 10 functionally independent bronchopulmonary segments that are the structural and surgical units of the lung. These segments have their own blood and nerve supply.

Each lung is located within a **pleural sac.** These serous membranes allow the lungs to move without friction. *Visceral pleura* covers the lung; the pulmonary capillaries lie between the alveoli of the lungs and the visceral pleura. *Parietal pleura* lines the pleural cavities and lies against the mediastinum medially.

On the mediastinal surface (Figure 42–7) are the structures of the *root* of each lung. The largest of these are the pulmonary veins, pulmonary arteries and the bronchi. The pulmonary arteries terminate as capillaries that surround the microscopic alveoli (Figure 42–8) and it is here that gaseous exchange takes place. The much smaller bronchial arteries and veins also enter the root of the lung to provide the blood supply for the bronchi, connective tissue of the lung, and the visceral pleura. Lymph vessels and nerves also enter the root of the lung.

Innervation of the bronchial tree is by way of the autonomic nervous system. Parasympathetic fibers from the vagus n. cause bronchoconstriction. Sympathetic fibers from the upper thoracic levels cause bronchodilation.

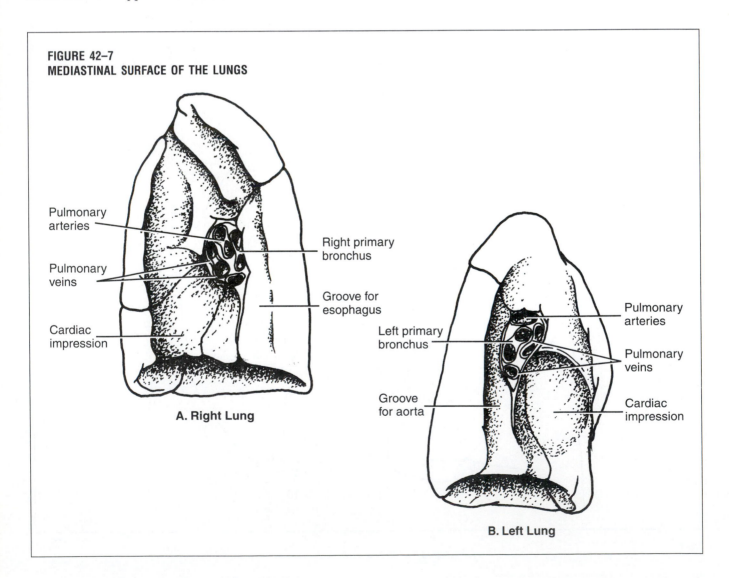

FIGURE 42–7
MEDIASTINAL SURFACE OF THE LUNGS

Pulmonary arteries

Pulmonary veins

Cardiac impression

Right primary bronchus

Groove for esophagus

A. Right Lung

Left primary bronchus

Groove for aorta

Pulmonary arteries

Pulmonary veins

Cardiac impression

B. Left Lung

FIGURE 42–8
MICROSCOPIC ILLUSTRATION OF BRONCHIOLES AND ALVEOLI

1. **Terminal bronchiole**—the last segment of the bronchial tree to contain cartilage.

2. **Respiratory bronchiole**—when the air reaches this portion of the tube there can be some exchange of gasses. The tubes contain no cartilage and have alveolar ducts and sacs.

3. **Alveoli**—the thin epithelium sacs that are the termination of the bronchial tree. They receive the air.

4. **Capillaries**—between the pulmonary arteries and pulmonary veins. Carbon dioxide in the blood is exchanged for oxygen from the alveoli.

5. **Pulmonary arteriole** bring poorly oxygenated blood from the right ventricle.

6. **Pulmonary venule** takes well-oxygenated blood back to the left atrium.

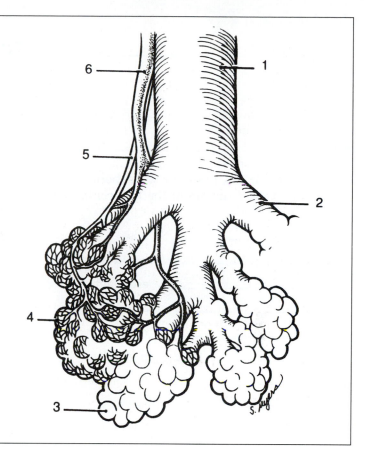

■ CLINICAL COMMENTS

In the United States, **lung cancer** is responsible for more cancer deaths than any other type of cancer. According to the American Cancer Society, smoking is responsible for 85–90% of all lung cancer cases; therefore, it is one of the most preventable types of cancer deaths.

■ Student Activities

1. In Figure 42–8, color the pulmonary arteriole blue; the pulmonary venule red. This is one site where arterial blood is poorly oxygenated.
2. In Figure 42–3 and 42–4, lightly color the nasopharynx blue, the oropharynx yellow, and the laryngopharynx green. **Remember:** The esophagus and the trachea start at the same level.
3. In Figures 42–4, 42–5B, and 42–6, color all visible laryngeal cartilages blue.
4. In Figure 42–6, use a yellow pencil to color a path from the trachea to a right tertiary bronchus.

Exercise Forty-Two

Name _____

1. Using anterior (A), posterior (P), superior (S), and inferior (I), indicate the relationship of the structure in the first column with that in the second (see *a.* for example):

   a. _____ A _____   nose   pharynx

   b. _____   hyoid bone   thyroid cartilage

   c. _____   esophagus   pharynx

   d. _____   cricoid cartilage epiglottis

   e. _____   oropharynx   nasopharynx

   f. _____   trachea   larynx

   g. _____   thyroid cartilage cricoid cartilage

   h. _____   larynx   esophagus

   i. _____   laryngopharynx   esophagus

   j. _____   torus tubarius   palatine tonsil

2. List, in order, the anatomical structures through which air passes:

   a. _____ Nose _____   In the space below, sketch the anatomical structures of the passageway of air from the nasal cavity to the alveolus.

   b. _____

   c. _____

   d. _____ Laryngopharynx _____

   e. _____

   f. _____

   g. _____

   h. _____

   i. _____

   j. _____

   k. _____

   l. _____ Alveolus _____

The Heart

The four-chambered heart is composed of two atria that receive blood and two ventricles that pump blood through arteries and veins. (Review Lesson 10.) In the adult there is no communication between the right side (pulmonary pump) and the left side (systemic pump) of the heart. The **right atrium** receives blood with high levels of carbon dioxide and sends it to the **right ventricle** to be pumped to the lungs. The **left atrium** receives highly oxygenated blood from the lungs and sends it to the **left ventricle** to be pumped to all the body systems.

■ OBJECTIVES

1. Orient the heart in the correct anatomical position.
2. Identify the major vessels supplying the heart muscle.
3. Describe the pathway of blood as it moves through the heart.
4. Identify each major vein that enters the atria and each major artery through which blood leaves the ventricles.
5. Identify and state the purpose of each structure located within the chambers of the heart.

■ METHODS

1. Using the heart models in the lab, identify each structure of the external and internal heart as described on the following pages.
2. Sketch the heart with its four chambers and each major vessel.
3. Trace the path of blood through the heart, naming each structure encountered until you do not need to refer to the text.

A. POSITION OF THE HEART

The heart lies in the mediastinum about 2/3 to the left of the midline. It is encased in a serous sac called the **pericardium.** The visceral pericardium (epicardium) covering the heart allows it to move against the parietal (fibrous) pericardium without causing friction. The fibrous, outer layer attaches to the diaphragm.

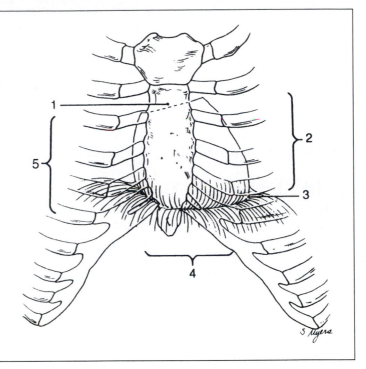

FIGURE 43-1
HEART IN THORAX (ANTERIOR VIEW)

1. **Base**—directed up and to the right. This is where the great vessels enter and leave. It is at the level of thoracic vertebrae 5–8.

2. **Left border**—formed largely by the left ventricle.

3. **Apex**—directed down and to the left. Mostly left ventricle, it is located at about the fifth left intercostal space.

4. **Inferior border**—formed largely by right ventricle.

5. **Right border**—formed largely by the right atrium.

■ **CLINICAL COMMENTS**

The most common cause of **heart disease** is diminished blood flow to the heart. This deprives the heart muscle of necessary oxygen and nutrients. When the heart is deprived of blood, pain **(angina pectoris)** may occur during activity because of the lack of oxygen. Usually this is a result of atherosclerosis in the coronary vessels. As the fatty plaque builds, blood flow slows and lack of oxygen can result in permanent heart damage. Sometimes there may be no warning and damaged muscle causes a sudden heart attack (myocardial infarction—MI).

B. BLOOD SUPPLY OF THE HEART

The first branches of the aorta are **coronary** arteries that supply oxygen to the muscle of the heart. The return vessels are called **cardiac veins.**

FIGURE 43–2
VESSELS OF THE HEART

1. **Superior vena cava (SVC)** brings venous blood to the right atrium from the upper body.

2. **Ascending aorta** contains blood being pumped by the left ventricle to all the systems of the body.

3. **Right coronary a.** leaves the base of the aorta to the right of the pulmonary trunk and lies in the fat-filled coronary sulcus as it passes to the posterior heart.

4. **Right auricle,** ear-like flap of atrium.

5. **Inferior vena cava** (IVC) enters the heart just after passing through the diaphragm.

6. **Ligamentum arteriosum** remnant of an embryonic vessel.

7. **Pulmonary trunk,** for blood being pumped by the right ventricle to the lungs for a fresh supply of oxygen.

8. **Left coronary a.** This vessel leaves the base of the aorta and turns to lie in the **coronary sulcus,** the depression between atria and ventricles.

9. **Circumflex a.**—the continuation of the left coronary a. to the posterior heart. It lies in the coronary sulcus.

10. **Anterior interventricular a.** (referred to as the left anterior descending **(LAD)** in clinical literature). This branch of the left coronary a. lies in the fat-filled **anterior interventricular sulcus,** the depression over the interventricular septum. It supplies blood to both ventricles.

11. **Great cardiac vein** lies in the anterior interventricular sulcus beside the artery. It continues by turning to lie in the coronary sulcus with the circumflex a. and then terminates on the posterior heart.

12. **Left auricle**—ear-like flap of left atrium.

13. **Pulmonary veins** take oxygenated blood into the left atrium.

14. **Coronary sinus**—termination of the great cardiac vein. It lies in the coronary sulcus and serves as a reservoir for the venous blood.

15. **Posterior interventricular artery** (direct continuation of the right coronary a.)—lies in the posterior interventricular sulcus.

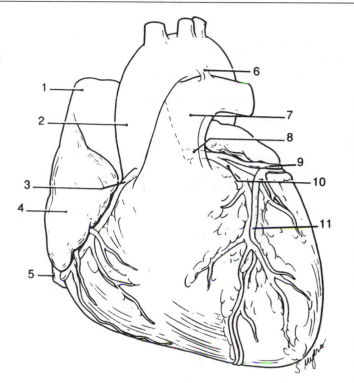

A. ANTERIOR VIEW

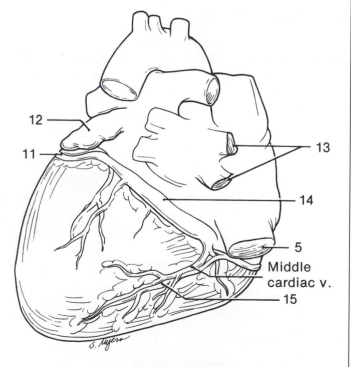

B. POSTERIOR VIEW

C. INTERNAL STRUCTURE OF THE HEART

Each structure of the heart will be discussed in the order in which it would be encountered as the blood moves through the heart. Find each structure in Figure 43–3.

FIGURE 43–3
INTERNAL STRUCTURE OF THE HEART

1. **Superior vena cava**—brings blood from the upper body.

2. **Inferior vena cava**—brings blood from the lower body.

3. **Opening of the coronary sinus**—brings blood used by the heart muscle.

4. **Right atrium**—pectinate muscles in its flaplike extension, the auricle. The wall of the atrium is smooth except for the ridges of muscle in the auricle.

5. **Fossa ovalis**—thin region of interatrial septum. Location of foramen ovale in the developing embryo.

6. **Tricuspid valve.** Three thin membranous flaps formed from **endocardium,** the lining tissue of the heart. It separates the right atrium from the right ventricle.

(Remainder of Key is on the next page.)

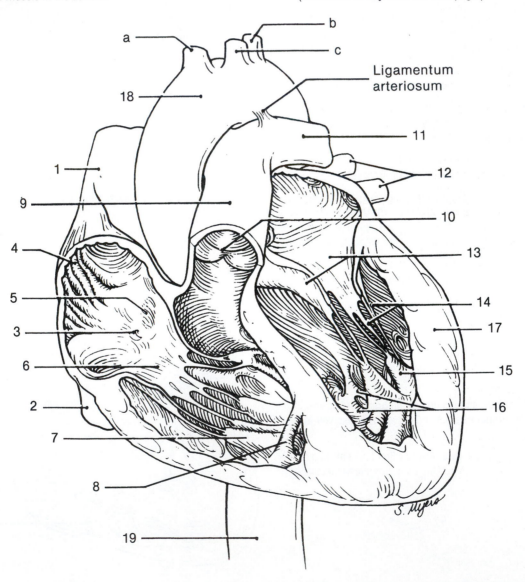

FIGURE 43–3
INTERNAL STRUCTURE OF THE HEART (CONTINUED)

7. **Papillary muscle**—specialized **trabeculae carnae**, the ridges of muscle in the ventricles.

8. **Moderator band**—another specialization of trabeculae carnae. Only found in the right ventricle, it extends from the interventricular septum to the right ventricular wall and carries part of the conduction system of the heart.

9. **Pulmonary trunk**—the elastic artery through which the blood is pumped by the right ventricle.

10. **Pulmonary semilunar valve**—prevents backflow of blood into the right ventricle. There is also an aortic semilunar valve (not seen here) at the entrance to the aorta; it prevents backflow of blood into the left ventricle.

11. **Left pulmonary artery.** The pulmonary trunk bifurcates to take blood to both the right and the left lungs via the pulmonary arteries.

12. **Left pulmonary veins** bring the highly oxygenated blood back to the left atrium. There are two on the left and two on the right.

13. **Bicuspid, mitral, or left atrioventricular valve.** Only two flaps separate the left atrium from the left ventricle. This valve works just like the right AV valve to prevent backflow

of blood into the left atrium when the left ventricle is pumping blood through the aorta.

14. **Chordae tendineae**—fibrous cords that attach from the apex of papillary muscles to atrioventricular valves. (See them in the right ventricle also.) The cords are passive restraints preventing the valves from being forced back into the atria when the ventricles contract.

15. **Papillary muscle**

16. **Trabeculae carnae**—general term for ridges of muscle in both ventricles.

17. **Myocardium,** muscle of the heart. Note that the muscle here is three times as thick as that of the right ventricle because the blood must be pumped over such a great area and distance.

18. **Arch of the aorta**— Label branches a, b, and c.

19. **Descending** (thoracic) **aorta.** The arch takes the aorta to the posterior heart, where it descends through the thorax.

■ CLINICAL COMMENTS

Mitral valve prolapse (MVP) is a common condition in which the AV valve flaps do not meet to completely close off the blood flow. This can be due to abnormally long or short chordae tendineae or to an irregularly shaped valve. The heart sound is not crisp due to some regurgitation of the blood and a heart murmur is heard. This condition is often undetected and people with minor valve anomalies live perfectly normal lives.

D. CONDUCTION SYSTEM OF THE HEART

The heart, which beats about 72 times per minute, has its own conduction system. This means that it does not require innervation from the CNS to initiate a heartbeat. The autonomic system does affect the rate of the heartbeat, but as long as there is sufficient oxygen and nutrition, the heart can continue to beat without the central nervous system.

The structures of the conduction system are not visible grossly, but they are illustrated and named in the schematic figure below. The **sinuatrial node,** often called the pacemaker, initiates the beat. The impulses move through the atrial muscle causing it to contract and pump the blood into the ventricles. The impulses converge on the **atrioventricular node,** are conducted through the **atrioventricular bundle,** and then to ventricular **Purkinje fibers,** which cause the muscles of the ventricles to contract. To prevent backflow of blood into the atria, the atrioventricular valves are forced to close, and the rapid change in pressure causes the first heart sound.

The ventricles force the blood into the pulmonary trunk and the aorta. After being stretched by the force of blood flow, the elastic fibers in these large conducting arteries recoil, forcing the blood along its way. The closing of the semilunar valves to prevent return of blood into the ventricles causes the second heart sound.

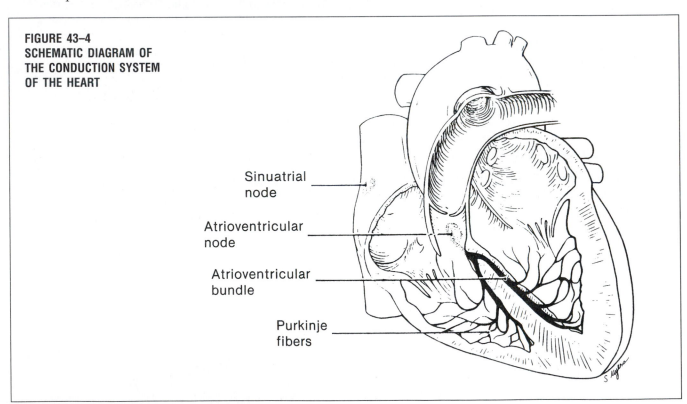

**FIGURE 43–4
SCHEMATIC DIAGRAM OF
THE CONDUCTION SYSTEM
OF THE HEART**

Sinuatrial node

Atrioventricular node

Atrioventricular bundle

Purkinje fibers

■ **Student Activities**

1. In Figure 43–2:
   a. Color the coronary arteries and their branches red; the cardiac veins and coronary sinus blue.
   b. Color the IVC and the SVC blue.
   c. Color the pulmonary trunk and the left pulmonary a. blue.
   d. Color the aorta red.
2. In Figure 43–3, color the vessels that carry highly oxygenated blood pink; color those that carry blood with a high level of carbon dioxide blue. Be careful!

43

Name _____

1. Draw arrows to indicate the direction of blood
   flow through each structure in the illustration.

   Use the following letters to label:

   a. tricuspid valve
   b. papillary m.
   c. pulmonary semilunar valve
   d. interventricular septum
   e. myocardium of left ventricle
   f. pulmonary v.
   g. superior vena cava
   h. inferior vena cava

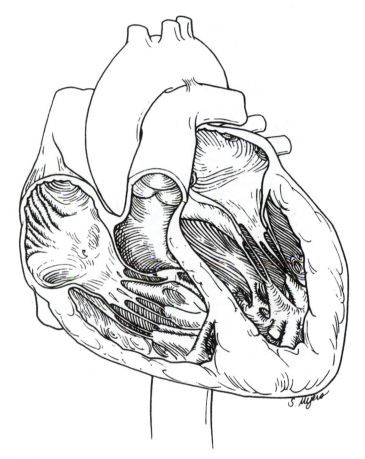

2. Place an X in front of the structure if it contains blood with a high concentration
   of carbon dioxide.

   a. _____ pulmonary   f. _____ aorta   k. _____ left atrium
               trunk

   b. _____ right atrium   g. _____ coronary   l. _____ superior
                                             sinus   vena cava

   c. _____ left ventricle   h. _____ cardiac vein   m. _____ coronary a.

   d. _____ inferior vena   i. _____ right auricle   n. _____ circumflex a.
               cava

   e. _____ right ventricle   j. _____ pulmonary   o. _____ left auricle
                                             vein

3. The three tissues of the heart from superficial to deep are:

a. _____ (the outer covering)

b. _____

c. _____

4. The valves that prevent backflow of blood into the atria are:

a. _____   b. _____

5. The valves that prevent backflow of blood into the ventricles are:

a. _____   b. _____

6. Beginning with the right atrium, name each structure through which the blood must flow to provide blood to the anterior heart muscle and return it to the right atrium.

a. _____right atrium_____

b. _____

c. _____

d. _____

e. _____

f. _____

g. _____

h. _____left ventricle_____

i. _____

j. _____

k. _____

l. _____

m. _____

n. _____right atrium_____

7. To take the blood to the upper limb or the lower limb, which named vessels from the list above would not be used? (Just list the appropriate letters.)

_____

Lesson 44

Fetal Circulation

Fetal circulation differs from adult circulation (1) because the fetus does not have functional lungs, and (2) because it cannot take in its own nutrition and get rid of its own wastes.

The **placenta,** an organ that develops within the uterus of the mother, serves as the communication between maternal and fetal blood. Oxygen and nutrients from the mother's body are carried to the placenta in the mother's blood; the *umbilical vein* originates in the placenta and carries this blood to the fetus. The waste products are returned to the placenta by **umbilical arteries.** The fetal vessels are contained within the **umbilical cord,** the connection between the placenta and the fetus.

■ OBJECTIVES

1. State the reasons why fetal and adult circulation differ.
2. Trace the pattern of blood through the fetal heart.
3. List the adult structures that remain after fetal circulation is no longer necessary.

■ METHODS

1. Study the information provided in this exercise.
2. Complete the indicated activities.

Included in Table 44–1 are the fetal structures with their function and the structures that remain after birth.

An important fact to remember in fetal circulation: The *umbilical vein* carries blood with high oxygen concentration because it is being carried *toward* the fetal heart; the *umbilical arteries* carry blood with high levels of *carbon dioxide* away from the fetal heart. The other system in which the arteries have high levels of carbon dioxide is the _____ .

TABLE 44–1. FETAL STRUCTURES, THEIR FUNCTION, AND NONFUNCTIONAL ADULT STRUCTURE

Fetal Structure	Purpose	Nonfunctional Adult Structure
Umbilical vein	To bring oxygen and nutrients to the fetus from the placenta.	Ligamentum teres hepatis
Ductus venosus	Shunts most of this blood through the liver, because it is already in a form to be used by the fetus.	Ligamentum venosum
Foramen ovale	Shunts blood from the right atrium directly to the left atrium to bypass nonfunctional lungs.	Fossa ovalis
Ductus arteriosus	Shunts blood from the pulmonary trunk directly into the aorta; therefore, most of the blood in the right ventricle bypasses the lungs.	Ligamentum arteriosum
Umbilical arteries	Return poorly oxygenated and waste-filled blood to the placenta.	Ligaments—lateral to the bladder

FIGURE 44–1
SCHEMATIC DIAGRAM OF FETAL CIRCULATION

1. **Umbilical vein**—carries blood going toward the fetal heart. *Place a red arrow in this vessel to indicate the direction of oxygenated blood moving toward the liver.*

2. **Ductus venosus**—shunts the blood through the liver since the maternal liver has already been involved in the preparation of nutrients for the fetus. Some blood needs to enter the fetal liver to help prepare it to take over when the baby is born. *Another red arrow should be drawn through the liver.*

3. **Inferior vena cava**—as all blood from the liver enters the IVC, so does this fetal blood. *Draw a red arrow entering the right atrium (RA).*

4. **Foramen ovale**—provides a way for oxygenated blood to avoid the pulmonary circulation since the fetal lungs are nonfunctional. This opening in the interatrial septum allows blood to cross into the left atrium (LA). *With a hashed line, draw an arrow from the right atrium into the left atrium. From the LA draw a red arrow into the left ventricle (LV).*

   Now this oxygenated blood is ready to be pumped through the aorta and to all body systems.

   Draw a red arrow into the aorta, out each major branch off the aortic arch and then to the descending aorta.

5. **Superior vena cava**—just as in the adult, this blood has supplied the upper body and is returning to the heart with high concentrations of carbon dioxide. *Draw a blue arrow from the SVC through the RA and into the RV.* This poorly oxygenated blood is now ready to be pumped through the pulmonary trunk and arteries into the lungs. *Draw a blue arrow through each pulmonary artery into each lung.* Since the lungs are nonfunctional, only enough blood goes into each to prepare it to function later.

6. **Ductus arteriosus**—shunts much of the blood from the RV directly into the aorta to bypass the nonfunctional lungs. *Draw a blue arrow through the ductus arteriosus and into the descending aorta.* Notice that the "best" blood fed the head before the blood from the RV was shunted into the aorta. Enough oxygen is left for the lower body.

7. **Umbilical arteries**—carry the used blood back to the placenta.

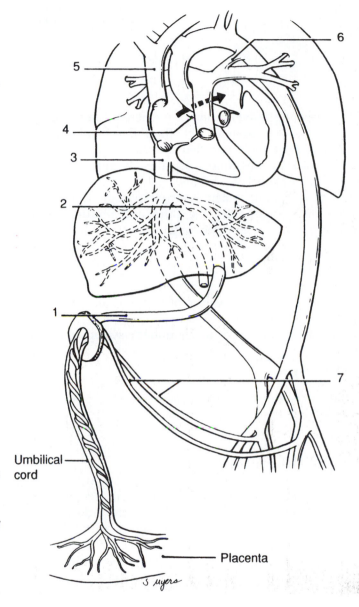

Umbilical cord

Placenta

J myers

Lesson 45

The Lymphatic System

The lymphatic system is often considered a part of the circulatory system. It is, however, a one-way system. The fluid that "leaks out" as the capillaries and cells exchange substances is called *intercellular,* or *interstitial, fluid.* Once the lymphatic vessels pick up this fluid it is called **lymph.** It is carried by lymph vessels to the right and left subclavian veins.

The lymphatic system is also important in helping prevent and fight infections. The lymph nodes filter the fluid and produce lymphocytes, white blood cells involved with the immune system.

■ OBJECTIVES

1. State the purpose of the lymphatic system.
2. Describe the major pattern of lymph drainage.
3. Define lymph node.
4. List the structures of the lymphatic system and describe their anatomical position.

■ METHODS

1. Study the information in this exercise.
2. Complete the indicated activities.

A. LYMPHATIC VESSELS

These vessels begin as blind capillaries in the periphery. As they anastomose they become larger and pass through **lymph nodes.** These small oval bodies contain **phagocytic** cells that clean the lymph of particulate matter such as dust from the lungs, bacteria, or other cellular debris. Another important function of the lymph nodes is the production of **lymphocytes,** white blood cells involved in defense against infection.

Lymph nodes are scattered throughout the body, usually in groups. Some areas where the groups are concentrated are: the popliteal fossa, the inguinal region, along the aorta, in the axillary region, and in the neck. Some can be palpated and, when enlarged, can indicate an area of infection.

The lymph vessels lead toward two major lymph ducts. The **thoracic duct** collects the lymph drainage from below the diaphragm and from the left half of the body above the diaphragm. It empties into the left subclavian vein. The **right lymphatic duct** collects the lymph fluid from the right side of the body above the diaphragm and drains into the right subclavian vein.

B. TONSILS (PHARYNGEAL, PALATINE, AND LINGUAL)

The tonsils are collections of lymphoid tissue. The tonsils produce lymphocytes and convey them to the bloodstream. They are involved in the body's immune response to infection.

C. THE THYMUS GLAND

This gland is located behind the sternum and anterior to the trachea. The thymus reaches its greatest size about puberty and then atrophies. Before it atrophies it has played a major role in the immune system by: (1) producing certain lymphocytes that migrate to other lymphoid tissue, and (2) producing hormones to stimulate the maturity of these cells.

D. THE SPLEEN

The spleen is the largest mass of lymphatic tissue in the body and is located between the fundus of the stomach and the diaphragm. The spleen is covered by a serous membrane, **peritoneum.** The spleen produces lymphocytes, but instead of filtering lymph fluid, it filters blood and phagocytizes bacteria and worn-out red blood cells. Products of red-cell destruction are carried to the liver.

An additional function of the spleen is the storage and release of blood in case of demand. Sympathetic impulses cause smooth muscle to contract and push out the blood. If the spleen is removed, the liver and bone marrow take over most of its functions.

■ CLINICAL COMMENTS

Edema is a condition in which a part of the body becomes swollen due to the buildup of fluid in the tissues. Fluid normally leaks into intercellular space from the capillaries; then, lymphatic vessels pick it up and return it to the cardiovascular system. Edema results when too much fluid enters the intercellular space, or when the lymphatic vessels do not pick up enough fluid.

FIGURE 45–1
THE LYMPHATIC SYSTEM

1. **Lymph vessels**

2. **Lymph nodes**

3. **Thoracic duct**—collects the lymph from the left half of the body above the diaphragm and all the lower body. It empties into the left subclavian vein.

4. **Right lymphatic duct**—collects the lymph from the right side of the head, neck, and thorax and the right upper extremity. It empties into the right subclavian vein.

5. **Tonsils**

6. **Thymus**

7. **Spleen**

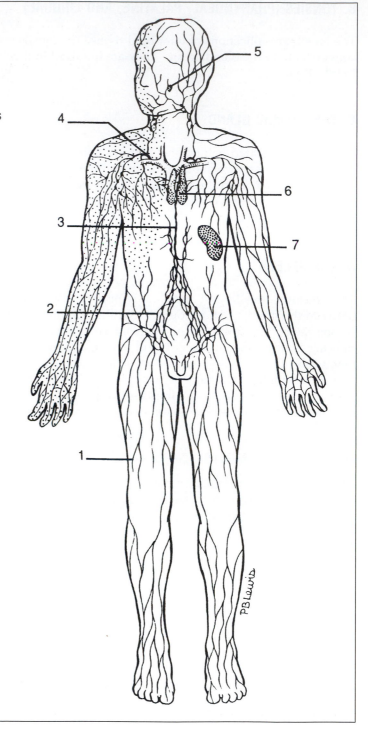

■ **Student Activities**

1. In Figure 45–1:
   a. Color the spleen and tonsils red.
   b. Color the thymus gland yellow.
   c. Place an arrow beside the thoracic duct to indicate the direction of flow of lymph.
2. Name the only lymph structure that does not produce lymphocytes.

Exercise 46

Review of Unit IV

I. In the illustration on the right, draw the following structures listed below. Label each with the appropriate letter. Use broken lines for any structure you must place behind another.

a. diaphragm (thoracic)
b. stomach
c. heart
d. lungs
e. pituitary gland
f. kidneys
g. liver
h. ovaries
i. spleen
j. adrenal gland
k. gall bladder
l. cecum
m. descending colon
n. thyroid gland
o. testes

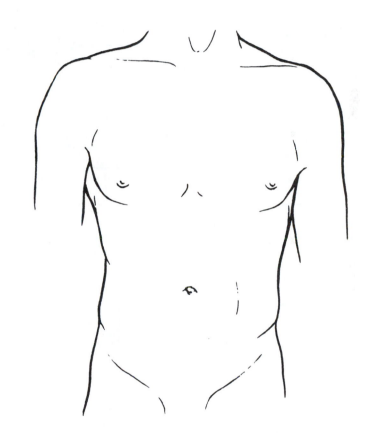

II. List below all the systems of the body represented in the list above.

a. _____   e. _____

b. _____   f. _____

c. _____   g. _____

d. _____   h. _____

III. Fill in the blank with the structure being described.

_____ a. Rolled under aponeurosis, which extends from the anterior superior iliac spine to the pubic tubercle.

_____ b. Vessel found just deep to rectus abdominis m. at the level of the iliac crest.

_____ c. Abdominal muscle that might help protect kidneys from a sharp blow.

_____ d. Located between the laryngopharynx and the stomach.

IV. Using illustrations shown here, color the arteries red and the veins blue; list correct name for the labeled vessels; answer the questions on the following page.

a. _____

b. _____

c. _____

d. _____

e. _____

f. _____

g. _____

h. _____

i. _____

j. _____

k. _____

l. _____

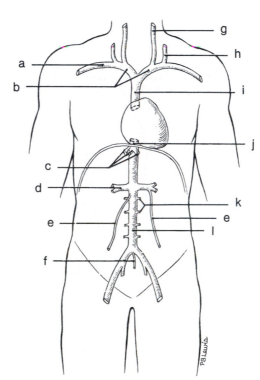

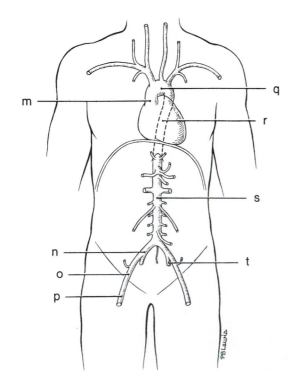

m. _____

n. _____

o. _____

p. _____

q. _____

r. _____

s. _____

t. _____

Name two large abdominal veins that have no artery of the same name. (One is not pictured. **Hint:** It carries intestinal blood.)

u. _____ and v. _____

w. Name one artery that has no vein of the same name. _____

V. Answer the following questions.
1. Name two structures that pass through the inguinal canal.
2. Name the layers of the digestive tube from superficial to deep.
3. What portion of the digestive tube receives the products from the accessory digestive organs?
4. Name the three accessory digestive organs located in the abdominal cavity.
5. Name the tubular structures in the path of urine.
6. Name the two structures that form the renal corpuscle.
7. Name three abdominopelvic organs that are largely storage vessels.
8. What is the peritoneal structure found between the diaphragm and the liver? Between the liver and the anterior abdominal wall?
9. Beginning at the mouth, list the structures through which water would pass before it could exit the urethra. How many body systems must be involved? What are they?
10. Name the muscle that is most important in respiration. What is its innervation?
11. What is the functional unit of the kidney? What is its function?
12. For each ligament listed below indicate whether it is a peritoneal structure (P) or a solid cord (C).

_____ falciform ligament _____ ligamentum teres hepatis

_____ ovarian ligament _____ broad ligament

_____ suspensory ligament of _____ ligamentum arteriosum
        ovary

_____ coronary ligament _____ round ligament of the uterus
13. Name each structure in the passageway of food from the mouth to the anus.
14. Name each structure in the passageway of air from the nose to the lungs.
15. Name the three serous sacs important in the proper functioning of viscera. In which body cavity are they located?
16. Name the pathway of blood from the heart to the intestines and back.
17. What are the common functions of the ovary and the testes?
18. Name the organ that would be suggested by each of the following:

glomerulus _____ seminiferous tubules _____

cystic _____ renal _____

hepatic _____ cardiac _____

alveoli _____ hemolymph _____

estrogen _____ mesenteric _____
19. Name the structures that would be encountered if you stuck a pin in the abdomen just superior to the anterior superior iliac spine.
20. Would it be possible for sperm to settle on the parietal peritoneum that lies between the uterus and the rectum? Explain.
21. Name the path of sperm from the testes to the penile urethra.
22. Sketch the anatomy of the hepatic portal system. Discuss its significance.
23. Name the vessels in the path of blood from the heart to the glomerulus.
24. Name the vessels in the path of blood from the heart to the spleen.
25. Name the tributaries of the inferior vena cava.
26. What autonomic fibers innervate the ascending colon? The descending colon?

27. What is the function of the vagal fibers to the colon?
28. What is the function of the sympathetic fibers to the colon?
29. Name the bones and muscles of the parietal thorax.
30. Describe the blood supply to the parietal thorax, giving both an anterior and posterior source of blood. What is the major venous structure?
31. What is the innervation of the parietal thorax?
32. What are the boundaries of the mediastinum?
33. Other than mediastinal structures, what is found in the thorax?
34. What is pleura?
35. Name the three largest structures that pass through the diaphragm.
36. Give the innervation of the diaphragm. What are the cord levels of origin?
37. Name the major sources of blood to the diaphragm.
38. Why are ventral rami of thoracic spinal nerves T1–T11 also called intercostal nerves? What is T12 called?
39. What is the major function of the respiratory system?
40. What is the contact between the respiratory system and the circulatory system?
41. What is the difference in bronchial vessels and pulmonary vessels?
42. List in order each anatomical structure the air would encounter from the nose to the alveoli.
43. Define pharynx. What is its direct continuation called?
44. Define larynx. List its four major cartilages.
45. What is the purpose of the larynx?
46. Where is the esophagus in relationship to the trachea?
47. If you climbed into the opening protected by torus tubarius, where would the passageway take you?
48. What cartilage helps protect the opening from the pharynx into the larynx?
49. What is the relationship of the true and false vocal folds?
50. What is the purpose of the right side of the heart?
51. Is there ever a direct communication between the right and left sides of the heart? Explain.
52. What vessels supply the blood to the heart muscle itself? What vessels are involved in the venous return?
53. What is the major purpose of the circulatory system?
54. What causes the first and then the second heart sound?
55. Name the two serous membranes of the thorax.
56. Name two places where veins contain high levels of oxygen.
57. Why is fetal circulation different from that of an adult?
58. Name two major purposes of the lymphatic system.
59. Name four structures of the lymphatic system other than vessels. Where is each located?
60. What lymphatic structure is involved in cleaning blood?
61. What is the major difference in the innervation of the parietal thorax and its viscera?

VI. Label the peritoneal structures in the illustrations:

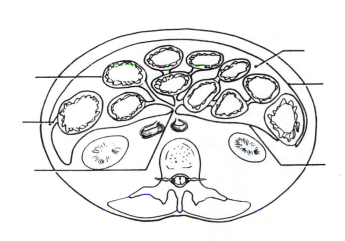

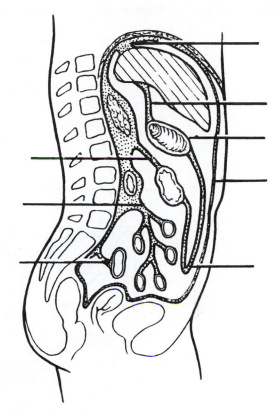

VII. In the illustration, sketch the appropriate location of the trachea, primary bronchi, lungs, heart, and diaphragm. On the left, list the major structures that would be found behind the heart.

1. _____

2. _____

3. _____

4. _____

5. _____

6. _____

7. _____

8. _____

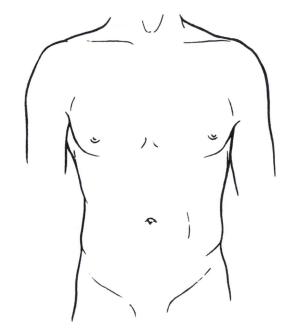

VIII. In the illustration, label all structures indicated. Place arrows indicating the direction of blood flow in all vessels and in each chamber.

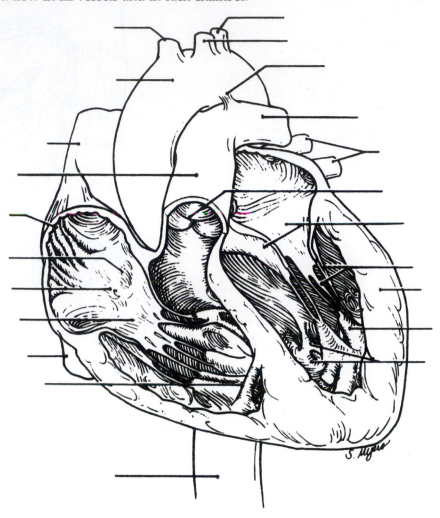

Appendix

Answers to Exercises and Student Activities

UNIT 1

STUDENT ACTIVITY, P 4

1. a. is distal to b;
   b. is proximal to a.

2. c. is proximal to b;
   b. is distal to c.

3. c. is proximal to a;
   a. is distal to c.

EXERCISE 1

1. a. Lateral view
   b. Anterior view

3. a. distal
   b. superior
   c. transverse
   d. superficial

EXERCISE 2

1. a. Posterior

2. a. Periosteum
   b. Compact bone
   c. Spongy bone
   d. Endosteum
   e. Yellow marrow

3. a. Epiphyseal plate
   b. Periosteum
   c. Diaphysis
   d. Osteoblast
   e. Osteon
   f. Red marrow
   g. Yellow marrow

EXERCISE 3

1. a. ischium
   b. ilium
   c. tibia; medial
   d. Femur
3. Right
4. a. P, femur
   b. P, tibia
   c. M, tibia
   d. P, femur
   e. P, femur
   f. L, fibula
   g. A, femur
   h. A, tibia

STUDENT ACTIVITY, P 32

   b. Extension of hip (thigh)
   c. Abduction of hip (thigh)
   d. Adduction of hip (thigh)
   e. Rotation of hip (thigh)
   f. Circumduction of hip
   g. Flexion of knee (leg)
   h. Extension of knee (leg)

EXERCISE 5

2. a. Tonus
   b. Skeletal
   c. Fascicle
   d. Epimysium
   e. Tendon
   f. Endomysium
   g. Skeletal
   h. Yes, the smooth muscle of vessels.
3. b. eight
   c. No
   d. Periosteum

FIGURE 6–2

1. Gluteus medius
2. Gluteus maximus

FIGURE 6–4. *SEE* EXERCISE 6.

FIGURE 6–9. *SEE* EXERCISE 6.

EXERCISE 6

3. Figure 6–4:
   a. Major action   extends knee
      Innervation   femoral n.
   b. Major action   adducts hip
      Innervation   obturator n.
   c. Major action   extends hip and flexes knee
      Innervation   tibial n.
   Figure 6–9:
   1. Gluteus medius
   2. Gluteus maximus
   3. Iliotibial tract
5. 1. f
   2. j
   3. h
   4. b, h
   5. i
   6. d
   7. g
   8. a
   9. e
  10. c
6. a. Adductor magnus or gracilis
   b. Iliopsoas
   c. Biceps femoris
   d. Flexed
   e. Quadriceps femoris
   f. Gluteus maximus or posterior femorals
   g. Extends hip

EXERCISE 7

6. a. Intrinsic
   b. Calcaneal tendon
   c. Eversion of foot
   d. Lateral
   e. Flexion of the knee (leg)
7. 1. Gastrocnemius, medial head
   2. Gastrocnemius, lateral head
   3. Soleus m.
   4. Calcaneal tendon
   5. Tibialis anterior m.
   6. Peroneus longus m.
   7. Gastrocnemius, medial head
   8. Extensor digitorum longus m.
   9. Extensor hallucis longus m.
  10. (Superior) extensor retinaculum

FIGURE 9–1

1. Femoral n. L2, 3, 4
2. Obturator n. L2, 3, 4
5. Sciatic n. L4, 5, S1, 2, 3

FIGURE 9–2

1. Gluteus medius
2. Gluteus minimus
3. Gluteus maximus
4. Piriformis

STUDENT ACTIVITIES, P 68

Muscle Group (Position)	Major Group Action	Major Group Innervation
Anterior Hip Muscles 1. iliacus 2. Psoas major	Flexes hip (trunk or thigh)	Femoral n.

Anterior Femoral Muscles
1. Sartorius
2. Quadriceps Femoris
  a. Rectus femoris b. Vastus medialis
  c. Vastus lateralis d. Vastus intermedius
	Extends leg (knee)	Femoral n.

Medial Femoral Muscles 1. Pectineus 2. Gracilis 3. Adductor longus 4. Adductor brevis 5. Adductor magnus	Adducts hip (thigh)	Obturator n.
Posterior Femoral Muscles 1. Biceps femoris 2. Semitendinosus 3. Semimembranosus	Extends hip; flexes knee	Tibial n. (some common peroneal n.)
Anterior Crural Muscles 1. Extensor digitorum longus 2. Tibialis anterior 4. Fibularis (peroneus) tertius 3. Extensor hallucis llongus	Inverts and dorsiflexes ankle; extends digits	Deep fibular (peroneal) n.
Lateral Crural Muscles 1. Fibularis (peroneus) longus 2. Fibularis (peroneus) brevis	Everts ankle (foot)	Superficial fibular (peroneal) n
Posterior Crural Muscles 1. Gastrocnemius 2. Plantaris 3. Soleus	Flexes knee; plantar flexes foot (ankle)	Tibial n.
Posterior Crural Muscles (Deep) 1. Tibialis posterior 2. Flexor digitorum longus 3. Flexor hallucis longus 4. Popliteus	Plantar flexes foot; inverts foot (ankle)	Tibial n.

EXERCISE 9

2. 1. d
   2. a
   3. f
   4. b
   5. e
   6. c
3. a. Superficial fibular (peroneal) n.
   b. Superior gluteal n.
   c. Sciatic n.

d. Deep fibular (peroneal) n.
   or common fibular (peroneal) n.
e. Obturator n.
f. Femoral n.
4. a. deep fibular (peroneal) n.
   b. femoral n.
   c. obturator n.
   d. sciatic n.
   e. tibial n.

EXERCISE 11

1. Walls are one cell thick.
2. a. Elastic conducting a.
   b. Muscular distributing a.
   c. Arterioles
   d. Capillaries
   e. Venules
   f. Veins
3. a. An **artery** is a vascular structure that takes blood away from the heart.
   b. A **vein** is a vascular structure that takes blood toward the heart.
4. a. Deep femoral a.
   b. Anterior tibial a.
   c. Popliteal a.
   d. Femoral a.
   e. Peroneal a.
5. a. Deep peroneal n.
   b. Tibial n.
   c. Superior gluteal n.
   d. Obturator n.
6. c. Common iliac a.
   d. External iliac artery
   e. Femoral a.
   f. Popliteal a.
   g. Anterior tibial a.
   i. Anterior tibial venae comitantes
   j. Popliteal v.
   k. Femoral v.
   l. External iliac v.
   m. Common iliac v.

STUDENT ACTIVITY, P 86

1. External iliac a.
2. Femoral n.
3. Superficial fibular (peroneal) n.
4. Deep fibular (peroneal) n.
5. Femoral a.
6. Obturator n.
7. Anterior tibial a.
8. Dorsalis pedis a.
9. Popliteal a.
10. Tibial n.
11. Fibular (peroneal) a.
12. Posterior tibial a.
13. Tibial n.
14. Medial plantar a.
15. Sciatic n.
16. Common fibular (peroneal) n.
17. Deep fibular (peroneal) n.
18. Superficial fibular (peroneal) n.
19. Lateral plantar n.

EXERCISE 12

a. Popliteal fossa
b. Femoral triangle

EXERCISE 13   REVIEW OF UNIT I

I.
1. Psoas major m.	20. Extensor digitorum longus m.
2. Iliopsoas m.	21. Fibularis (peroneus) brevis m.
3. Pectineus m.	22. Extensor retinaculum
4. Sartorius m.	23. Gluteus medius m.
5. Gracilis m.	24. Adductor magnus m.
6. Vastus lateralis m.	25. Semitendinosus m.
7. Tibialis anterior m.	26. Iliotibial tract
8. Extensor digitorum longus m.	27. Semimembranosus m.
9. Soleus m.	28. Plantaris m.
10. Extensor hallucis longus m.	29. Gastrocnemius m.
11. Extensor digitorum brevis m.	30. Soleus m.
12. Iliacus m.	31. Gluteus maximus m.
13. Tensor fasciae latae m.	32. Biceps femoris m.
14. Adductor longus m.	33. Semimembranosus m.
15. Adductor magnus m.	34. Gracilis m.
16. Rectus femoris m.	35. Gastrocnemius m.
17. Vastus medialis m.	36. Plantaris tendon
18. Gastrocnemius m.	37. Calcaneal tendon
19. Fibularis (peroneus) longus m.	

II. Asterisks indicate the most important muscles; parentheses indicate the least important muscles.

Muscles that act on the hip to:

Flex	**Extend**	**Abduct**
1. Psoas major*	1. Gluteus maximus*	1. Gluteus minimus*
2. Iliacus*	2. Semimembranosus*	2. Gluteus medius*
3. Sartorius*	3. Semitendinosus*	3. Tensor fasciae latae
4. Rectus femoris*	4. Biceps femoris*	4. Obturator internus
5. Tensor fasciae latae	(Gluteus medius)	(Gemelli)
(Adductor longus)	(Adductor magnus)	
(Adductor brevis)		
(Pectineus)		

Adduct	**Medially rotate**	**Laterally rotate**
1. Pectineus	1. Tensor fasciae latae	1. Gluteus maximus*
2. Gracilis	2. Gluteus medius	2. Piriformis
3. Adductor longus	3. Gluteus minimus	3. Sartoris
4. Adductor brevis	(Adductor magnus)	4. Quadratus femoris
5. Adductor magnus	(Adductor longus)	5. Gemelli
		6. Obturator internus
		and externus
		(Adductor longus)
		(Adductor magnus
		and brevis)

Muscles that act on the knee to:

Flex	Extend
1. Biceps femoris*	1. Rectus femoris
2. Semitendinosus*	2. Vastus lateralis
3. Semimembranosus*	3. Vastus intermedius
4. Gastrocnemius*	4. Vastus medialis
5. Plantaris	
6. Sartorius	
7. Gracilis	
8. Popliteus	

Muscles that act on the ankle and intertarsal joints to:

Dorsiflex	Plantar flex	Invert
1. Tibialis anterior	1. Gastrocnemius*	1. Tibialis anterior*
2. Extensor digitorum longus	2. Soleus*	2. Tibialis posterior*
3. Extensor hallucis longus (Fibularis tertius)	3. Plantaris	3. Extensor hallucis longus
	4. Tibialis posterior	4. Flexor hallucis longus
	5. Flexor hallucis longus	
	6. Flexor digitorum longus	
	7. Fibularis (peroneus) longus	
	8. Fibularis (peroneus) brevis	

Evert

1. Fibularis (peroneus) longus*
2. Fibularis (peroneus) brevis*
   (Fibularis tertius)
   (Extensor digitorum longus)

Muscles that act on the metatarsophalangeal and interphalangeal joints to:

Flex digits	Extend digits	Abduct digits
1. Flexor hallucis longus	1. Extensor hallucis longus	1. Abductor hallucis
2. Flexor hallucis brevis	2. Extensor digitorum longus	2. Abductor digiti minimi
3. Flexor digitorum longus	3. Extensor digitorum brevis	3. Dorsal interossei
4. Flexor digitorum brevis		

Adduct digits

1. Adductor hallucis
2. Plantar interossei

III. Answers to questions:

1. **Gross anatomy**—the study of large structures that can be seen with the naked eye
   Histology—microscopic study of cells and tissues
   Embryology—study of the developing organism from the time of fertilization to birth
   Neuroanatomy—study of the structure of the nervous system
2. Epithelial, connective, muscle, nerve
3. The body is standing erect, face toward observer, with feet together and parallel, the arms at the sides and the palms directed forward
4. **inferior**—superior is nearer the head end than that which is inferior.
   superficial—deep structures are not as near the surface of the body as those which are more superficial.
   lateral—medial structures are nearer the midline than those which are lateral.
   proximal—distal structures are farther from the attached end than those which are more proximal.
5. **Sagittal**—a vertical plane that divides the body into right and left portions
   Coronal—a vertical plane that divides the body into anterior and posterior portions
   Transverse—a horizontal plane that cuts the body into superior and inferior portions
6. The skeleton provides support, protection, leverage in movement, production of blood cells, and storage for minerals.
7. The **diaphysis** is the long shaft of the bone; the **epiphysis** is the end of the bone.
8. Periosteum
9. Osteocyte; osteoblast
10. **Osteon**—composed of Haversian canal, lamellae, lacunae, osteocytes, canaliculi
11. **Process**—rough bony prominence   *Example:* tibial tuberosity
    Spine—pointed projection of bone   *Example:* ischial spine
    Foramen—a hole in a bone   *Example:* obturator foramen
    Crest—a prominent border, which may be rough   *Example:* iliac crest
    Fossa—a saucer-like depression   *Example:* iliac fossa
    Condyle—a smooth, concave or convex structure for articulation with other bone   *Example:* medial condyle of femur
    Facet—a smooth surface for articulation   *Example:* fibular facet on tibia
12. Sacrum
13. Ilium, ischium, pubis
14. *See* Figure 3–4 (lateral view).
15. The **false pelvic cavity** is bounded by the flared portion of the iliac bones; the **true pelvic cavity** is inferior to the false and is surrounded by pelvic bones. The **pelvic brim** separates these regions.
16. *See* Figure 3–6.
17. **Patella**—It is located within the tendon of the quadriceps femoris muscles and on the anterior aspect of the knee. It serves as a fulcrum for the quadriceps muscles and helps protect the knee joint.
18. Fibula, tibia
19. Crest of tibia, calcaneal tendon, medial malleolus, lateral malleolus, plantar aspect of foot
20. **femur:** proximal = os coxae;   distal = tibia and patella
    tibia: proximal = femur and fibula; distal = fibula and talus
    fibula: proximal = tibia;   distal = tibia and talus

21. Cuboid
22. **Synarthrosis**—tibia to fibula
    Amphiarthrosis—pubic symphysis
    Diarthrosis—knee
23. Production of movement, production of heat, maintenance of posture
24. Cardiac, smooth (visceral), skeletal
25. Endomysium, perimysium, epimysium
26. *See* "Actions Produced by Skeletal Muscle" and Figure 5–3.
27. Antagonist
28. a. Extension of hip, flexion of knee
    b. Extension of knee
    c. Plantar flexion of ankle, flexion of knee
    d. Abduction of hip
29. a. Inguinal ligament
    b. Sacrospinous ligament
    c. Inguinal ligament
30. **Fascia lata** is the deep fascia that invests the thigh. The **iliotibial tract** is a thickened strip of fascia lata on the lateral thigh.
31. Adductor magnus m.; vastus lateralis (or tensor fascia lata if superior)
32. Gluteus maximus
33. Rectus femoris, vastus lateralis, vastus medialis, vastus intermedius
34. Biceps femoris
35. Extensor digitorum longus and flexor digitorum longus
36. **Intrinsic foot muscles** include extensor digitorum brevis and any from Table 7–6.
    Extrinsic foot muscles include all those muscles with bellies on the leg and tendons to the foot. *See* Tables 7–1, 7–2, 7–3, and 7–4.
37. Two
38. A **retinaculum** is a strip of fascia with a greater collagen fiber density than the crural fascia. This band holds tendons close to the joint.
39. Tibialis anterior; gastrocnemius
40. Interosseous membrane
41. Gastrocnemius and soleus
42. Tendons of tibialis posterior, flexor digitorum longus, posterior tibial artery, tibial nerve, tendon of flexor hallucis longus
    Tendon of fibularis (peroneus) brevis then tendon of fibularis (peroneus) longus
43. Extensor digitorum brevis m.
44. Interosseous muscles between the metatarsal bones
45. A **neuron** is a functional nerve cell.
46. Anterior horn of gray matter in the spinal cord
    Dorsal root ganglia
47. Brain, spinal cord
48. A **nerve** is a bundle of nerve cell *processes* held together in a fascial sheath. A **mixed nerve** contains both motor and sensory processes.
49. A **nerve plexus** is an intermingling of the nerve cell processes of spinal nerves from different cord levels of origin. The lower limb plexuses are the lumbar and sacral.
50. Lumbar plexus = T12, L1, 2, 3, 4
    Sacral plexus = L4, 5 and S1, 2, 3, 4
51. Femoral n. and obturator n.
52. Sacral only
53. Common fibular (peroneal) n. Inability to dorsiflex the ankle; eversion of the foot would also be almost totally eliminated.

54. Sciatic n., superior and inferior gluteal nerves (plus other sacral plexus nerves to the posterior gluteal m.)
55. Nerves that are sensory to the skin (no motor fibers); dorsal root ganglia
56. The cardiovascular system is the transportation system delivering nutrients and removing wastes from all body tissues.
57. The right side of the heart receives poorly oxygenated blood and pumps it to the lungs—the **pulmonary pump.** The left side of the heart receives well-oxygenated blood and pumps it to the entire body—the **systemic pump.**
58. From superficial to deep: tunica externa, tunica media, tunica intima
59. **Arteries** have thicker walls, smaller diameter, and no valves. **Veins** are more numerous, have a greater number of anastomoses, and contain valves.
60. Muscular distributing
61. Typically one cell thick, the **capillary** provides the thin wall needed for exchange of nutrients and wastes between the circulatory system and the body cells.
62. **Anastomoses** occur when structures open into each other by connecting channels. In **collateral circulation,** there is more than one source of blood to the same area.
63. Veins
64. Aorta, common iliac a., external iliac a., femoral a., popliteal a., anterior tibial a., dorsalis pedis a.

    Aorta, common iliac a., external iliac a., femoral a., popliteal a., posterior tibial a., medial plantar a.
65. Inguinal ligament; adductor hiatus; ankle
66. Deep peroneal nerve; tibial nerve; obturator nerve
67. medial
68. popliteal surface; popliteal muscle
69. An opening in the tendon of adductor magnus muscle
70. The muscles—and their deep fascia
71. The **greater saphenous vein** arises on the medial side of the foot, ascends on the medial leg and thigh to move antero-laterally and empty into the femoral vein at the femoral triangle.

    The **lesser saphanous vein** arises on the lateral side of the foot and ascends on the posterior leg to enter the popliteal fossa and empty into the popliteal vein.
72. Sartorius
73. Soleus
74. Forked—having two branches
75. Two veins accompanying one artery

    They are found largely in the leg and forearm.

76. Completed chart

Innervation	Muscle (or group)	Bone Marking (attachment)	Artery that supplies blood	Figure # of marking used
Femoral n.	Quadriceps femoris	tibial tuberosity (distal)	femoral a.	3-8
Obturator n.	medical femoral m.	medial pelvis [pubis] (proximal)	obturator a.	3-1 or 3-4
Superior gluteal n.	gluteus medius & minimus	greater trochanter (distal)	superior gluteal a.	3-6
Inferior gluteal n.	gluteus maximus	gluteal tuberosity (distal)	inferior gluteal a.	3-6
Tibial div. of sciatic (above split)	posterior femoral m.	ischial tuberosity (proximal)	deep femoral n.	3-4 or 3-5
Tibial n. (below split)	posterior crural m.	calcaneus and bones of foot (distal)	posterior tibial a.	
Femoral n.	Ant. hip muscle	lesser trochanter (distal)	external iliac and femoral a. [some common and internal iliac]	3-6

UNIT II

FIGURE 14–4.

See Exercise 14.

FIGURE 14–5.

See Exercise 14.

FIGURE 14–6

See Figure 3–2

EXERCISE 14

FIGURE 14–4:

3. Intervertebral foramen
6. Intervertebral disc
7. Vertebral body

FIGURE 14–5:

4. Vertebral body
4. a. Scoliosis
   b. Lordosis
   c. Kyphosis
5. a. Axis
   b. Lumbar vertebra
   c. Cervical vertebra
   d. Atlas
6. 1. e
   2. c
   3. d
   4. a
   5. g
   6. h
   7. b
   8. f

STUDENT ACTIVITIES, P 103

2. a. axial
   b. three
   c. dorsal rami of spinal nerves
   d. extension and rotation of vertebral column and head

FIGURE 16–6

2. Middle phalanx of 5th digit
3. Proximal phalanx of 5th digit

STUDENT ACTIVITIES, P 109

2. humerus, ulna, scaphoid, lunate

EXERCISE 16

1. a. scapula
   b. ulna
   c. radius
      scaphoid
      lunate
   d. humerus
   e. radius
3. 1. L, humerus
   2. P, humerus
   3. A, humerus
   4. A, ulna
   5. A, scapula
   6. M, humerus
   7. P, humerus
   8. M, ulna *or*
      L, radius

STUDENT ACTIVITY, P 111

diarthroses

FIGURE 18–4

2. Serratus anterior

FIGURE 18–6

1. Supraspinatus m.
2. Infraspinatus m.
3. Teres minor m.

FIGURE 18–10

1. Supraspinatus m.
2. Infraspinatus m.
3. Teres minor m.
4. Teres major m.
5. Deltoid m.

STUDENT ACTIVITIES, P 121

3. medial head

EXERCISE 18

1. a. Trapezius and latissimus dorsi
   b. Levator scapulae and rhomboids
   c. Subscapularis
   d. Pectoralis minor, short head biceps, and coracobrachialis
   e. Brachialis
2. 1. f, b
   2. c, i
   3. e
   4. a, h (g, f)
   5. a, h, j (f)
   6. g
   7. c (f)
   8. d (f)
3. a. Trapezius
   b. Deltoid
   c. Pectoralis major
   d. Serratus anterior
   e. Biceps brachii
   f. Supraspinatus
   g. Infraspinatus
   h. Teres major
   i. Deltoid
   j. Teres minor

EXERCISE 19

2. medial epicondyle
4. Opponens pollicis, opponens digiti minimi, and adductor pollicis
5. a. Brachioradialis—radial n.—flexes elbow
   b. Flexor retinaculum
   c. Medial epicondyle
   d. Pronator teres—median n.—pronator of hand
   e. Palmar aponeurosis
6. a. Extend digits
   b. Abduct digits
   c. Pronation
   d. Supination

TEXT, P 134

1. Radial n. (cord levels) C5, 6, 7, 8, T1
2. Axillary n. (cord levels) C5, 6
3. Musculocutaneous n. C5, 6, 7
4. Median n. C5, 6, 7, 8, T1
5. Ulnar n. C8, T1

EXERCISE 20

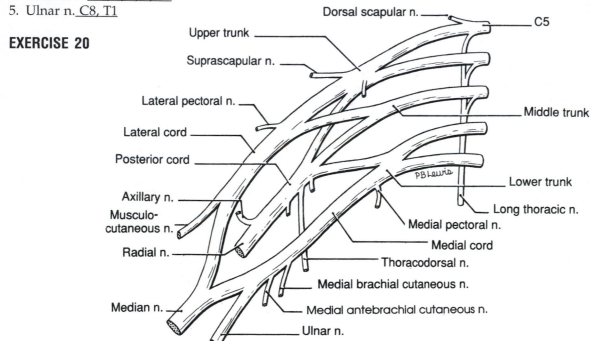

2. a. CN XI, accessory n.
   b. Axillary n.
   c. Medial and lateral pectoral nerves
   d. Long thoracic n.
   e. Musculocutaneous n.

3. Completed chart:

Name	Muscle Innervated	Origin
Axillary n.	1. Deltoid	Posterior cord
Radial n.	1. Triceps brachii 2. (group) All posterior arm All posterior forearm	Posterior cord
Musculocutaneous n.	1. Coracobracialis 2. Biceps brachii 3. Brachialis	Lateral cord
Median	1. (group) Anterior forearm 2. (group) Thenar eminence	Medial and lateral cord
Ulnar	1. (group) Most hand m.	Medial cord

4. a. radial n.
    b. musculocutaneous and radial nerves
    c. median n.
    d. ulnar n.
    e. CN, XI, accessory n.

EXERCISE 21

5. 1. Right brachiocephalic vein
   2. Left brachiocephalic vein
   3. Superior vena cava
6. a. brachial a.
   b. radial a.

STUDENT ACTIVITIES, P 145

2. Circumflex scapular a.; posterior circumflex humeral a. and axillary n.

STUDENT ACTIVITIES, P 146

4. 1. axillary a.
    2. axillary n.
    3. anterior circumflex humeral a.
    4. musculocutaneous n.
    5. radial n.
    6. deep brachial a.
    7. radial a.
    8. deep palmar arterial arch
    9. ulnar n.
    10. brachial a.
    11. median n.
    12. ulnar a.
    13. ulnar n.
    14. superficial palmar arterial arch
    15. medial cord
    16. ulnar n.
    17. upper trunk
    18. lateral cord
    19. posterior cord
    20. axillary n.
    21. radial n.
    22. deep brachial a.
    23. radial n.
    24. posterior interosseous a.

EXERCISE 23   REVIEW OF UNIT II

I.

1. Deltoid m.
2. Latissimus dorsi m.
3. Biceps brachii m.
4. Brachialis m.
5. Pronator teres m.
6. Brachioradialis m.
7. Flexor retinaculum m.
8. Thenar eminence m.
9. Pectoralis major m.
10. Serratus anterior m.
11. Hypothenar eminence m.
12. Trapezius m.
13. Latissimus dorsi m.
14. Deltoid m.
15. Triceps brachii m.
16. Extensor retinaculum

II. Asterisks indicate the most important muscles; parentheses indicate the least important muscles.

Muscles that act on the shoulder (glenohumeral) joint to:

Flex the arm

1. Pectoralis major
2. Deltoid* (anterior fibers)
3. Coracobrachialis*
4. Biceps brachii

Extend the arm

1. Latissimus dorsi*
2. Deltoid (posterior fibers)
3. Teres major
4. Triceps brachii

Abduct the arm

1. Supraspinatus
2. Deltoid

Adduct the arm

1. Pectoralis major*
2. Latissimus dorsi*
3. Teres major
4. Coracobrachialis (Infraspinatus)

Medially rotate arm

1. Pectoralis major*
2. Latissimus dorsi*
3. Deltoid (anterior fibers)
4. Subscapularis
5. Teres major

Laterally rotate arm

1. Deltoid (posterior fibers)
2. Infraspinatus (Teres minor)

Muscles that act on the elbow to:

Flex forearm

1. Biceps brachii*
2. Brachialis*
3. Brachioradialis* (Pronator teres)

Extend forearm

1. Triceps brachii* (Anconeus)

Supinate

1. Biceps brachii
2. Supinator

Pronate

1. Pronator teres
2. Pronator quadratus (Flexor carpi radialis)

Muscles that act on the wrist to:

Flex

1. Flexor carpi radialis
2. Palmaris longus
3. Flexor carpi ulnaris
4. Flexor digiti superficialis
5. Flexor digiti profundis
6. Flexor pollicis longus

Extend

1. Extensor carpi radialis longus
2. Extensor carpi radialis brevis
3. Extensor digitorum communis
4. Extensor carpi ulnaris
5. Extensor digiti minimi
6. Extensor indicis

Abduct

1. Flexor carpi radialis
2. Extensor carpi radialis longus
3. Extensor carpi radialis brevis
4. Abductor pollicis longus (Extensor pollicis brevis) (Extensor pollicis longus)

Adduct

1. Flexor carpi ulnaris
2. Extensor carpi ulnaris

Muscles that act on the metacarpophalangeal and interphalangeal joint to:

Flex digits

1. Flexor digitorum superior
2. Flexor digitorum profundis
3. Flexor pollicis longus
4. Flexor pollicis brevis
5. Flexor digit minimi
6. Lumbricales [metacarpophalangeal]

Extend digits

1. Extensor digitorum [communis]
2. Extensor digiti minimi
3. Extensor pollicis brevis
4. Extensor pollicis longus
5. Extensor indicis
6. Lumbricales [interphalangeal]

Abduct digits

1. Abductor pollicis longus
2. Abductor pollicis brevis
3. Abductor digiti minimi
4. Dorsal interossei

Adduct digits

1. Adductor pollicis
2. Palmar interossei

III.

Name of Nerve				
1. Musculo-cutaneous	2. Median	3. Ulnar	4. Radial	5. Axillary
a. Coraco-brachialis m. b. Biceps brachii m. c. Brachialis m.	a. Pronator teres m. b. Pronator quadratus m. c. All other anterior forearm m. except flexor carpi ulnaris and ulnar 1/2 flexor digitorum profundus d. Thenar eminence (3) m. and lubricales 1 and 2	a. Flexor carpi ulnaris m. b. Ulnar half, flexor digitorum profundus c. Hypothenar eminence m. d. All hand m. except thenar eminence and lumbricales 1 and 2	a. Triceps brachii m. b. Brachio-radialis m. c. Supinator m. d. All posterior forearm muscles	a. Deltoid m. b. Teres minor

IV. Answers to Questions 1–46.
1. *See* Table 14–1, p 96
2. **Primary**—thoracic and sacrococcygeal
   Secondary—cervical and lumbar
3. Scoliosis
4. They do not attach to anything anteriorly.
5. Just lateral to the spines of the vertebrae
   They are the major extensors of the vertebral column and are innervated by dorsal rami of spinal nerves.
6. Sternoclavicular, acromioclavicular, and glenohumeral
7. *See* Figure 16–2, pp 105 and 106
8. Thirty
9. *See* Figure 16–3, p 107
10. **Medial**—Ulna,   Proximal = humerus and radius
                     distal = radius
    Lateral—Radius, proximal = humerus and ulna
                     distal = ulna, scaphoid, and lunate
11. Radius
12. Sternoclavicular joint
13. Supraspinatus and deltoid; anconeus and triceps brachii
14. Extension of the elbow; radial n.
15. Pronation of the hand
16. Trapezius; levator scapulae
17. Winged scapula
18. Trapezius, infraspinatus, subscapularis, serratus anterior
19. Trapezius, rhomboids (major and minor)
20. Subscapularis, supraspinatus, infraspinatus, teres minor
    As a group, they help hold the humerus into the glenoid fossa and help prevent dislocation of the shoulder joint.
21. Long head of biceps brachii
22. Median n. and ulnar n.
23. Radial n.
24. Thenar eminence; hypothenar eminence
25. Biceps brachii, brachialis, brachioradialis
    Two nerves—musculocutaneous and radial
26. In the radial (spiral) groove
    They are between the medial and lateral heads of the triceps brachii.
27. In the medial, anterior forearm
28. Radial a.
29. Brachial a.; brachial a.; brachial a.
30. Brachioradialis
31. Extension of wrist and fingers
32. Flexion of the thumb
33. Median n. and ulnar n.; median nerve
34. Median n. and radial n.
35. Deep anterior forearm and deep posterior forearm m.
36. Lumbricales
37. The brachiocephalic trunk exists on the right only. The blood to the left side branches directly off the arch of the aorta.
38. Superior vena cava
39. Cephalic vein
40. Radial a.
41. Combine Figures 21–2 and 20–1. (Check with Figures 22–4A and B.)

42. Flexor pollicis longus, abductor pollicis longus, extensor pollicis brevis, extensor pollicis longus, abductor pollicis brevis, opponens pollicis, flexor pollicis brevis, adductor pollicis
43. a. Behind the medial epicondyle of the humerus
    b. In the cubital fossa
    c. In the cubital fossa
    d. Over the cervical vertebrae
44. Because it is important in extension, adduction, and medial rotation of the arm, all actions are used in swimming.
45. Trapezius, CN XI
46. *See* Exercise 20, p 136

UNIT III

STUDENT ACTIVITIES, P 161

1. Cribiform plate
2. Optic foramen
3. Superior orbital fissure
4. Foramen rotundum
5. Foramen ovale
6. Foramen spinosum
7. Foramen lacerum
8. Jugular foramen
9. Internal acoustic meatus
10. Stylomastoid foramen
11. Hypoglossal canal
12. Foramen magnum
13. Carotid canal

EXERCISE 24

2. 1. c
    2. j
    3. i
    4. d
    5. a
    6. h
    7. b
    8. f
    9. g
    10. e

EXERCISE 25

2. Check your own labels using Figure 25–3.
3. 1. g
    2. j
    3. a
    4. h
    5. b
    6. d
    7. c
    8. f
    9. i
    10. e

4. 1. V
    2. M
    3. M
    4. M
    5. V
    6. M
    7. D
    8. L
    9. L
    10. V
5. a. nuclei
    b. cerebral cortex
6. a. Third
    b. Fourth
    c. Lateral

7. Lobes

1. Frontal
2. Parietal
3. Occipital
4. Temporal

Gyri

1. Precentral
2. Postcentral

Fissures and sulci

1. Longitudinal
2. Central
3. Calcarine
4. Lateral

8. frontal; parietal
9. A group of nerve cell bodies in the central nervous system

STUDENT ACTIVITIES, P 178

2. pons

EXERCISE 26

2. a. middle cerebral a.
    b. posterior cerebral a.
    c. anterior cerebral a.
3. a. Posterior communicating a.
    b. Anterior cerebral a.
    c. Middle cerebral a.
    d. Anterior communicating a.
    e. Posterior cerebral a.
6. 1. f
    2. d
    3. h
    4. a
    5. g
    6. b
    7. c
    8. e

STUDENT ACTIVITIES, P 183

1. Paracentral lobule; parietal lobe (postcentral gyrus)
2. 3,1,2

EXERCISE 27

1. a. Sight
   b. Left upper limb and face; same
   c. Right lower limb
   d. More nerve fibers are involved for more sensitivity of touch and for fine motor control.
2. Paracentral lobule
3. Frontal lobe, precentral gyrus

FIGURE 28–1

1. Ventral horn
2. Dorsal horn
3. Dorsal root
4. Dorsal root ganglion
5. Ventral root
6. Spinal nerve
7. Dorsal ramus
8. Ventral ramus

FIGURE 28–3

4. Dorsal root ganglion
5. Ventral root
6. Subarachnoid space
7. Ventral horn of gray matter

FIGURE 28–8

1. Longitudinal fissure
4. Thalamus

EXERCISE 28

1. 1. Subarachnoid space
   2. Central canal
   3. Dorsal root ganglion
   4. Ventral root
   5. Fasciculus gracilis
   6. Fasciculus cuneatus
   7. Dorsal root
   8. Spinal n.
   9. Ventral horn
2. 1. c
   2. e
   3. g
   4. h
   5. b
   6. a
   7. d
   8. f
3. a. Lateral spinothalamic; pain and temperature
   b. fasciculus cuneatus
   c. fasciculus gracilis
4. a. On left side of body
   b. Left lower extremity
5. Flaccid paralysis

STUDENT ACTIVITY, P 195

Sensory	Motor	Mixed
1. CN I	1. III	1. V
2. CN II	2. IV	2. VII
3. CN VIII	3. VI	3. IX
	4. XI	4. X
	5. XII	

EXERCISE 29

2. a. Ophthalmic n.
   b. Maxillary n.
   c. Mandibular n.
4. CN VII, facial n.
5. In the order of occurrence, from top of illustration to bottom: CN I, II, III, IV, V, VI, VII, VIII, IX, X, XII, and XI.

TEXT, P 203

A. CN I; cribriform plate; ethmoid
B. optic n.; optic foramen

EXERCISE 30

1. Nerves that carry a *special sense,* the sensations they control, the foramen through which they pass, and, where indicated, the lobe of the brain involved.

Nerve	Sensation	Foramen	Brain Structure
a. Olfactory	Smell	Cribriform plate	—
b. Optic	Sight	Optic foramen	Occipital lobe
c. Facial	Taste	Internal acoustic meatus	—
d. Vestibular	Equilibrium	Internal acoustic meatus	—
e. Cochlear	Hearing	Internal acoustic meatus	Temporal lobe
f. Glossopharyngeal	Taste	Jugular foramen	—

2. a. CN XII
   b. CN IV
   c. CN XII
   d. CN III
   e. CN VI
   f. CN XII
3. Malleus, incus, stapes
4. Four; trigeminal, facial, glossopharyngeal, hypoglossal
5. 1. g
   2. c
   3. f
   4. d
   5. a
   6. h
   7. e
   8. b

FIGURE 31–5

3. Right subclavian a.
4. Right common carotid a.

EXERCISE 31

2. a. Occipitalis
   b. Frontalis
   c. Orbicularis oculi
   d. Orbicularis oris
   e. Buccinator
   f. Platysma
   g. Temporalis
   h. Masseter
   i. Medial pterygoid
   j. Lateral pterygoid
   k. Trapezius
   l. Sternocleidomastoid
3. a. Mylohyoid
   b. Digastric
   c. Stylohyoid
   d. Geniohyoid
   e. Sternohyoid
   f. Omohyoid
   g. Sternothyroid
   h. Thyrohyoid
4. a. Temporalis
   b. Masseter
7. a. Frontalis, VII
   b. Orbicularis oculi, VII
   c. Buccinator, VII
   d. Orbicularis oris, VII
   e. Platysma, VII
   f. Masseter, V3
   g. Occipitalis, VII
   h. Temporalis, V3
8. a. Heart
   b. Aorta
   c. Brachiocepalic trunk
   d. Right common carotid a.

   a. Masseter muscle
   b. Maxillary v.
   c. External jugular v.
   d. Subclavian v.
   e. Brachiocephalic v.
   f. Superior vena cava
   g. Right atrium
9. *See* Figure 31–6 and the subsequent text: "B. Carotid Sinus and Carotid Body."

STUDENT ACTIVITIES, P 223

1. Splanchnic
3. III, VII, and IX; X
4. 1. Sympathetic trunk
   2. Rami communicantes
   3. Sympathetic ganglion
   4. Lateral horn (of gray matter)

EXERCISE 33   REVIEW OF UNIT III

I. The eight bones of the cranial vault:

frontal	occipital
parietal (2)	temporal (2)
ethmoid	sphenoid

II. *See* Figures 24–1 and 24–2, pp 153 and 154

III. The Cranial Nerves

Number	Name	Mixed, Motor, Sensory	Distribution	Sensation
I	Olfactory	Sensory	Nasal mucosa	Smell
II	Optic	Sensory	Eye (retina)	Sight
III	Oculomotor	Motor	Eye muscles	None
IV	Trochlear	Motor	Superior oblique m.	None
V	Trigeminal	Mixed	Face, head, tongue Muscles of mastication	General
VI	Abducens	Motor	Lateral rectus m.	None
VII	Facial	Mixed	Anterior 2/3 tongue Muscles facial expression	Taste
VIII	Vestibulo-cochlear	Sensory	Ear	Equilibrium Hearing
IX	Glossopharyngeal	Mixed	Tongue (posterior 1/3) Muscles of pharynx	Taste and general sensations
X	Vagus	Mixed	Viscera of thorax, abdomen; larynx	General sensations
XI	Accessory	Motor	Larynx, pharynx, sternocleidomastoid m., and trapezius m.	None
XII	Hypoglossal	Motor	Tongue	None

IV. *See* Figures 25–2 and 25–3 in Lesson 25 to check your answers.

V. *See* Figures 31–1, 31–2, and 31–3 to check your answers.

VI. Answers to questions:

1. Ascending aorta; brachiocephalic trunk; common carotid artery; external carotid artery; facial artery
2. Orbicularis oculi, orbicularis oris, buccinator
3. Temporalis, masseter, medial pterygoid, lateral pterygoid
4. choroid plexus
5. *See* section entitled "Ventricles of the Brain" preceding Figure 25–7.
6. Interventricular foramen, third ventricle, cerebral aqueduct, fourth ventricle, subarachnoid space, arachnoid granulations (or villi)
7. A **suture** is the line of fusion between two cranial bones. **Coronal, squamosal, lambdoidal,** and **sagittal** are four sutures.
8. Dura mater, arachnoid, pia mater
9. Falx cerebri, tentorium cerebelli
10. They provide reservoirs to collect venous blood from the brain and take it toward the jugular foramen.
11. Internal jugular vein

12. **Paranasal sinuses** are the cavities within bones of the skull. They contain air unless the mucous membrane lining has produced mucus.
   Ethnoid, sphenoid, maxillary, and frontal
13. No. It innervates only the muscles of mastication; you smile with muscles of facial expression.
14. Difficulty chewing because the mandibular nerve is injured
15. Perpendicular plate of ethmoid bone, vomer bone
16. Carotid canal; foramen lacerum
17. Mandible; temporomandibular joint
18. frontal lobe
   temporal lobe
   cerebellum
19. CN VII, facial n.
20. Elevation and depression, retraction and protraction of the hyoid bone
   Talking and **swallowing** are made possible.
21. Trapezius and sternocleidomastoid
   accessory CN XI
22. The **carotid body** detects oxygen content in blood.
   Carotid sinus is sensitive to blood pressure.
They are both near the bifurcation of the common carotid a.
23. Maxillary a.
24. You will need to include the internal and external jugular veins to provide a pathway from the internal and external head. *See* Figure 31–7.
25. See Figure 26–6.
   vertebral arteries and **internal carotid** arteries
26. Functional areas of the brain were assigned numbers by a neurologist named Brodmann. He assigned the number **4** to the primary motor cortex located on the precentral gyrus and **3,1,2** to the primary sensory area on the postcentral gyrus.
27. A **homunculus** is a small complete body representation such as that drawn on the precentral and postcentral gyri, to indicate body distribution of nerve cells.
28. Postcentral; middle cerebral artery
29. The right lower limb
30. Lateral corticospinal
31. Pain and temperature; left
32. Commissural; projection
33. The left side of the brain controls the right side of the body and the right side of the brain controls the left side of the body.
34. In the cerebral cortex and in nuclei
   In the central gray matter
35. At about the level of the first lumbar vertebra
   Conus medullaris
   The extension of the pia mater, innermost meningeal layer
36. The **upper motor neuron** cell body is in the brain; the **lower motor neuron** cell body is located in the spinal cord.
37. The ciliary muscles are in the ciliary body surrounding the lens of the eye and contract to change the shape of the lens for accommodation. The muscles of the iris of the eye change the size of the pupil to admit differing amounts of light.
38. *See* Figures 30–1 and 30–6.
39. CNs III, VII, IX, and X
40. Sympathetic and parasympathetic
41. *See* Table 32–1.
42. Hypothalamus and medulla oblongata

VII. *See* Figure 30–4.

VIII. a. Lateral rectus m.
  b. Superior rectus m.
  c. Medial rectus m.
  d. Inferior rectus m.
  e. Optic nerve
  f. Anterior horn of gray matter
  g. Anterior roots
  h. Dorsal ramus
  i. Ventral ramus
  j. Dorsal column of white matter
  k. Dorsal roots
  l. Dorsal root ganglion
  m. Rami communicantes
  n. Sympathetic ganglion
  o. Lateral horn of gray matter

UNIT IV

STUDENT ACTIVITIES AND EXERCISE 34, P 235

6. a. T7–L2
  b. Somatic
  c. external abdominal oblique m., internal abdominal oblique m., and transverse abdominus
  d. Anterior rectus sheath, rectus abdominis m., and posterior rectus sheath

FIGURE 35–1

1. a. Liver
  b. Gall bladder
  c. Hepatic flexure
2. a. Spleen
  b. Splenic flexure
  c. Stomach
  d. Pancreas
3. a. Cecum
  b. Vermiform appendix
4. a. Sigmoid colon

FIGURE 35–12

2. Common bile duct

EXERCISE 35

1. a. Liver
  b. Gall bladder
  c. Vermiform appendix
  d. Esophagus
  e. Stomach
  f. Spleen
  g. Pancreas
  h. Small intestine
2. 1. g
  2. i
  3. c
  4. e
  5. a
  6. j
  7. b
  8. d
  9. h
  10. f

3. a. Epiploic appendages
   b. Haustra coli
   c. Tenia coli
4. a. Mesentery proper
   b. Visceral peritoneum
   c. Greater omentum
   d. Falciform ligament
   e. Lesser omentum
   f. Mesocolon
   g. Parietal peritoneum
   h. Coronary ligament
5. Ligamentum teres hepatis; obliterated umbilical v.
6. a. Mouth
   b. Esophagus
   c. Stomach
   d. Small intestine
   e. Large intestine
   f. Mouth
   g. Stomach
   h. Mouth
   i. Stomach
   j. Small intestine
   k. Small intestine
   l. Anus

TABLE 36–1

TABLE 36–1. BLOOD SUPPLY AND INNERVATION OF THE ABDOMEN

	Parietal supply	**Visceral supply**
Vessels	Anterior–superior and inferior epigastic arteries Posterior–lumbar, inferior phrenic, median sacral arteries Return to IVC	Single midline trunks: celiac, superior mesenteric, and inferior mesenteric a. Bilateral arteries: renal, gonadal RETURN to PORTAL vein and IVC

Nerves	Ventral rami T7–L2	Autonomics:
		  sympathetic splanchnics
		  parasympathetic–vagus and S2-4

FIGURE 36–5

a. subclavian v.
b. brachiocephalic v.
c. gonadal v.
d. external iliac v.
e. femoral v.
f. internal jugular v.
g. external jugular v.
h. superior vena cava
i. internal iliac v.

STUDENT ACTIVITIES, P 256

Aorta
Superior mesenteric a.
Capillaries
Superior mesenteric v.
Portal v.
Capillaries
Hepatic v.
Inferior vena cava
Right atrium

EXERCISE 36

1. 1. j
    2. g
    3. h
    4. i
    5. b
    6. f
    7. a
    8. d
    9. e
    10. c
2. a. 1. Splenic v.
    2. Superior mesenteric v.
    3. Inferior mesenteric v.
    4. Left gastric v.
    b. Products of digestion must be taken to the liver.

3. **Sympathetic**   **Parasympathetic**

   a. Celiac ganglion   Vagus
   b. Superior mesenteric   Vagus
   c. Inferior mesenteric   S2–4
   d. Superior mesenteric   Vagus
   e. Celiac   Vagus
   f. Celiac   Vagus
   g. Inferior mesenteric   S2–4
   h. Superior and inferior mesenteric   Vagus and S2–4

STUDENT ACTIVITIES, P 263

2. Renal pelvis/ureter
   Renal vein

EXERCISE 37

1. a. Glomerulus
    b. Bowman's capsule
    c. renal corpuscle
2. a. Urinary bladder
    b. Ureter
    c. Renal pyramid
    d. Urethra
    e. Nephron
    f. Renal pelvis
    g. Hilus

3. a. Kidney
   b. Inferior vena cava
   c. Urethra
   d. Renal v.
   e. Ureter
   f. Urinary bladder
   g. Minor calyx
   h. Major calyx
   i. Renal cortex
   j. Renal pyramid
   k. Renal pelvis
   l. Ureter

FIGURE 38–5

3. Symphysis pubis
8. Epididymis
9. Testis
10. Seminal vesicle

STUDENT ACTIVITIES, P 268

2. a. Prostatic urethra
   b. Membranous urethra
   c. Penile urethra

EXERCISE 38

1. a. Ductus deferens
   b. Duct of seminal vesicle
2. Testis
3. a. Seminal vesicle
   b. Prostate gland
   c. Bulbourethral gland
4. a. Production of sperm
   b. Production of testosterone
5. a. Seminiferous tubules
   b. Efferent ductules
   c. Epipidymus
   d. Ductus deferens
   e. Ejaculatory duct
   f. Prostatic urethra
   g. Membranous urethra
   h. Penile urethra
6. 1. g
   2. j
   3. e
   4. f
   5. a
   6. i
   7. b
   8. c
   9. h
   10. d

FIGURE 39–3

2. Ovary
3. Ovarian ligament
4. Broad ligament

STUDENT ACTIVITIES, P 277

1. **Peritoneal Structures**
   a. Suspensory ligament of ovary
   b. Broad ligament
2. a. Peritoneal sac
   b. Infundibulum of uterine tube
   c. Ampulla of the uterine tube
   d. Isthmus of uterine tube
   e. Uterus
   f. Cervix
   g. Vagina

Solid Cords
a. Round ligament of uterus
b. Ovarian ligament

EXERCISE 39

1. 1. f
    2. a
    3. e
    4. j
    5. c
    6. d
    7. i
    8. b
    9. g
   10. h
2. Scrotum—Labia majora
   Testis—Ovary
   Penis—Clitoris
3. a. Perimetrium
   b. Myometrium
   c. Endometrium
4. a. Infundibulum
   b. Fimbriae
   c. Ampulla
   d. Isthmus

STUDENT ACTIVITIES, P 281

1. Pancreas
2. a. Ovary
   b. Testis

STUDENT ACTIVITIES, P 288

4. Trachea
5. Posterior
6. Heart
7. Inferior vena cava

FIGURE 42–4
1. Frontal sinus
2. Crista galli
3. Middle nasal concha
7. Genioglossus m.
8. Geniohyoid m.
14. Sphenoid sinus

FIGURE 42–6
1. Thyroid cartilage
2. Cricoid cartilage

EXERCISE 42
1. a. A
   b. S
   c. I
   d. I
   e. I
   f. I
   g. S
   h. A or S
   i. S
   u. S
2. b. Nasopharynx
   c. Oropharynx
   e. Larynx
   f. Trachea
   g. Primary bronchus
   h. Secondary bronchus
   i. Tertiary bronchus
   j. Bronchiole
   k. Respiratory bronchiole

EXERCISE 43

2. You should have an X in front of the following: a, b, d, e, g, h, i, and l.
3. a. Pericardium
   b. Myocardium
   c. Endocardium
4. a. Tricuspid
   b. Bicuspid
5. a. Aortic semilunar
   b. Pulmonary semilunar
6. a. right atrium
   b. right ventricle
   c. pulmonary trunk

    d. pulmonary arteries
    e. pulmonary capillaries
    f. pulmonary veins
    g. left atrium
    h. left ventricle
    i. aorta
    j. left coronary a.
    k. anterior interventricular a. (LAD)
    l. great cardiac v.
    m. coronary sinus
    n. right atrium
7. j, k, l, and m

TEXT, P 308

The other system in which the arteries have high levels of carbon dioxide is the pulmonary system.

STUDENT ACTIVITY, P 312

2. Lymph vessels

EXERCISE 46   REVIEW OF UNIT IV

  I. *See* Figures 35–2, 37–1, and 40–1.
 II. Respiratory, digestive, cardiovascular, endocrine, urinary, female reproductive, male reproductive, lymphatic
III. a. Inguinal ligament
    b. Inferior epigastric a.
    c. Quadratus lumborum
    d. Esophagus
 IV. *See* Figures 11–1, 11–3, 36–2, and 36–5 to check your answers.
    u. Inferior vena cava
    v. portal vein
    w. aorta
  V. Answers to questions:

  1. Spermatic cord; round ligament of the uterus
  2. Visceral peritoneum (not on esophagus), muscularis, submucosa, mucosa
  3. Duodenum
  4. Liver, gall bladder, pancreas
  5. Minor calyx, major calyx, renal pelvis, ureter, (bladder), urethra
  6. Glomerulus, Bowman's capsule
  7. Stomach, gall bladder, urinary bladder
  8. Coronary ligament
    Falciform ligament
  9. Pharynx, esophagus, stomach, small intestine, superior mesenteric vein, portal vein, liver sinusoids (capillaries), hepatic vein, inferior vena cava, right atrium, right ventricle, pulmonary trunk, pulmonary artery, pulmonary capillaries, pulmonary veins, left atrium, left ventricle, aorta, renal artery, interlobar a., arcuate a., interlobular a., afferent arteriole, glomerulus, nephron, collecting duct, minor calyx, major calyx, renal pelvis, ureter, bladder, urethra
    Three body systems must be involved. They are: digestive, cardiovascular, urinary
10. Diaphragm; phrenic n.
11. Nephron; produces urine

12. | P | C |
    | C | P |
    | P | C |
    | P | C |

13. Mouth, pharynx, esophagus, stomach, duodenum, jejunum, ileum, ascending colon, transverse colon, descending colon, sigmoid colon, rectum, anal canal

14. Nose, pharynx, larynx, trachea, primary bronchus, lung (secondary bronchus, tertiary bronchus, bronchiole, respiratory bronchiole, alveoli)

15. Pleura—thorax; pericardium—thorax; peritoneum—abdomen

16. Left ventricle, aorta, superior mesenteric a. (or inferior mesenteric a.), capillaries, superior mesenteric vein, portal vein, liver sinusoids (capillaries), hepatic v., inferior vena cava, right atrium

17. Production of hormones and germ cells

18. | kidney | testis |
    | gall bladder | kidney |
    | liver | heart |
    | lung | spleen |
    | ovary | intestines |

19. Skin, fascia, external abdominal oblique muscle, internal abdominal oblique muscle, transverse abdominis muscle, parietal peritoneum, visceral peritoneum, intestine

20. Yes. The sperm could enter the vaginal canal, the cervix, the uterine body, and the uterine tube, then exit the infundibulum to enter the peritoneal sac and then move to the region between the uterus and rectum.

21. *See* Exercise 38.

22. *See* Figure 36–6. Blood containing digested food products must be taken to the liver to be metabolized, stored, and/or converted into usable products to be taken to the body cells.

23. *See* answer to question 9, beginning with left ventricle.

24. Left ventricle, aorta, celiac trunk, splenic artery

25. Common iliac, lumbar, renal, hepatic, gonadal, inferior phrenic, and median sacral veins

26. **Ascending colon:** *sympathetic fibers,* which synapsed in the superior mesenteric ganglia, and *parasympathetic fibers* from the vagus nerve
    Descending colon: *sympathetic fibers,* which synapsed in the inferior mesenteric ganglion, and parasympathetic fibers from the *sacral level (S2-4) parasympathetics*

27. Stimulates muscle contraction, for peristalsis, and elaboration of mucus by the mucous membrane

28. Inhibition of the functions listed in answer 27, above

29. **Bones:** thoracic vertebrae, ribs, sternum
    Muscles: external and internal intercostal muscles and diaphragm

30. **Anterior source:** anterior intercostal arteries from the internal thoracic a.
    Posterior source: posterior intercostal arteries largely from the thoracic aorta.
    Diaphragm: musculophrenic artery, superior and inferior phrenic arteries
    Major venous structure: azygos vein

31. Intercostal nerves 1–11—or ventral rami T1-T11

32. Anterior—sternum; inferior—diaphragm; lateral—pleural sacs; posterior—thoracic vertebrae; superior—root of neck

33. Lungs and pleura

34. A serous sac that covers the lungs

35. Esophagus, inferior vena cava, aorta

36. Phrenic nerve; C3, 4, 5

37. *See* answer to 30, above.

38. Because they lie in the costal grooves and are between ribs
    T12 is the subcostal nerve because there is no rib below T12
39. Exchange of waste gases (mainly carbon dioxide) for a fresh supply of oxygen in the blood
40. The alveoli of the respiratory system are in contact with the capillaries of the pulmonary arteries of the circulatory system.
41. **Bronchial vessels** supply the bronchial tree with oxygen and nutrients and remove the waste products of metabolism within the cells of the lung; **pulmonary vessels** are taking the systemic blood to the alveoli of the lungs for a fresh supply of oxygen that will be taken directly to the heart
42. *See* the answer to question 14.
43. The **pharynx** is a posteriorly positioned fibromuscular tube that is used in both respiration and digestion; it continues as the esophagus.
44. The **larynx** is a cartilaginous box located between the pharynx and the trachea. Four main cartilages are: epiglottis, thyroid, cricoid, arytenoid.
45. The larynx is for passage of air and production of the voice.
46. Posterior to the trachea
47. Into the middle ear
48. Epiglottis
49. False folds are superior to the true folds.
50. It receives "used blood" and pumps it to the lungs.
51. Yes. In fetal circulation the lungs are not functional and there is no need for the blood to be sent there. The **foramen ovale** is an opening in the interatrial septum that allows the blood going directly to the left side of the heart to be pumped to the systems.
52. Coronary arteries; cardiac veins
53. Transportation of nutrients and oxygen to all body cells
    Removal of waste products from the cells
54. 1st heart sound: closing of the atrioventricular valves
    2nd heart sound: closing of the semilunar valves
55. Pericardium; pleura
56. Pulmonary and fetal circulation
57. The fetal lungs and digestive systems are not functional.
58. Return of interstitial fluid to the cardiovascular system; helps the immune system fight infections
59. **Lymph nodes:** along the path of lymph vessels—particularly in areas such as popliteal fossa, inguinal region, along the anterior aorta, axilla, neck
    Tonsils: found in the pharynx, at the base of the tongue
    Thymus gland: found anterior to the trachea and behind the sternum
    Spleen: in the upper left quadrant of the abdomen
60. Spleen
61. **Parietal innervation** is by way of regular somatic nerves
    Visceral innervation is by way of autonomic nerves
VI. *See* Figures 35–3 and 35–4.
VII. *See* Figure 40–1.
    a. Descending aorta
    b. Esophagus
    c. Azygos vein
    d. Thoracic duct
    e. Thoracic vertebrae
    f. Sympathetic trunk
VIII. *See* Figure 43–3.

Index

Notes . . .

Notes . . .

Notes . . .

Notes . . .

Notes . . .

Notes . . .

Notes . . .

Notes . . .

Notes . . .

Notes . . .